THE

PAIN
CLINIC
MANUAL

SECOND EDITION

THE

PAIN CLINIC MANUAL

SECOND EDITION

EDITORS

STEPHEN E. ABRAM, M.D.
Professor and Chair of Anesthesiology
and Critical Care Medicine
University of New Mexico,
Health Sciences Center—School of Medicine
Albuquerque, New Mexico

J. DAVID HADDOX, D.D.S., M.D., D.A.B.P.M.
Atlanta, Georgia;
Consultant in Pain Medicine
Pain and Policy Studies Group
University of Wisconsin
Madison, Wisconsin

With 32 Contributors

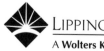 LIPPINCOTT WILLIAMS & WILKINS
A **Wolters Kluwer** Company
Philadelphia · Baltimore · New York · London
Buenos Aires · Hong Kong · Sydney · Tokyo

Acquisitions Editor: R. Craig Percy
Developmental Editor: Alexandra T. Anderson
Production Editor: Emily Lerman
Manufacturing Manager: Kevin Watt
Cover Designer: Mark Lerner
Compositor: Circle Graphics
Printer: Edwards Brothers

© 2000 by LIPPINCOTT WILLIAMS & WILKINS
530 Walnut Street
Philadelphia, PA 19106-3780 USA
LWW.com

Printed in the USA

Library of Congress Cataloging-in-Publication Data

The pain clinic manual / editors, Stephen E. Abram, J. David Haddox. — 2nd ed.
    p.   cm.
    Includes bibliographical references and index.
    ISBN 0-7817-1253-X (alk. paper)
    1. Pain—Treatment Handbooks, manuals, etc. 2. Analgesia Handbooks, manuals, etc. 3. Pain clinics Handbooks, manuals, etc.
I. Abram, Stephen E. II. Haddox, J. David.
    [DNLM: 1. Pain—therapy. 2. Pain—diagnosis.   WL 704 P14442 1999]
RB127.P332176   1999
616'.042—dc21
DNLM/DLC
for Library of Congress   99-31928
                                               CIP

10 9 8 7 6 5 4 3

Contents

Part V: Cancer Pain Management

Part VI: Techniques

Appendices

Contributing Authors

Stephen E. Abram, M.D.
Professor and Chair of Anesthesiology and
  Critical Care Medicine
University of New Mexico, Health
  Sciences Center—School of Medicine
2701 Frontier NE, Surge Building
Albuquerque, New Mexico 87131
Chapter 1, Pain Clinic Organization and
  Staffing
Chapter 2, Pain Pathways and Mechanisms
Chapter 12, Electrical Stimulation of the
  Nervous System
Chapter 16, Systemic Opioid Therapy for
  Noncancer Pain
Chapter 37, Epidural Steroid Injections
Chapter 38, Sympathetic Blocks

Nabil M. K. Ali, M.D.
Director, The New Mexico Center for Pain
  Management;
Partner, Anesthesia Specialists of
  Albuquerque;
St. Joseph Healthcare
St. Joseph Medical Towers
500 Walter NE, Suite 409
Albuquerque, New Mexico 87102
Chapter 22, Acute Herpes Zoster and
  Postherpetic Neuralgia

Doralina L. Anghelescu, M.D.
Department of Anesthesiology
St. Jude Children's Research Hospital
332 North Lauderdale
Memphis, Tennessee 38101
Chapter 30, Chronic Pain in Children
Chapter 31, Substance Abuse and
  Addiction

David M. Biondi, D.O.
Associate Neurologist
Michigan Head, Pain, and Neurological
  Institute
3120 Professional Drive
Ann Arbor, Michigan 48104;
Assistant Clinical Professor of Medicine
Department of Neurology
Michigan State University College of
  Osteopathic Medicine
East Lansing, Michigan 48824
Chapter 24, Facial Pain
Chapter 25, Headache

Daniel Brookoff, M.D., Ph.D.
Associate Director
Methodist Comprehensive Pain Institute
Methodist Healthcare
1211 Union Avenue, Suite 225
Memphis, Tennessee 38104
Chapter 26, Chronic Pelvic Pain

Stanley L. Chapman, Ph.D.
Associate Professor of Anesthesiology
Division of Pain Medicine
Emory University School of Medicine;
Center for Pain Medicine
Section of Anesthesiology
The Emory Clinic, Inc.
1365 Clifton Road NE
Atlanta, Georgia 30322
Chapter 7, The Pain-Focused
  Psychologic Evaluation
Chapter 9, Pain Rehabilitation Programs

Margaret Charsley, M.D.
Assistant Professor of Anesthesiology
Department of Anesthesiology and Critical
  Care Medicine
University of New Mexico, Health
  Sciences Center—School of Medicine
2701 Frontier NE, Surge Building
Albuquerque, New Mexico 87131
Chapter 27, Postdural Puncture Headache
Chapter 31, Substance Abuse and
  Addiction

Penney L. Cowan
Founder and Executive Director
The American Chronic Pain Association
Rocklin, California 95677
Chapter 3, Pain: The Patient's Perspective

Oscar A. deLeon-Casasola, M.D.
Associate Professor of Anesthesiology
Roswell Park Cancer Institute
Elm and Carlton Streets
Buffalo, New York 14263
Chapter 36, Neurolytic Blocks and Other
Neuroablative Procedures for Cancer
Pain

Kenneth A. Follett, M.D., Ph.D.
Associate Professor of Neurosurgery
The University of Iowa Hospitals and
   Clinics
200 Hawkins Drive
Iowa City, Iowa 52242
Chapter 28, Central Pain Syndromes

Walter B. Forman, M.D.
Professor of Medicine
University of New Mexico, Health
   Sciences Center—School of Medicine
2211 Lomas Boulevard NE
Albuquerque, New Mexico 87131
Chapter 34, Palliative Care of the
Terminally Ill Patient

Antonio M. Goncalves, Ph.D.
Clinical Psychologist
Cancer Research/Treatment Center
University of New Mexico, Health
   Sciences Center—School of Medicine
900 Camino De Salud NE
Albuquerque, New Mexico 87131
Chapter 33, Psychologic Assessment and
Treatment of Patients With Cancer Pain

Martin Grabois, M.D.
Professor and Chairman of Physical
   Medicine and Rehabilitation
Baylor College of Medicine
1333 Moursund Avenue
Houston, Texas 77030
Chapter 20, Myofascial Pain Syndrome

M. Alexander Gupta, M.D.
Attending Anesthesiologist
Critical Care Health Systems,
Carolina Pain Consultants
P.O. Box 18139
Raleigh, North Carolina 27619
Chapter 21, Complex Regional Pain
Syndromes and Sympathetically
Maintained Pain

J. David Haddox, D.D.S., M.D.,
D.A.B.P.M.
Atlanta, Georgia;
Consultant in Pain Medicine
Pain and Policy Studies Group
University of Wisconsin
Madison, Wisconsin
Chapter 21, Complex Regional Pain
Syndromes and Sympathetically
Maintained Pain
Chapter 24, Facial Pain

James E. Heavner, D.V.M., Ph.D.
Professor of Anesthesiology and
   Physiology
Director of Anesthesia Research
Texas Tech University Health Sciences
   Center
3601 Fourth Street
Lubbock, Texas 79430
Chapter 13, Principles of Clinical
Pharmacology

David J. Hewitt, M.D.
Assistant Professor of Neurology
Emory University;
Co-director
Section of Neurology
The Emory Clinic, Inc.
1365 Clifton Road NE, Suite A4100
Atlanta, Georgia 30322
Chapter 23, Painful Peripheral
Neuropathies

Quinn H. Hogan, M.D.
Associate Professor of Anesthesiology
Clinic and Fellowship Director
Pain Management Center
Medical College of Wisconsin
9200 West Wisconsin Avenue
Milwaukee, Wisconsin 53226
Chapter 8, Diagnostic and Prognostic
Nerve Blocks
Chapter 19, Back Pain and Radiculopathy

Margaret B. Hopwood, Ph.D.
Assistant Professor of Anesthesia and
   Director of Clinical Research
The University of Iowa Hospitals and
   Clinics
200 Hawkins Drive
Iowa City, Iowa 52242
Chapter 4, Collection of Historical Data

Nora A. Janjan, M.D., F.A.C.P.
Professor of Radiation Oncology
The University of Texas M.D. Anderson
  Cancer Center
1515 Holcombe Boulevard
Houston, Texas 77030
*Chapter 35, Radiation Therapy for Cancer
  Pain*

William L. Johnson, M.D.
Assistant Professor of Anesthesiology
University of New Mexico, School of
  Medicine
1127 University Boulevard NE
Albuquerque, New Mexico 87102
*Chapter 1, Pain Clinic Organization and
  Staffing*

Pushpa Nambi Joseph, M.D.
Assistant Professor of Anesthesiology
Kansas University Medical Center
3901 Rainbow Boulevard
Kansas City, Kansas 66160
*Chapter 36, Neurolytic Blocks and Other
  Neuroablative Procedures for Cancer
  Pain*

John W. Luckwitz, M.D.
Staff Anesthesiologist
Mountain West Anesthesia
2040 Murray Holladay Road, 106
Salt Lake City, Utah 84117
*Chapter 29, Management of Painful
  Medical Diseases*
Chapter 39, Peripheral Nerve Blocks
Chapter 40, Head and Neck Blocks

N. Timothy Lynch, Ph.D.
Associate Clinical Professor of
  Anesthesiology
Medical College of Wisconsin
9200 West Wisconsin Avenue
Milwaukee, Wisconsin 53226
*Chapter 1, Pain Clinic Organization and
  Staffing*

Donald C. Manning, M.D., Ph.D.
Assistant Professor of Anesthesiology
University of Virginia
Charlottesville, Virginia 22906;
Novartis Pharmaceuticals Corp.
59 Route 10
East Hanover, New Jersey 07936
Chapter 18, Adjuvant Analgesics

Richard B. Patt, M.D.
President and Chief Medical Officer
The Patt Center for Cancer Pain
  and Wellness
7120 Cecil Street, Suite B
Houston, Texas 77030
Chapter 32, Oncologic Pain Management

Srinivasa N. Raja, M.D.
Professor of Anesthesiology and Critical
  Care Medicine
The Johns Hopkins University School
  of Medicine;
Department of Anesthesiology and Critical
  Care Medicine
Division of Pain Medicine
Johns Hopkins Hospital
600 North Wolfe Street, Osler 292
Baltimore, Maryland 21287
*Chapter 21, Complex Regional Pain
  Syndromes and Sympathetically
  Maintained Pain*

Arun Rajagopal, M.D.
Assistant Professor of Anesthesiology
Departments of Anesthesiology and
  Symptom Control and Palliative Care
The University of Texas M.D. Anderson
  Cancer Center
1515 Holcombe Boulevard
Houston, Texas 77030
*Chapter 12, Electrical Stimulation of the
  Nervous System*

Christian R. Schlicht, D.O.
Department of Anesthesiology
University of New Mexico, Health
    Sciences Center—School of Medicine
2701 Frontier NE, Surge Building
Albuquerque, New Mexico 87131
*Chapter 14, Local Anesthetic
    Pharmacology*
Chapter 15, Local Anesthetic Toxicity

**Donna Marie Schramm-Bloodworth,
    M.D.**
Assistant Professor of Physical Medicine
    and Rehabilitation
Baylor College of Medicine
6550 Fannin, Suite 1421
Houston, Texas 77030
*Chapter 10, Physical Therapy in the Pain
    Clinic Setting*

Denice C. Sheehan, M.S.N.
Instructor of Nursing
The Breen School of Nursing
Ursuline College
2550 Lander Road
Pepper Pike, Ohio 44124
*Chapter 34, Palliative Care of the
    Terminally Ill Patient*

Mary Lou Taylor, Ph.D.
Assistant Professor of Anesthesiology
Medical College of Wisconsin
9200 West Wisconsin Avenue
Milwaukee, Wisconsin 53226
*Chapter 6, Psychological Assessment of
    Patients Experiencing Chronic Pain*
*Chapter 11, Psychological Strategies for
    Managing Chronic Pain*

Sridhar V. Vasudevan, M.D.
Clinical Professor of Physical Medicine
    and Rehabilitation
Medical College of Wisconsin
19333 West North Avenue
Brookfield, Wisconsin 53045
*Chapter 5, Physical Examination of the
    Patient Experiencing Pain*

Mark S. Wallace, M.D.
Associate Professor of Anesthesiology
University of California, San Diego—
    School of Medicine
9500 Gilman Drive
La Jolla, California 92093
*Chapter 17, Chronic Intrathecal Drug
    Delivery*

Preface

Although the purpose of the second edition of *The Pain Clinic Manual* has not changed, the content has been greatly expanded and updated. Rather than selecting authors from a single institution, we attempted to choose the most appropriate contributors for each chapter and have solicited contributions from all over the United States. Although we have added material about interventional treatment methods, the manual continues to address multimodal patient management, focusing on comprehensive assessment and using social and vocational, psychological, rehabilitative, and medical interventions where appropriate.

We anticipate publication of this volume as we approach the twenty-first century. We have learned a great deal during the past quarter century about how to manage patients with severe, persistent pain and have incorporated a wide range of therapeutic methods into effective treatment paradigms. For many patients, we know what to do and how to do it.

The question we now face is: Can we afford to do it? In the current environment of cost savings and the shift of resources from patient care to corporate profits, it is becoming increasingly difficult to provide the coordinated services that are so important to treatment success. The likelihood that workers' compensation plans or HMOs will pay a flat fee for a comprehensive treatment program is decreasing each year. Many carriers are willing to pay for expensive surgical procedures, infusion devices, or spinal stimulation, but refuse to support the rehabilitative, psychological, and drug detoxification services that may be much more important for a given patient. Nevertheless, we must provide those services that have been shown to be effective and we must document resulting improvement in outcome and overall cost savings.

We believe that this volume will provide a good foundation for physicians who wish to provide effective pain management services for their patients. We hope that our health care systems will encourage those physicians to provide appropriate and effective care throughout the next century.

Stephen E. Abram, M.D.

Preface to the First Edition

It is the purpose of this manual to provide the reader with some approaches to the management of some common pain management problems. It is by no means a definitive reference, for it contains limited information about the pathophysiology of the painful disorders presented, and does not detail the technical aspects of treatment. References to such information are provided at the end of each section. The book does provide the reader with diagnostic criteria and management protocols for a fairly wide range of pain syndromes. Treatment algorithms are based on review of available literature, discussions with recognized authorities, and experience from the Medical College of Wisconsin Pain Clinics.

Treatment suggestions presented in this volume are by no means uniformly effective. Many of the pain syndromes discussed are exceedingly resistant to medical intervention. All of the therapeutic options presented have had some degree of success, and the authors have made an effort to provide an honest assessment of the likelihood that a particular modality will be beneficial. For most pain syndromes, there is an inverse relationship between the duration of symptoms and the chance of success. Social, psychological, and vocational factors may further reduce the likelihood of benefit from treatment.

The list of treatment options presented is not entirely comprehensive. Many of the painful disorders discussed are extremely common. Others are relatively rare, but are included because they are likely to respond dramatically to fairly simple interventions.

For generations, the emphasis of the medical community has been on a purely medical approach to acute and chronic pain management. With chronic pain problems, the success of medical and surgical interventions is limited, hence there has been a tendency for patients to seek care by practitioners whose treatment may have little or no scientific basis. Acupuncturists, chiropractors, Rolfers, faith healers, Shen therapists and a host of other practitioners offer little insight and even less long-term benefit to patients with long-standing pain. Fortunately, the mainstream of health care professionals and scientists is developing treatment programs that effectively address the physical and psychological impairment that develops among chronic pain patients. The emphasis in chronic pain is on physical rehabilitation, development of coping strategies, psychological support, and modification of counterproductive behaviors.

There is considerable disagreement within the scientific community about when pain becomes chronic. When do we continue with nerve blocks, surgery, and pharmacological interventions, and when do we decide that a chronic pain management program is needed? Such decisions should not be based upon the duration of pain but upon the nature of the painful process and the patient's psychosocial responses to the pain. A patient with a 3-year history of painful osteomyelitis may have a purely nociceptive process, whereas a patient with a 3-month history of work-related back pain may demonstrate problems that require predominantly psychological and rehabilitative interventions.

Any practitioner who deals with pain problems must be aware of the entire range of pathophysiological and psychopathological problems that are commonly encountered, and must have access to a reasonable range of medical, physical, and psychological therapies. The practitioner who applies a single modality to the entire range of painful conditions, whether he is an anesthesiologist, chiropractor, surgeon, or psychologist, is costing his patients and society dearly, both in financial costs and in personal suffering.

Stephen E. Abram, M.D.

PART I

Introduction

The Pain Clinic Manual, Second Edition,
edited by Stephen E. Abram and J. David Haddox.
Lippincott Williams & Wilkins,
Philadelphia, © 2000

1

Pain Clinic Organization and Staffing

William L. Johnson, Stephen E. Abram, and N. Timothy Lynch

W. L. Johnson: Department of Anesthesiology,
University of New Mexico, School of Medicine,
Albuquerque, New Mexico 87102.
S. E. Abram: Department of Anesthesiology and Critical Care Medicine,
University of New Mexico, Health Sciences Center—School of Medicine,
Albuquerque, New Mexico 87131.
N. T. Lynch: Department of Anesthesiology, Medical College of Wisconsin,
Milwaukee, Wisconsin 53226.

I. CLASSIFICATION OF PAIN CENTERS

A. Multidisciplinary Pain Clinic

The characteristics and structure of a pain center depend on the personnel and resources available as well as the patient population to be served. The ideal multidisciplinary/interdisciplinary pain clinic should represent a balanced program of patient care as well as a diverse collection of medical specialists and office support personnel. This multidisciplinary model provides extensive diagnostic, therapeutic, and rehabilitative services as outlined in Table 1-1. In some centers a major comprehensive pain center for both inpatient and outpatient facilities is impossible in one setting. As long as the full spectrum of services is available on a consultation basis in a timely fashion, the clinic can function adequately.

B. Syndrome-Oriented Clinic

Limiting the practice of a clinic to management of a specific pain problem (headache, cancer pain, low back pain) reduces the range of services and personnel required. The type of health care providers needed will vary greatly according to the syndrome being treated. A few types of syndrome-oriented clinics and the typical staffing requirements are listed in Table 1-2.

C. Modality-Oriented Clinic

Modality-oriented clinics offer a single type of treatment or a limited range of treatment options. Nerve block clinics that are staffed by anesthesiologists are common in both private and teaching hospitals. Psychologists often provide behavioral and cognitive management protocols as a sole means of treatment. Physiatrists typically offer physical therapeutic and psychosocial

TABLE 1-1. *Services of a multidisciplinary pain clinic*

I. Diagnostic
  A. History
    1. Questionnaire
    2. Verbal
  B. Physical examination by staff physician
  C. Psychologic testing and interpretation
  D. Psychologic interview (psychiatrist or psychologist)
    1. Interview with patient
    2. Interview with family members
  E. Laboratory
    1. Clinical laboratory
    2. Radiographs, computed tomography, magnetic resonance imaging, bone scan, etc.
    3. Special tests (thermography, EMG, evoked potentials)
II. Therapeutic
  A. Pharmacologic (analgesics, psychotropics, antiinflammatory, muscle relaxants, drug detoxification)
  B. Cognitive (coping strategies, biofeedback, and relaxation)
  C. Medical modalities (nerve blocks, steroid injections, neurosurgical ablation, neurolysis, neural stimulation, orthopedic surgery)
  D. Physical modalities (strengthening, and range of motion exercises, heat, cold, ultrasound)
  E. Vocational retraining
  F. Other support services (dietary, social services)

interventions without any medical treatment. Modality-oriented clinics are the most likely pain clinics to offer inappropriate or unnecessary services to their patients. To function in an effective manner, modality-oriented clinics must meet the criteria outlined in Table 1-3.

  D. Other Models
    Many clinics do not exactly fit the description above. A common type, organized around a small group of physicians who offer a restricted range of

TABLE 1-2. *Types and staffing of syndrome-oriented clinics[a]*

Clinics	Staff
Headaches	Neurology
Low back pain	Orthopedics, physical medicine and rehabilitation, neurosurgery, anesthesiology
Cancer	Oncology, radiation therapy, anesthesiology, neurosurgery, orthopedic surgery
Facial pain	Oral surgery, ENT, neurology
Arthritis pain	Rheumatology, orthopedic surgery
Spinal cord injury centers	Neurology, rehabilitation, anesthesiology

[a] In addition to the specialties noted, psychology, psychiatry, and nursing are involved in almost all types of clinics.

TABLE 1-3. *Criteria for effective operation of a modality-oriented clinic*

1. Physician director familiar with a wide range of pain syndromes and therapeutic options
2. Comprehensive evaluation by a physician
3. Recognition of pain syndromes likely to respond to available treatment by clinic staff and referring physicians
4. Rapid, easy access to other treatment options
5. A willingness *not* to treat referred patients who are unlikely to respond to treatments

modalities, might best be described as "oligodisciplinary." The composition of such a clinic might consist of an anesthesiologist, a psychologist, physiatrists, physical therapist, and nurses. Such a group would be capable of handling a reasonable range of pain problems but would depend fairly heavily upon consultants for services required by their patients.

  E. Admission Criteria for Pain Management Programs
    1. No surgically correctable pathology
    2. Failure to respond to conventional medical or physical therapy approaches
    3. Possible psychologic component to pain syndrome
    4. Unable to return to gainful employment because of pain
    5. No active drug or alcohol abuse
    6. Agreeable to program's expressed treatment principles
  F. Pain Management Program Treatment Objectives
    1. Increase physical function, endurance, and strength.
    2. Develop insight into obstacles to recovery.
    3. Begin realistic vocational plan.
    4. Foster independence from entitlement.
    5. Initiate long-term medication use plan.
    6. Improve sleep patterns.

II. STAFFING
  A. Medical Director
  One of the most important and essential factors in the successful organization of a pain center is the medical director. The medical director should be a physician who possesses medical, scientific, and administrative leadership.
    1. Role of the medical director
      a. The medical director must be familiar with a wide range of painful disorders. A sound knowledge of the neurophysiology of pain perception; the pharmacology of analgesic, psychotropic, and neuropharmacologic agents; and the psychologic mechanisms of acute and chronic pain is essential. The director should be aware of the entire spectrum of treatment options available for pain management so that the broadest range of treatment modalities can be utilized either directly or by consultation.

b. The most important attribute of the director is a firm commitment to caring for this difficult group of patients. The director must apply sound pain management principles in dealing with patients and their family members and must ensure that the pain clinic staff is educated in the use of these principles. Financial motivations should not be allowed to interfere with patient care. One must avoid the temptation to use costly procedures if the likelihood of success is low.

c. The director's specialty will often depend on the type of patients being treated. An oncologist is a rational choice to direct a cancer pain clinic; a neurologist may be best qualified to direct a headache clinic. Anesthesiologists are often best qualified to manage acute to subacute posttraumatic pain disorders.

2. Credentials of a medical director. To meet the Commission on Accreditation of Rehabilitation Facilities (CARF) accreditation standards, the medical director must

a. Be American Board of Medical Specialities (ABMS) Board certified in his or her specialty area.

b. Have at least 2 years of experience in the interdisciplinary management of chronic pain.

c. Be a member of a regional or national pain society.

d. Participate in pain-related Continuing Medical Education (CME) programs at least yearly.

e. Be able to serve as team leader to provide direction to treating staff, including occupational therapist (OT), physical therapist (PT), *and* nursing personnel.

3. Responsibilities of the medical director:

a. Medical approval of all patients admitted to ensure that admission is appropriate

b. Acquisition of appropriate diagnostic tests

c. Assumption of medical management of patients admitted: provide prescriptions and physician orders

d. Communication with referring physicians

e. Explanation of treatment protocols and rationale for specific therapies to patient; communication of the diagnosis and prognosis to the patient

f. Procural of appropriate consultations

g. Participation in regular staffing conferences

h. Provision of education to the treating team

i. Provision of public relations activity for the program

B. MD Specialists

1. Physicians who provide regular staffing of pain clinics should possess knowledge of the general principles of acute and chronic pain management in addition to training in their specialty.

2. A multidisciplinary pain management unit should have direct staffing by, or at least rapid access to, physicians of the following specialties: psychiatry, anesthesiology, physiatry, neurosurgery, orthopedic surgery, neurology, and rheumatology. A close working association with members of the specialties discussed in the following paragraphs.

C. Psychologist

1. The psychologist is a member of the pain management team for patients with acute, chronic, and cancer pain. The patient's affective status, stressful factors that influence pain, and underlying coping mechanisms are assessed. Psychogenic pain, "conversion hysteria," or motivation related to secondary gain are occasionally seen. Less than 5% of chronic pain patients, however, are found to have hysterical or conversion disorders. More frequently, increased patient understanding of chronic pain and related symptoms is needed.

2. Role of the psychologist

   a. Patients must be made aware of lifestyle changes, counterproductive behavior, anxiety, and fear of reinjury, all of which may aggravate and contribute to the pain cycle.

   b. Inconsistency of response should be noted during physical examination and sources of secondary gain identified as well as family, vocational, and interpersonal contributions to the pain cycle.

   c. Muscle relaxation through such methods as progressive relaxation, biofeedback-assisted relaxation, and hypnotic relaxation is used to decrease the cycle of pain/spasm/pain.

   d. Counseling about appropriate coping mechanisms is provided along with education and insight into the contributions of stress to the pain cycle.

   e. Adjunct biofeedback (electromyogram) can be useful with instruction in stress management and muscle relaxation. Biofeedback may also assist in providing patients with a sense of control over muscle activity and, once mastered, can assist in counteracting perceptions of helplessness and hopelessness often associated with chronic painful conditions.

   f. Cognitive factors, beliefs, and previous experience with pain are assessed and treated.

   g. Psychologic testing is often performed at the time of admission to the clinic. The psychologist reviews the testing results, looking for disabling psychologic factors, the patient's attitudes toward pain, presence of anxiety or depression, coping abilities, environmental contributors to pain behaviors, and underlying personality disorders or major psychopathology.

   h. A screening interview provides added depth of information and allows the psychologist to uncover specific problems that must be addressed. Individual or group psychotherapy is often recommended on the basis of the screening session.

D. Neurologist

Provides complete neurologic consultation and examination of patients with neurologic disease. This individual should also possess expertise in the management of the wide spectrum of cephalgia; painful neuropathies; central pain syndromes; and diseases involving the spinal cord.

E. Nursing

Nursing personnel must possess unique qualifications. It is important to be able to deal compassionately with a demanding and, at times even hostile, group of patients. A list of duties frequently performed by pain clinic nurses is presented in Table 1-4. The pain clinic nurse must have a sound knowledge of hospital and community resources available to pain patients and must be skilled in the recognition and immediate management of adverse reactions to treatments performed in the clinic.

F. Duties of a Nurse Case Manager

In addition to responsibilities of a pain management nurse noted earlier, a nurse case manager has responsibilities as follows:

1. Schedule daily treatments.
2. Arrange transportation to and from treatment areas.
3. Administer medications while the patient is in the program.
4. Assist in data collection for program evaluation and research.
5. Observe patient behavior and compliance.
6. Participate in team conferences.
7. Arrange and participate in patient follow-up visits.

TABLE 1-4. *Duties of the pain clinic nurse*

I. Patient data collection
  A. Administer and review pain questionnaire.
  B. Administer psychologic testing.
  C. Collect follow-up data.
  D. Take a verbal pain history from patients and family.
II. Patient Education
  A. Discuss principles of pain control with patients and family.
  B. Provide written or audiovisual materials.
  C. Provide instructions for home treatments.
III. Assistance with office treatment
  A. Assist with nerve blocks, other injections.
  B. Monitor patients after procedures; initiate resuscitative measures.
  C. Apply certain therapeutic modalities [transcutaneous electrical nerve stimulation units (TENS) biofeedback, intramuscular injections, cold, heat therapy].
IV. Maintenance of supplies, medications
V. Arrangement for services outside the clinic
  A. Home nursing care.
  B. Medical devices (e.g., TENS, infusion pumps, needles, and syringes).
  C. Social and vocational services.

G. Office Support Services

Office support services must be performed by separate individuals unless the clinic is very small.

1. Receptionist
   a. The receptionist has one of the most important jobs in the clinic. The job involves frequent telephone and personal contact with patients and referring physicians and requires good diplomatic and personal interactive skills.
   b. The receptionist must be familiar with clinic policies regarding referral policies and patient preparation. The receptionist must also be able to recognize inappropriate referrals and determine which patient phone calls require immediate physician attention. Many patient questions can be handled by a knowledgeable receptionist. Answers to patient questions must reflect a certain familiarity with basic pain management principles.
   c. A certain amount of decision making regarding timing of patient scheduling is required of the receptionist, who must have some knowledge of which pain consultations require prompt attention.

2. Secretary
   a. The secretary is responsible for ensuring that patient records are available and kept up to date. Transcription is an essential skill.
   b. If daily records are handwritten, legible treatment summaries must be provided periodically.
   c. The secretary should ensure that referring physicians are provided with treatment and progress reports in a timely fashion.
   d. The secretary must also keep track of insurance and billing data. In particular, prior authorization must often be arranged before the patient's clinic appointment. In many instances, if third-party payors do not provide a "prior authorization number" services provided in the pain clinic may not be reimbursed. The secretary must also be able to provide records to insurance companies, attorneys, and other physicians in a timely fashion.

III. DIAGNOSTIC FACILITIES

To function optimally, the multidisciplinary pain clinic requires adequate space for patient assessment and the appropriate equipment for therapeutic interventions. A patient care conference room is essential. This can facilitate patient care conferences with members of the multidisciplinary team as well as patient/staff seminars and lectures. A nerve block/procedure room should be available and include all the pertinent drugs and equipment necessary for interventional blocks. Resuscitative supplies and equipment for patient monitoring should also be present. The range of diagnostic tools needed in the clinic varies considerably with the type of services provided. A list of diagnostic procedures frequently carried out in pain clinics is provided in Table 1-5. Table 1-6 outlines some frequently ordered tests that are generally available outside of the clinic.

TABLE 1-5. *Diagnostic tests often available in pain clinics*

1. Skin temperature monitoring (surface thermistors, thermography)
2. Joint range of motion (goniometer)
3. Pain tolerance and threshold (ischemic tourniquet test, ice water immersion test, Von Frey hairs)
4. Muscle strength testing (dynamometer)
5. Sensory testing (cold, pinprick, two-point discrimination position, vibration)
6. Skin conductivity, skin potential (sympathogalvanic reflex)
7. Muscle tension (surface electromyogram)
8. Diagnostic nerve blocks

IV. TREATMENT EFFICACY

Given the current level of concern regarding efficient use of medical services and resultant financial resources, the issues of efficacy and long-term outcome become very important. In general, the success rates of a multidisciplinary pain center often appear to be conflicting from center to center, despite numerous treatment outcome studies demonstrating the overall efficacy of multidisciplinary pain centers in treating patients with chronic refractory pain.

A. Outcome Variables that Influence Program Treatment Success
1. Patient characteristics
   a. Patients treated in a multidisciplinary program tend to have very different characteristics compared with those treated in a conventional medical setting.
   b. Specific patient characteristics typical of individuals involved in a multidisciplinary pain center often include higher levels of emotional distress, greater utilization of health care resources, greater functional impairment, increased opiate usage, and a high prevalence of surgical interventions.
   c. Multidisciplinary program patients appear to be at an increased risk of failure with any treatment. As a result, defining treatment outcome becomes difficult.
2. How outcomes are measured varies greatly from one study to the next.

TABLE 1-6. *Frequently ordered diagnostic tests available outside the pain clinic*

1. Plain radiographs
2. Myelography
3. Computerized tomography
4. Magnetic resonance imaging
5. Bone scan (including three-phase) and tomographic (SPECT) bone scans
6. Electromyography and nerve conduction studies
7. Sensory and motor evoked potentials

V. TREATMENT OUTCOME
   A. Many epidemiologic studies have evaluated the efficacy of multidisciplinary
      pain centers. Using many criteria, many of these surveys have included the
      following treatment outcome variables:
      1. Return to work
      2. Decreased health care utilization
      3. Increased physical activity
      4. Reduction of opiate medication
      5. Resolution of workman's compensation claims
      6. Improved role functioning at home
   B. Cost of Inadequate Treatment of Pain
      1. It is important to utilize multiple criteria. For example, a patient may
         exhibit excellent reduction in pain without returning to work.
      2. It has been estimated that the annual cost for lower back pain after
         occupational injury is $7.2 billion for workman's compensation and
         medical expenditures plus another $6 to $11 billion annually in lost
         production.
      3. Disability payments add another tremendous expenditure to the cost to
         society. It is estimated that more than 5 million Americans are perma-
         nently disabled by chronic back pain and that the average cost for each
         patient receiving permanent disability payments for job-related back
         injuries is $300,000.
      4. Multiple literature reviews coupled with estimated cost savings suggest
         that the multidisciplinary pain center model is not only clinically sig-
         nificant in treating patients with chronic pain, but also cost-effective.
         The estimated savings from expansion of multidisciplinary treatment to
         the entire population who are appropriate for such management is about
         $700 million.

RECOMMENDED READING

Lynch NT, Hegman KT. Organization of pain management in the clinical and workplace settings. In: Abram SE, ed. *Atlas of Anesthesia,* vol 6: *Pain Management.* Philadelphia: Current Medicine, 1998:12.1–12.13.

The Pain Clinic Manual, Second Edition,
edited by Stephen E. Abram and J. David Haddox.
Lippincott Williams & Wilkins,
Philadelphia, © 2000

2

Pain Pathways and Mechanisms

Stephen E. Abram

*S. E. Abram: Department of Anesthesiology and Critical Care Medicine,
University of New Mexico, Health Sciences Center—School of Medicine,
Albuquerque, New Mexico 87131.*

The systems associated with pain perception are highly complex and adaptable. Sensitivity of many neural components of the pain projection system can be reset by a variety of physiologic and pathologic as well as psychologic conditions. Injury to neural elements under certain circumstances may result in loss of ability to perceive pain and under other conditions may cause spontaneous pain, allodynia (pain evoked by normally nonpainful stimuli) or hyperalgesia (exaggerated pain from a normally painful stimulus).

An understanding of acute pain requires knowledge of the physiology of receptors that respond to tissue-threatening stimuli, the anatomy of peripheral and central nervous system pathways that are activated, and the mechanisms by which various components of the pain projection system can be sensitized or suppressed. Mechanisms responsible for chronic pain states are still more complex. Persistent noxious stimulation or neural injury may lead to irreversible alterations in nociceptor sensitivity, to spontaneous firing of peripheral or central pain projection fibers, and to dramatic changes in the reaction of the central nervous system to sensory inputs. This chapter will provide an overview of the anatomic pathways, the physiologic modulating mechanisms, and the pathologic alterations that are important to the perception of pain.

I. PERIPHERAL MECHANISMS
    A. Nociceptors (Receptors that Respond Exclusively to Intense, Potentially Tissue-Damaging Stimuli)
        1. Cutaneous nociceptors
            a. Characterized by the fiber type involved (thinly myelinated and unmyelinated) and by the types of stimuli to which they respond.
                (1) High-threshold mechanoreceptors: thinly myelinated (A-delta), respond only to intense mechanical stimuli.
                (2) C-polymodal nociceptors: unmyelinated (C) fibers, respond to intense mechanical or thermal stimuli and to a variety of chemical irritants.

          (3) C-fiber and A-fiber mechano-heat nociceptors: respond to noxious mechanical and noxious heat stimuli.

          (4) A-delta high-threshold mechanoreceptors: respond to strong pressure; may respond to high temperatures following heat sensitization.

  2. Nociceptors in other somatic structures

    a. Muscle, tendon, fascia

      (1) A-delta and C fibers

      (2) Poor response to normal stretching or contraction

      (3) Many C fibers respond to chemical irritants, high heat, and strong pressure; some respond to strong contraction, ischemia; others respond to muscle stretching.

      (4) Some A-delta fibers respond best to chemicals, such as bradykinin, others to pressure, stretch, muscle contractions.

    b. Joints

      (1) Small myelinated and unmyelinated fibers terminate in free nerve endings.

      (2) A-delta: widespread plexus in capsules, fatpads, ligaments. Respond to noxious stimuli, intracapsular bradykinin.

      (3) Nociceptive responses are enhanced by prostaglandins.

    c. Cornea

      (1) Most stimuli to corneal epithelium are sensed as pain.

      (2) Innervation mainly by A-delta fibers, with fine terminals devoid of Schwann cell covering. Response characteristics similar to C-polymodal nociceptors.

    d. Tooth pulp

      (1) Afferents respond to a variety of chemical stimuli, strong heating, cooling, and pressure.

      (2) Electrical stimulation produces almost exclusively painful sensations.

  3. Visceral pain receptors

    a. Little evidence that specialized pain receptors exist in visceral structures.

    b. Many damaging stimuli (e.g., cutting, burning, or clamping) produce no pain when applied to visceral structures.

    c. Inflammation, ischemia, mesenteric stretching, or dilation or spasm of hollow viscera may produce severe pain.

    d. For most visceral organs pain perception is a function of visceral afferent (sometimes termed *sympathetic afferent*) fibers.

      (1) Accompanying sympathetic efferent axons in the sympathetic chain and intraabdominal and intrathoracic plexuses

      (2) Cell bodies in dorsal root ganglia, synapse with dorsal horn neurons

e. Pain perception in the gut
  (1) There are probably no nociceptive-specific fibers.
  (2) Pain is thought to result from intense activation of afferent fibers that serve other functions, such as stretch receptors.
  (3) High-frequency activation of visceral afferents activates dorsal horn neurons, producing pain perceived within cutaneous referral sites.
  (4) Referred pain results from viscerosomatic convergence (a single spinothalamic tract neuron can be activated by either visceral or somatic stimuli). Pain is poorly localized.
f. Cardiac pain
  (1) C and A-delta cardiac afferents fire at high rates in response to coronary occlusion or to intracoronary bradykinin.
  (2) Cardiac afferents that respond vigorously to noxious stimuli probably have physiologic functions under normal circumstances.
  (3) Viscerosomatic convergence probably occurs with these fibers.
g. Other visceral structures
  (1) Pain from the upper esophagus mediated by vagal afferents
  (2) Pain of urethral origin transmitted via sacral roots rather than sympathetic afferents
4. Nociceptor sensitization
  a. Results from inflammation or repeated tissue injury
  b. Mediated by several endogenous chemical substances
    (1) 5-hydroxytryptamine
    (2) Histamine
    (3) Bradykinin
  c. Prostaglandins do not produce pain, but they potentiate the action of bradykinin and act as sensitizers of nociceptors.
    (1) Cell membrane phospholipids are acted on by phospholipase A_2 to form arachidonic acid.
    (2) Arachidonic acid is transformed by cyclo-oxygenase to cyclic endoperoxides.
    (3) Cyclic endoperoxides are transformed to prostacyclin and to prostaglandin E_2 and F_{2a}.
    (4) Prostacyclin potentiates bradykinin and histamine-induced edema.
    (5) Prostaglandin E_2 potentiates pain induced by histamine, bradykinin.

II. DORSAL HORN MECHANISMS
  A. Neurons Responsive to Noxious Stimuli
    1. Nociceptive specific (NS)
      a. Located in lamina I

      b. Responsive only to noxious stimuli

   2. Wide dynamic range (WDR)

      a. Located mainly in lamina V

      b. Responsive to either noxious or innocuous stimuli

   3. Both types of neurons give rise to spinothalamic tract axons.

B. Activation of the Dorsal Horn Projection System

   1. Excitatory amino acids (EAAs) such as glutamate and aspartate are the principal nociceptive neurotransmitters.

   2. Excitatory amino acid receptors are in the dorsal horn.

      a. α-amino-3-hydroxy-5-methylisozole-4-proprionic acid (AMPA) receptor responds briefly (milliseconds) to glutamate release.

      b. *N-methyl D-aspartate* (NMDA) receptor results in more prolonged (seconds to minutes) postsynaptic potentials.

         (1) Normally unresponsive to EAAs

         (2) Enabled by repetitive glutamate release or substance P

         (3) Responsible for "windup" (phenomenon of progressive increase in response to repeated electrical stimulation)

   3. Long-term potentiation

      a. Prolonged increase in sensitivity of spinal cord in response to ongoing nociceptor activation.

      b. Possibility of lasting hours to days

      c. Initiated via NMDA and other (e.g., metabotropic) EAA receptors

      d. Mediated by several intracellular mechanisms:

         (1) Increased intracellular calcium

         (2) Activation of protein kinases

         (3) Production of nitric oxide

         (4) Production of prostaglandins

         (5) Early immediate gene transcription, increased production of excitatory neuromodulator peptides

      e. Prolonged excitation and release of EAAs can lead to neuronal damage, possibly producing irreversible dysfunction

C. Modulation of Dorsal Horn Neuron Function

   1. Excitatory modulators

      a. Tachykinins—substance P (SP), neurokinin A

         (1) Enhance excitability by reducing potassium efflux

         (2) Enable NMDA receptor

      b. Dynorphin—endogenous opioid that, in certain concentration ranges, is antianalgesic

   2. Inhibitory modulators

      a. Glycine—intrathecal strichnine, a glycine antagonist, causes intense hyperalgesia, allodynia.

      b. Gamma-amino butyric acid (GABA)

         (1) $GABA_A$—produces hyperpolarization via chloride channel activation; no clinically available direct agonists; benzodiazepines enhance action of GABA on receptor.

  (2) $GABA_B$—G-protein-mediated inhibitory effect; baclofen is a receptor agonist.

 c. Enkephalins—leucine enkephalin, methionine enkephalin.

  (1) Endogenous opiates released near primary afferent nerve terminals in dorsal horn

  (2) Presynaptic: inhibiting release of EAAs, SP from nerve terminal

  (3) Postsynaptic: G-protein-mediated activation of potassium channel; hyperpolarization of WDR, NS neurons

  (4) Prolonged activation of opiate receptor by exogenous opioids causes increase in protein kinase C, which interferes with action of opiate receptor and increases effect of NMDA receptor activation, resulting in tolerance, hyperalgesia.

 d. Serotonin, or 5-hydroxytryptamine (5HT)

  (1) Analgesic when injected intrathecally

  (2) Serotonin antagonist methysergide is involved in descending pain control mechanisms that originate in the midbrain and medulla.

  (3) Analgesic effect of some antidepressants may be related to an increase in serotonin availability in the central nervous system.

 e. Norepinephrine

  (1) Important neurotransmitter in descending inhibitory pathways

  (2) Spinal analgesic effect mediated by alpha-2 adrenergic receptors

  (3) Alpha-2 agonists clonidine and dexmedetomidine analgesic when injected spinally; alpha-2 antagonists yohimbine and idazoxan block their analgesic effects.

 f. Adenosine receptors modulate dorsal horn nociceptive transmission.

  (1) Two receptor subtypes: A_1 inhibits adenylcyclase activity, A_2 stimulates it.

  (2) Adenosine receptors may play a role in spinal opioid analgesia and analgesia induced by transcutaneous electrical nerve stimulation (TENS).

  (3) Adenosine agonists reverse intrathecal (IT) strichnine-induced tactileallodynia; may prove effective in certain hyperalgesic states.

III. ASCENDING PATHWAYS

 A. Spinothalamic Tract (STT)

 Considered the most important pain projection pathway to the brain; not the only pathway

  1. Neurons in laminae I and V that respond to noxious stimulation are cells of origin of the STT.

  2. Majority of STT fibers cross near their spinal level of origin.

  3. Two functionally distinct divisions of the STT

   a. Neospinothalamic tract

(1) Lateral portion of the spinothalamic tract

(2) Discriminative functions—distinct information regarding location, intensity, duration of noxious stimulus

(3) Projects to posterior nuclei of thalamus

   b. Paleospinothalamic tract

(1) Medial portion of the pathway

(2) Autonomic and unpleasant emotional aspects of pain

(3) Projects to medial thalamic nuclei

(4) Stimulation of the tract in patients with denervation dysesthesia reproduces the burning pain these patients experience.

  B. Spinoreticular Tract

    1. Cells of unknown origin

    2. Thought to produce arousal associated with pain perception

    3. Probably mediates motivational, affective, autonomic responses to pain

  C. Spinomesencephalic Tract

    1. Projects to the midbrain reticular formation.

    2. Evokes nondiscriminative painful sensations.

    3. May be important in the activation of descending antinociception.

  D. Spinocervical Tract

    1. Located in the dorsolateral funiculus

    2. Fibers ascend uncrossed to the lateral cervical nucleus, which serves as a relay, sending fibers to the contralateral thalamus.

  E. Dorsal Columns

    1. Mainly associated with nonpainful sensation

    2. Evidence that some fibers are responsive to noxious stimuli

IV. DESCENDING CONTROL

  A. Electrical Stimulation of Periaqueductal Gray (PAG)

Stimulation of this area of the midbrain produces widespread analgesia in animals and humans.

  B. Microinjection of Morphine

Morphine into that area produces generalized analgesia.

  C. Descending Pain Inhibitory Pathways

    1. Anatomic connections from PAG area to nucleus raphe magnus (NRM) and medullary reticular formation (RF)

    2. Adrenergic and serotonergic fibers from NRM and RF descend via the dorsolateral funiculus to spinal dorsal horn cells.

    3. Serotonin and norepinephrine analgesic when injected spinally

    4. Other neurotransmitters likely to be involved in descending inhibition

  D. Multiple Environmental Factors Affect Descending Pain Control Mechanisms

    1. Nociceptive inputs, physical stress activate inhibitory pathways.

    2. Anxiety, depression, emotional distress can reduce pain threshold.

V. NEUROPATHIC PAIN
  A. Spontaneous Discharge from Injured Peripheral Nerves
    1. Demonstrated to arise from experimentally induced neuromas
      a. Activity generated at site of injury and at dorsal root ganglion (DRG)
      b. Activity enhanced by sympathetic stimulation or norepinephrine
        (1) Blocked by phentolamine
    2. Increased number of sodium and calcium channels at site of injury
      a. Possibly different qualitatively from other ion channel types
    3. Increased number of adrenergic receptors at site of injury
    4. Spontaneous activity suppressed by low systemic levels of lidocaine
       and by high-frequency electrical stimulation
  B. Ephaptic Transmission
    1. Loss of myelin from A fibers and loss of Schwann cell sheath from
       C fibers allow spread of electrical activity between axons.
      a. Sympathetic efferent discharge may activate nociceptors.
      b. Mechanoreceptor afferents may activate nociceptors.
      c. Abnormal neuronal activity spreads both proximally and distally.
        (1) Anterograde transmission releases substance P and other vaso-
            active and sensitizing substances peripherally.
  C. Denervation Dysesthesia
    1. Intact peripheral nerve pathways essential for normal function of dor-
       sal horn pain projection neurons and inhibitory interneurons
    2. Following loss of peripheral nerve activity, there may be increased sen-
       sitivity or onset of spontaneous activity in STT neurons.
      a. Loss of large afferents may decrease the activity of inhibitory neu-
         rons in SG.
      b. Spontaneous or heightened activity may also occur more centrally.
    3. Thalamic cells may be sensitized following cord injury or CVA.
    4. Central sensitization may also occur after peripheral nerve injuries.
VI. SYMPATHETICALLY MAINTAINED PAIN
  A. Sympathetic Nervous System Influences on Pain Perception
    1. Norepinephrine, sympathetic stimulation increase spontaneous firing in
       injured nerves.
    2. Central dysregulation of autonomic function
      a. Sympathetic efferents that control skin vasoconstriction are ordina-
         rily under hypothalamic control.
      b. After experimental nerve injury in animals, skin vasoconstrictors
         no longer respond to thermoregulatory influences and come
         under medullary control, as with muscle vasodilator nerves.
    3. Cross-talk between sympathetic efferents and nociceptor axons
      a. Associated with focal demyelination or Schwann cell sheath injury
    4. Sympathetic mediated sensitization of sensory receptors
      a. There is little evidence that sympathetic discharge sensitizes peri-

pheral nociceptors.

b. There is evidence for sympathetically mediated sensitization of mechanoreceptors.

   (1) Sympathetic fiber anatomically contacts mechanoreceptors.

   (2) Sympathetic stimulation reduces firing threshold of mechano-receptors.

c. It has been postulated that a combination of peripheral mechano-receptor sensitization plus sensitization of WDR neurons in the dorsal horn is responsible for some cases of mechanical allodynia associated with sympathetic dystrophy.

RECOMMENDED READING

Basbaum AI. Spinal mechanisms of acute and persistent pain. *Reg Anesth Pain Med* 1999;24:59–67.

Cervero F, Laird JM. Visceral pain. *Lancet* 1999;353:2145–2148.

Coderre TJ, Katz J, Vaccarino AL, Melzack R. Contribution of central neuroplasticity to pathological pain: Review of clinical and experimental evidence. *Pain* 1993;52:259–285.

Raja SN, Meyer RA, Campbell JN. Peripheral mechanisms of somatic pain. *Anesthesiology* 1988;68:571.

Roberts WJ. A hypothesis on the physiological basis for causalgia and related pains. *Pain* 1986;24:297.

Sorkin LS, Wallace MS. Acute pain mechanisms. *Surg Clin North Am* 1999;79:213–229.

Wall PD, Devor M. Sensory afferent impulses originate from dorsal root ganglia as well as from the periphery in normal and nerve injured rats. *Pain* 1983;17:321.

Wilcox GL. Excitatory neurotransmitters and pain. In: Bond MR, Charlton JE, Woolf CJ, eds. *Proceedings of the VIth World Congress on Pain.* Amsterdam: Elsevier, 1991:97–117.

Willis WD. The origin and destination of pathways involved in pain transmission. In: Melzack R, Wall PD, eds. *Textbook of Pain.* New York: Churchill Livingstone, 1984:88.

Woolf CJ, Mannion RJ. Neuropathic pain: aetiology, symptoms, mechanisms, and management. *Lancet* 1999;353:1959–1964.

The Pain Clinic Manual, Second Edition,
edited by Stephen E. Abram and J. David Haddox.
Lippincott Williams & Wilkins,
Philadelphia, © 2000

3

Pain: The Patient's Perspective

Penney L. Cowan

P. L. Cowan: The American Chronic Pain Association, Rocklin, California 95677.

People today focus on what is black and white, wanting yes or no answers. They believe either that something is working according to expectations or that it is not and must be replaced. Either you are sick or you are well. Health care providers know that chronic pain exists in a very gray area of medicine. There may be no evidence of disease or injury. All attempts to determine the cause of the pain may be unsuccessful. The surgery may have been successful, but the person may still have pain. The disease process may have ended, but the pain may remain. The injury may be completely healed, but the pain may still be with the patient. Although pain is not life-threatening, the person with pain feels as if it is.

It is important to drop any preconceived notions you may have about chronic pain and look at what it can do to the lives of those who must live with it and their families.

With all that medicine has to offer today, it is not logical that one would have to live with pain so severe that it can completely control a person. But it happens. Some 80 million Americans live with chronic pain. The task is to help them manage the pain. Before you can do that, it is important to understand what the person with pain must endure. There is much more to chronic pain than the pain.

I. THE BEGINNING OF CHRONIC PAIN
   What actually happens to the person who is sick or injured and fails to find a means to alleviate pain?
   A. Modern medicine is expected to be able to fix, cure, or heal any health problem.
   B. The person with pain willingly undergoes a variety of tests to determine its cause. The tests are frightening. The patient has no reason to believe that the doctor will not identify the cause of the pain and treat it effectively.
   C. When all the tests come back negative, patients with pain experience many emotions.
      1. Disappointment in the doctor and in themselves for not finding a quick fix

    2. Fear
       a. Fear of the pain getting worse
       b. Fear that the diagnosis is so terrible the doctor is not telling them
       c. Fear that they may die because of the pain
       d. Fear that they will be unable to live with such overwhelming pain
    3. Self-doubt about their pain and their ability to endure it
       a. Is the pain real or imaginary?
       b. Are they simply weak and have no endurance for the pain?
    4. Anger
       a. Anger at what caused their pain
         (1) Person who caused their injury
         (2) Accident that began the pain
         (3) Employer that was neglectful
       b. Anger at the doctor for not doing his job properly, not caring, or not believing how much pain he or she really had
       c. Anger at themselves for their inability to make family, friends, and health care providers understand the extent to which they were suffering

D. Searching for a diagnosis and a cure begins. Millions of dollars are spent annually by chronic pain sufferers who believe the next doctor will be able to cure their pain.
    1. The person with pain begins by seeking one doctor after another in an attempt to find out what is causing the pain. Unfortunately, this often becomes an exercise in futility.
    2. People with pain may willingly exhaust financial resources looking for a cure.
    3. With each new doctor, the person with pain becomes more desperate and thus more willing to try anything that promises relief.
       a. Repeating painful and expensive tests
       b. Agreeing to repeated surgeries, hoping that the next one will make the pain go away
       c. Willing to take any medications, regardless of the effects
    4. As doctor shopping and ineffective treatments fail, the person with pain reaches a new level of frustration.
       a. The patient questions the skill and knowledge of the doctors he or she has seen.
       b. Self-doubt may be the patient's most difficult struggle at this point. Patients are unsure if they are imagining their pain. They begin to think that if the pain were real, the medical community would have been able to cure them.
       c. Patients begin to question their mental ability. Are they losing touch with reality? Is the pain really imagined?

    d. Throughout this process the person with pain alienates friends, family, and many health care providers, increasing his or her frustrations.

II. ACCEPTANCE OF THE PAIN

Accepting the pain is without a doubt the most difficult part of chronic pain. With all the miracles in medicine today, it is not logical that pain cannot be relieved. It may be very difficult for people with pain to accept that they will have pain for the rest of their lives.

    A. What does accepting the pain mean to people with pain?

        1. They think it means that they are to give up their search for a cure.

        2. They believe that they will have to accept the same level of pain for the rest of their life. They have no way of knowing that they can reduce their sense of suffering at this point.

        3. They are afraid that the medical community will no longer be available to treat them. They feel abandoned by the health care system.

    B. What do people with pain need from the medical community at this point?

        1. They need to know that there is hope. They need to be told that it is possible to reduce their sense of suffering and improve the quality of their life.

        2. They need to know that the health care community is willing to work with them to find a way to reduce their suffering.

        3. They need to understand the role of pain medications in treating chronic pain.

        4. They need to understand that there may be no treatment or surgery that will alleviate their pain completely.

    C. The person with pain must face many emotions when trying to accept pain.

        1. Confusion

        2. Anger

        3. Frustration

        4. Guilt

        5. Betrayal

        6. Abandonment

III. LOSSES

Many losses accompany a life of chronic pain. In addition to the pain, there are many personal and professional losses that the person must cope with. This is a part of chronic pain that is not recognized by others, unless they have first-hand experience with chronic pain.

    A. The greatest loss of all is the loss of oneself. The person that he or she used to be no longer exists.

        1. A large number of people with pain are overachievers and base their value on their ability to achieve.

        2. Their identity is in what they accomplish. Pain significantly reduces that ability and thus takes away their identity.

3. They fear they have outlived their value because they can no longer contribute anything of value. Their pain has taken complete and total control of their lives.

B. The demands of working become impossible to fulfill and the person with pain is forced to take a leave of absence or apply for disability. Sometimes people are fired because they cannot perform their jobs as required. This in turn results in more losses.

   1. Loss of medical insurance
   2. Loss of income
   3. Loss of future security
   4. Loss of self-esteem and sense of personal value

C. Friends quickly become weary of hearing how much the person with pain hurts. They avoid contact with the person until he or she no longer has a support system from friends.

D. Family may be the only support system people with pain have or can depend on. But family can also find the person with pain too difficult to deal with and abandon him or her. Some of the problems in the family unit because of chronic pain are

   1. Reduction of financial security
   2. Isolation from coworkers who are tired of hearing about their family problems
   3. Loss of any future with the pain person. Dreams are no longer within reach (e.g., retirement or starting a family).
   4. Additional responsibility as family members take on the pain person's jobs.
   5. The members of the family have no support system to help them cope.
   6. Family members experience exactly the same issues as the person with pain; they just do not feel the pain.

IV. OVERCOMING THE STIGMA

Overcoming the stigma of chronic pain may be the most important hurdle in chronic pain. There are many misconceptions about chronic pain today. Only when a person with pain is treated with respect will he or she be receptive to any suggestions offered by the medical community.

A. It is impossible to believe what we do not see; pain is invisible.

B. The phrase "It's all in your head" is by far the most damaging one. Explaining that one experiences pain in both mind and body at the same time will go a long way in providing positive treatment.

C. Explain that depression is a part of any life crisis. It is not necessarily the depression that is causing the pain, but it is an issue that must be addressed.

D. People with pain experience days when they cannot do anything at all. They also experience days when they feel good enough to be more active than normal. It is difficult for everyone to understand their varying level of functioning.

1. Questions about a person's level of pain are asked, such as, "If he can work today, why can't he work every day?"
2. To avoid these types of questions, the person with pain simply stops doing everything, even on good days.
3. People with pain become defensive about their pain. They believe that they constantly must prove their suffering.
4. The end result is that the person with pain becomes more out of shape, experiences increased pain, and is unwilling to do anything that requires physical activity.

V. LEARNING TO LIVE WITH THE PAIN

Learning to live with pain means that the person with pain must become part of the treatment team. This is a complete reversal of any type of medical treatment in the past, so it is necessary to explain how that can be accomplished.

A. People with pain need to understand exactly what to expect from their bodies. They need to know what is normal and what is not.

B. They need to learn what their physical limits are and what type of exercise they are expected to do. Reassurance that pain will increase initially is vital if they are to work to a place where they can exercise without making their pain worse.

C. They need to understand the dynamics of multidisciplinary pain management.

1. Exercise. Patients must realize that inactivity will increase their pain level and that exercise will increase their ability to manage their pain.
2. Biofeedback and the effect that stress has on their pain. People with pain will be defensive about this initially, believing that their pain is all in their head.
3. Assertiveness training, so that they realize they have the right to be who they are instead of trying to be what they think others want them to be. Many of the people with chronic pain are people pleasers and need to stop such behavior.
4. Self-awareness and personal growth is vital if they are going to accept part of the responsibility for their recovery.
5. Communication skills are important so that they can express their needs clearly without resorting to pain behaviors.
6. Recognition of emotions and the connection between the mind and body is important. People with pain need to understand that they are not responsible for their pain, but their emotions have a direct effect on their level of pain. They are very sensitive about their pain and their role in causing it.

VI. HELP FROM THE MEDICAL COMMUNITY

The medical community can do a number of things to help the person in pain.

A. The need to be validated by the medical community is by far the most important need.

       1. The person with pain simply wants others to listen to what he or she is saying and to believe that the pain is real.

       2. The feeling of being labeled can create or add to the depression the person with pain is feeling.

       3. People with pain want the doctor to understand how much they want to get better instead of being made to feel as if they chose their pain to avoid responsibilities in life.

       4. Health care workers may not know what is causing the pain but should at least let the person know they believe their pain is real.

  B. If the doctor accepts the person as having pain, then the patient can accept the pain much more easily and will be willing to work as part of the treatment team.

       1. If you take away the person's defense of trying to continually prove the pain, he or she is more likely to get involved.

       2. When people with pain are referred for counseling, they usually take that to mean that the physician making the referral thinks their pain is imagined.

       3. The physician should help them to focus on their abilities rather than on their disabilities.

VII. RESOURCES YOU NEED TO KNOW ABOUT

  A. American Chronic Pain Association (ACPA) is a self-help organization for persons with chronic pain (telephone: 916-632-0922).

  B. There is a new manual for family members. The *American Chronic Pain Association Family Manual* is available through the ACPA. There are times when the patient is not willing to be treated but the family members are looking for help and support.

  C. Various self-help groups exist that are designed for specific illnesses. They can provide additional information and peer support.

Academy for Guided Imagery

P.O. Box 2070
Mill Valley, CA 94942
(800) 726-2070

ACHE Headache Support Group

875 Kings Highway, Suite 200
Woodbury, NJ 08096-3172
(609) 423-0043

American Academy of Neurology

1080 Montreal Avenue
St. Paul, MN 55116-2325
(651) 695-1940

American Council for Headache Education

875 Kings Highway, Suite 200
Woodbury, NJ 08096
(800) 255-2243

Ankylosing Spondylitis Association

511 North La Cienegra Boulevard, #216
Los Angeles, CA 90048
(800) 777-8189

Arachnoiditis Support Group

Valerie Kruser
2322 Imperial Lane
Waukesha, WI 53188
(414) 896-0095

Arthritis Foundation

P.O. Box 19000
Atlanta, GA 30326
(800) 283-7800

ARMS—information on Carpal Tunnel

P.O. Box 471973
Aurora, CO 80047-1973
(303) 369-0803
www.certifiedpst.com/arm

Chronic Fatigue Syndrome (CFIDS)

P.O. Box 220396
Charlotte, NC 28222-0398
(800) 442-3437

Crohn's and Colitis Foundation

444 Park Avenue South
New York, NY 10018
(800) 932-2423

Fibromyalgia Network

P.O. Box 31750
Tucson, AZ 85751-1750
(800) 853-2929

International Endometriosis Association

8585 North 76th Place
Milwaukee, WI 53223
(800) 992-3636
(414) 355-2200

Interstitial Cystitis Association

P.O. Box 1553
Madison Square Station
New York, NY 10159
(800) 435-7422

Lupus Foundation of America, Inc.

4 Research Place, #180
Rockville, MD 20805-3226
(800) 558-0121

National Chronic Pain Outreach

P.O. Box 274
Millboro, VA 24460
(540) 862-9437

National Foundation for Depressive Illness, Inc.

P.O. Box 2257
New York, NY 10116
(800) 248-4344

National Headache Foundation

428 West St. James Place, 2nd Floor
Chicago, IL 60614-2750
(888) 643-5552
www.headaches.org

National Institute of Health

www.nih.gov
(301) 496-4000

National Multiple Sclerosis Society

733 3rd Avenue
New York, NY 10017-3288
(800) 344-4867

National Osteoporosis Foundation

1150 17th Street NW, #500
Washington, DC 20036-4603
(202) 223-2226

Overactive Bladder Hotline

300 West Pratt Street, Suite 40
Baltimore, MD 21201
(800) 828-7866

Peripheral Neuropathy

P.O. Box 2055
Lennox Hill Station
New York, NY 10021
(800) 247-6968

Phantom Pain Information

(410) 614-2010

Reflex Sympathy Dystrophy

116 Haddon Avenue, #D
Haddonfield, NJ 08033
(609) 795-8845

Sickle Cell Disease Association of America, Inc.

200 Corporate Pointe, Suite 495
Culver City, CA 90230-7633
(800) 421-8453

TMJ Association, Ltd.

5418 West Washington Boulevard
Milwaukee, WI 53213
(414) 259-3223

Trigeminal Neuralgia Association

P.O. Box 340
Barnegat Light, NJ 08006
(609) 361-1014

Vulvar Pain Foundation

P.O. Drawer 177
Graham, NC 27253
(336) 226-0704

VZV Information Line

Shingles & PHN
40 East 72 Street
New York, NY 10021
(800) 472-8478

PART II

Patient Assessment

The Pain Clinic Manual, Second Edition,
edited by Stephen E. Abram and J. David Haddox.
Lippincott Williams & Wilkins,
Philadelphia, © 2000

4

Collection of Historical Data

Margaret B. Hopwood

M. B. Hopwood: Department of Anesthesia, The University of Iowa Hospitals and Clinics, Iowa City, Iowa 52242.

I. IMPORTANCE OF PATIENT HISTORY

As in other fields of medicine, a thorough patient history is an important part of a pain clinic's patient evaluation. In taking such a history, factors influencing a patient's current status can be elucidated and taken into account when planning treatment. It is easiest to obtain historical information by constructing a questionnaire that may be sent to the patient prior to the first visit or administered at the time of clinic entry. Use of such a questionnaire does not, of course, obviate the need for a direct evaluation of the patient, which affords the physician the opportunity to assess verbal and nonverbal cues. The following items are considered essential history.

II. PERSONAL HISTORY

A. General Information

General items required are name, sex, age, and birth date. Address and telephone numbers should also be obtained to facilitate all contact with and follow-up of the patient.

B. Education

The level of the patient's education may influence the response to treatment. It appears that the higher the level of education, the more likely the patient is to benefit from treatment.

C. Occupation

This is also a factor in treatment response, with blue-collar workers showing less favorable responses to treatment than white-collar workers or professionals.

D. Current Employment Status

Employment appears to have a strong influence on treatment outcome. Those who are working full or part time are far more likely to benefit from treatment than those on sick leave or unemployed as a result of pain.

E. Marital Status

This is important both for legal reasons and for assessment of the patient's support systems. Current status should be evaluated, as should previous divorce/relationship patterns.

F. Marital Relationship Rating

This again is a means of assessing support for the patient and of determining the impact of pain on the patient's life.

G. Family Environment

Is the patient living in a nuclear family or with friends? Has he any family members with chronic illness or pain problems? Responses to such questions also reveal the nature of the support system or the possibility of conditioning toward chronicity.

H. Ethnic Origin

Ethnicity of the patient has long been shown to be a strong influence on the patient's perception of and response to pain.

I. Religious Belief

The patient may refuse various treatments or may have an altered perception of his pain due to his particular belief.

III. PAIN HISTORY

Characterization of the patient's pain and of the patient's response to pain is one of the key elements in treatment. By determining the location, quality, duration, and intensity of the pain; how the patient deals with it; and what psychosocial factors are part of the patient's coping mechanisms, the physician can decide how best to treat the patient.

A. Site of Pain

Localization and distribution of the pain help determine the type of pain the patient has (i.e., central versus peripheral).

B. Pain Drawing

Frequently, patients are vague on localization of their pain. Having them shade in the appropriate parts on a full-body drawing is helpful in determining distribution.

C. Duration

Patients who have had pain less than 6 months appear to respond best to medical interventions, whereas those who have had pain for more than 2 years are unlikely to respond to certain treatments. If pain is chronic, the clinician should ascertain if there has been a recent change in severity or quality of pain.

D. Place of Onset

Work-related injuries have a negative correlation with successful treatment outcome. Treatment response may also be negatively affected if the pain had a postsurgical onset or is related to a motor vehicle accident.

E. Pain Characteristics

Time of pain occurrence as well as pain intensity, quality, and radiation give clues to diagnosis and potential treatment.

F. Response of Pain to Activity
Determining which activities improve the patient's pain and which ones exacerbate it will provide clues to the source of pain and to potential treatments.

G. Associated Symptoms
Are other symptoms associated with the patient's pain? Does he have numbness or paresthesia, weakness, bowel or bladder dysfunction, decreased temperature, increased sweating, cyanosis, or edema? Is there local tenderness, hyperesthesia, or hyperalgesia?

IV. MANAGEMENT HISTORY

A. Prior Treatment
Frequently, the patient comes to a pain clinic as a last resort after a long series of treatments in a multitude of settings. By compiling a treatment history, it is possible to avoid both the expense and the frustration of repetitive treatment. What has been tried, and which treatments have helped?

B. Prior Surgery
If the patient has had prior surgery specifically for the pain, he is less likely to have a positive outcome. In fact, an increasing number of surgeries is negatively correlated with successful outcome, and certain operations may complicate subsequent treatment regimens. For instance, lumbar fusion may make epidural injections difficult or impossible.

C. Medications
To determine drug usage (or abuse), interaction, or efficacy of treatment, it is imperative that the clinician know what types of pain medication or other medication a patient is taking. Record the amount of relief and duration of benefit from analgesics, as well as side effects from past and present medications. Note which pain medications have not been helpful.

D. Review of Systems Checklist
Determine if there is any interplay between the pain complaint and other medical conditions. Preexisting medical conditions may complicate or contraindicate certain treatments.

E. Diagnostic Tests
All previous radiologic and laboratory investigations should be reviewed at or before admission.

V. SUBSTANCE ABUSE

A. Alcohol Use
Assess the degree of use/abuse and whether alcohol is used to relieve the patient's pain. Any type of substance abuse poses a serious barrier to successful treatment.

B. Smoking History
Certain disorders, particularly vasospastic problems, may be aggravated by tobacco.

VI. OTHER FACTORS AFFECTING TREATMENT OUTCOME
  A. Job Characteristics
     Delineation of the type of job—such as light, moderate, or heavy physical work—helps to determine the degree to which the job may have contributed to the patient's pain or whether it is realistic to expect a patient to return to his job.
  B. Compensation/Disability
     If a patient is receiving some form of financial remuneration related to his pain, he may have a vested interest in not responding to treatment.
  C. Litigation
     As with compensation, there is a vested interest in not improving when there is potential for remuneration through litigation.
  D. Sleep Disruption
     Insomnia and frequent awakening commonly result from persistent pain or from the anxiety and depression that accompany pain.
  E. Activity Scales
     Pain has a multidimensional effect on the patient that is reflected in changes in vocational, social, recreational, and sexual activities. Measurement of uptime and ability to perform activities of daily living are important elements in a patient history.
  F. Treatment Expectations
     What does the patient expect from treatment: complete relief of pain or reduction to a more tolerable level?

The Pain Clinic Manual, Second Edition,
edited by Stephen E. Abram and J. David Haddox.
Lippincott Williams & Wilkins,
Philadelphia, © 2000

5

Physical Examination of the Patient Experiencing Pain

Sridhar V. Vasudevan

S. V. Vasudevan: Department of Physical Medicine and Rehabilitation, Medical College of Wisconsin, Brookfield, Wisconsin 53045.

Physical examination of the pain patient requires the physician to understand anatomy and the underlying pathophysiology, and to be skillful in neuromusculoskeletal examination. Although pain can arise from several sources, this chapter focuses on the physical examination of the neuromusculoskeletal system. It is important to follow the appropriate procedure for assessment of visceral pain through both clinical and laboratory examination.

I. FOCUS OF THE PHYSICAL EXAMINATION

A systematic approach to the physical examination will provide the most valuable information within the time frames frequently available at a pain clinic. A conceptual framework for the physical examination should include the following.

A. Data Selection

The physician/examiner should predetermine the most important elements that need to be examined. For example, symptoms pertaining to the lumbosacral region (low back pain) require a thorough examination of the lumbosacral spine, lower-extremity reflexes, and neurologic status. For patients presenting with widespread diffuse pain and whose history suggests a possible generalized disorder, such as fibromyalgia/myofascial pain syndrome, a more thorough examination of peripheral joints; the cervical, thoracic, and lumbosacral spine; and gait analysis and neurologic examination is required. Thus the most important step of the physical examination is the selection of appropriate data to collect.

B. Data Collection

The examiner then proceeds systematically to collect the required data. Ongoing assessment is necessary to detect additional abnormalities that may need further study. As an example, finding hyperreflexia in the lower extremities may then result in the need to evaluate for other corticospinal involvement, such as Babinski signs, and other posterior column involvement, for which studies of proprioception and vibration sense would be necessary. In this practical and systematic approach, data are obtained in different stages and different patient postures. For example, some information can be obtained while the patient is initially sitting on the examination table, then with the patient standing, and finally while observing the gait.

C. Data Integration/Analysis

As data are collected in different stages, the examiner needs to integrate the information, look for consistencies, and outline a pattern that corresponds with the historical information, and then find the possible pathophysiology to explain it. Any discrepancies at this stage may require the examiner to collect additional data. For example, an examiner may find atrophy of a group of muscles wherein there were no corresponding neurologic abnormalities during the initial assessment. A more thorough assessment of other muscle groups innervated by the same peripheral nerve or nerve root supplying the atrophied muscle may be indicated to determine if there is a pattern of neurologic atrophy or if this simply represents a disuse atrophy.

D. Problem Identification

The purpose of the physical examination is to obtain the appropriate data and correlate the findings with the historical information. The eventual goal of the examiner is to identify and diagnose the underlying problem.

Following the diagnosis, the additional steps include solution identification and solution implementation.

II. GENERAL PRINCIPLES

A. Reviewing Patient History

By the time the physical examination has commenced, the examiner should have a sufficiently detailed history obtained directly from the patient or supplemented with a data collection system, such as a pain questionnaire. The examiner should review all available medical records and ask the patient about his responses on the questionnaire, noting conflicts and discrepancies in history. The patient's version of the history is noted, as well as the affect and attitude of the patient during the history taking and examination. Historical information should include not only the medical aspect of the chief complaint, history of present illness, and previous medical care, but also the physical, social, psychologic, vocational, and lifestyle changes that have resulted from the persistent pain and the present status of the patient.

B. Examination Protocol

Physical examination should be done systematically. Each examination situation is different. In all examinations, however, the patient is undressed to the point where most of the body part that needs to be examined is clearly accessible and visible. The patient should either be observed while undressing, which can provide significant information, or be clearly instructed to remove outer clothing, including shoes and socks. The patient should wear a comfortable gown that affords privacy while providing opportunity for the physician to examine the most symptomatic body parts.

C. Observing Patient Affect

The physician/examiner observes the affect. Does the patient have a flat affect? Is it inappropriate? Is it consistent? Observe the emotional tone with which the history is provided and how the patient cooperates. Is the patient demonstrating exaggerated behaviors in an attempt to demonstrate and to legitimize the long-standing history of pain, as if no one in the past has addressed her symptoms? Is the patient demonstrating inappropriate, inconsistent, and nonphysiologic responses? Frequently, this is observed in situations wherein minimal palpation evokes severe withdrawal with marked contortions of the body, which in itself would be anticipated to produce more pain. Similarly, a patient may be observed to use a cane at times and at other times reveal an exaggerated pain behavior, demonstrating an outside "badge" to prove the disability. The body language of the patient is a valuable tool to the physician because it can demonstrate acceptance, anger, mistrust, or anxiety needing clarification for a diagnosis and treatment plan.

D. Musculoskeletal Examination

The musculoskeletal examination consists of evaluating the joints of the part involved by inspecting them for swelling, discoloration, warmth, and tenderness. Each joint's range of motion should be evaluated and reported in degrees. Then an assessment of muscles is performed by palpating for tenderness, trigger points, and twitch response over nodular muscles. Muscle length or shortening of muscles, such as the gastrocnemius and hamstrings, can frequently be observed and measured. Posture of the spine and any exaggeration or flattening of the normal curves or any lateral curves, such as scoliosis, need to be observed and reported, indicating the vertebral level at which convexities are noted in the scoliotic curve.

E. Neurologic Examination

Peripheral neurologic examination consists of evaluating muscle strength, deep tendon reflexes, superficial reflexes, and sensory modalities. Central nervous system findings, including mental status and cognitive and cranial nerve functioning, may need to be recorded in detail, depending on the underlying symptoms and pathophysiology.

1. Muscle strength

Muscle strength should be graded using a standardized protocol. The neurologic system that is based on a scale of 0 to 5 or a word system using a zero to normal scale can be used.

2. Reflexes

The examiner should clearly state which deep tendon reflexes were examined and the results of their grading on a 1+ to 4+ scale: 1+ is when deep tendon reflexes are obtained with reinforcement, 2+ is normally obtainable, 3+ is hyperactive reflexes, and 4+ is clonus.

3. Sensory examination

Similarly, sensory examination should be more specific and indicate the areas examined, such as the dermatomes, and what method was used for testing. Thus the examiner attempting to assess a lumbar radiculopathy may indicate "sensory examination to pinprick and touch over the L_5 to S_1 dermatome on the right is normal."

4. Recording data

The examiner is cautioned to avoid using global statements such as "DTRs and sensations are physiologic." Such a report does not give any indication to a colleague or a subsequent examiner as to what specific reflexes and sensations were examined and in what location, and thus causes difficulty when comparing one examination with another.

F. Gait Analysis

The examination of a patient's gait provides valuable information. A neurologic examination should be combined with the musculoskeletal examination for the assessment of gait. Muscle weakness that may not be noticed in a static position may become evident in dynamic gait assessment. Similarly, proprioceptive and joint position loss and coordination difficulties, such as dysmetria due to cerebellar problems, may become evident.

In addition to the formal gait assessment performed in the examination room, it is helpful for the physician to observe the patient's gait as she enters the examination room, as she leaves the examination room, and as she leaves the clinic.

1. Gait consists of two phases

a. The stance phase includes heel strike, foot flat, midstance, and pushoff. During the stance phase, pain on an extremity may result in a decreased stance phase, a quick withdrawal after stance phase, or a lateral bending of the whole body on the side where the patient steps. All these signs suggest an antalgic or painful gait.

The stance phase should consist of a smooth heel strike and flat foot placement, with the toe as the most weight-bearing part of the foot. On midstance, weakness of gluteus medius may cause a lurching toward the involved side, resulting in a gluteus medius lurch or waddling gait.

b. The swing phase includes acceleration, midswing, and deceleration. During acceleration, the ankle is dorsiflexed, the knee is flexed, and the hip joint is flexed. During deceleration, the hamstring muscles contract to slow down the swing phase and the knee extends to begin the heel strike.

2. Gait abnormalities
   a. Wide gait

   The physician should observe the base width, which should not exceed 2 to 4 inches from heel to heel.

   A wide gait suggests instability and can be seen in sensory loss, such as with peripheral neuropathy, and proprioceptive loss, such as with posterior column problems, or with cerebellar dysfunction. The average length of a step is approximately 15 inches. With a painful extremity, unilaterally painful spine, or muscle weakness, step length may be shorter on one side.

   b. Causes of abnormalities

   Gait abnormalities can occur as a result of muscle weakness, instability, or pain. The patient can be asked to walk on his heels and toes to assess lower-extremity strength and stability. Squatting and returning 10 times or getting up on the toes 10 times may be a good indicator of any asymmetry and weakness of the quadriceps or plantar flexor (gastrocnemius—soleus muscle groups). Specifically, asymmetry would become evident with these activities.

   (1) Muscle weakness examples include weakness of ankle dorsiflexors in L_4 or L_5 radiculopathy, causing a drop foot gait; weakness of L_5 muscles, causing weakness of the gluteus medius and a gluteus medius lurch; or weakness of the quadriceps, causing a locking of the knee into extension during the stance phase.

   (2) Instability examples are widening of the gait owing to peripheral neuropathy, an ataxic gait owing to cerebellar dysfunction, and buckling of the knee owing to internal derangement of the knee.

   (3) Pain examples include an antalgic gait or exaggerated nonphysiologic gait in patients with chronic pain.

III. A PRACTICAL SCHEMA

A systematic examination of a patient's spine and major extremities is described herein. For specific joints such as pain in the ankle, knee, or shoulder, the examiner is referred to the Recommended Readings.

A. Patient in the Sitting Position

After obtaining the patient history and deciding on the appropriate data to be selected, the examiner begins collecting the following information with the patient in the sitting position.

1. Joint range of motion. Joint mobility should be assessed passively by the examiner. A joint could be limited in active motion because of weakness or pain inhibition. Look for symmetry between like joints, and note any asymmetry in the passive motion between the joints in the upper extremities. In the sitting position, the following can be examined.

    a. Fingers. All the fingers should be able to touch the distal wrist crease. The thumb should be able to oppose to touch the tip of the little finger and the base of the little finger.

    b. Wrist. Wrist flexion and extension, radial and ulnar deviation

    c. Radial ulnar joint. Pronation and supination with the elbow at 90° of flexion

    d. Elbow extension and flexion

    e. Shoulder. Forward flexion, abduction, external and internal rotation of the shoulder with shoulder held at 90° of abduction, extension of the shoulder

    f. Ankle. Dorsiflexion and plantarflexion

    g. Knee. Extension and flexion

    h. Hip. Flexion, external and internal rotation. Hip extension needs to be examined in the supine, standing, or prone position.

2. Muscle strength testing. In the sitting position the major muscle groups of the upper and lower extremities can be evaluated for static strength, as shown in the following chart:

Muscle Grading Chart

Muscle gradations	Description
5—Normal	Complete range of motion against gravity with full resistance
4—Good	Complete range of motion against gravity with some resistance
3—Fair	Complete range of motion against gravity
2—Poor	Complete range of motion with effect of gravity eliminated
1—Trace	Evidence of slight contractility. No joint motion
0—Zero	No evidence of contractility

    a. The upper-extremity strength assessment can provide indirect evidence of nerve root involvement.

    b. Shoulder abductors and elbow flexors provide information about the C_5 nerve root.

    c. Elbow flexors and wrist extensors, especially the extensor carpi radialis, provide information about the C_6 nerve root.

    d. Elbow extension and wrist extensors provide information about the C_7 nerve root.

    e. Finger flexors, interossei muscles by finger abduction and adduction, provide information about the C_8 nerve root.

    f. Finger abduction also provides information about the T_1 nerve root.

    g. Tibialis anterior strength with ankle dorsiflexion provides information about the L_4 and L_5 nerve roots, predominantly the L_5 and the peroneal nerve.

h. The extensor hallucis longus strength provides information about the L_5 deep peroneal nerve.

3. Deep tendon reflexes

Deep tendon reflexes can be examined in a sitting position and provide the following information.

a. Biceps reflex provides information about the C_5 nerve root.
b. Brachioradialis reflex provides information about the C_6 nerve root.
c. Triceps reflex provides information about the C_7 nerve root.
d. The patellar reflex provides information about the L_4 nerve root.
e. The achilles reflex provides information about the S_1 nerve root.
f. The posterior tibial and hamstring reflex provides information about the L_5 nerve root.
g. Babinski reflex can provide information about the corticospinal tract and any upper motor neuron involvement.

4. Sensation

A sitting position provides good opportunity to assess sensation to pin-prick and touch.

a. Sensory examination over the lateral upper arm provides information about the C_5 nerve root and the axillary nerve.
b. Sensory examination of the lateral forearm, thumb, index, and half of the middle finger provides information about the C_6 nerve root and sensory branches of the musculocutaneous nerve.
c. The middle finger provides information about the C_7 nerve root.
d. The ring and little finger provide information about the ulnar nerve and the C_8 nerve root.
e. The medial part of the arm provides information about the medial brachial cutaneous nerve and the T_1 nerve root.
f. In the lower extremity, the web space between the first and second toes can provide information about the L_5 nerve root.
g. The lateral aspect of the foot provides information about the S_1 nerve root.
h. The anterior thigh provides information about the L_2 and L_3 nerve roots.
i. The anterior part of the lower leg provides information about the L_4 nerve root.
j. The anterior lateral aspect of the thigh provides information about the lateral femoral cutaneous nerve (meralgia paresthetica).

5. Cervical spine range of motion

The sitting position is excellent for assessing the cervical spine range of motion in flexion, extension, and lateral rotation and bending to either side.

6. Special tests

Again, the sitting position provides an ideal opportunity to assess joint position sensation of the lower extremities and vibratory sensation of upper and lower extremities.

The sitting position also provides opportunity to perform the straight-leg raising test, which can later be corroborated with the supine straight-leg raising test.

A positive straight-leg raising test consists of radiation of the pain in the peripheral nerve distribution, usually extending below the knee, and should be described as such. Complaints of pain in the low back or grimacing during straight-leg raising is not, however, a positive result. The physician should instead record the exact symptoms the patient describes, such as pain behind the knee or pain in the lumbar area.

Other specific tests such as cranial nerve examination and palpation of the scapular, cervical paraspinal, thoracic paraspinal, and lumbar paraspinal areas requiring a relaxed position could be done in the sitting position. Cerebellar heel-to-shin, finger-to-finger, and finger-to-nose testing; dysdiadochokinesia testing, with rapid alternating movement of the fingers to the thumb; and dysmetria assessment, using alternate patting of the plantar and dorsal aspect of the hand on the thigh can also be performed in the sitting position.

Muscle tone could be assessed in this position for hypertonia, suggesting upper motor neuron pathology or localized muscle spasm. Always look for asymmetry when using any of the preceding tests.

B. Patient in a Supine Position

After the patient is comfortably examined in a sitting position, he should be placed in a supine position. The following tests are conducted in this position.

1. Straight-leg raising
2. Patrick's test is a test for hip joint and sacroiliac pathology. This involves *f*lexion, *ab*duction, *e*xternal *r*otation, and *e*xtension of the hip joint. This is referred to as the *fabere sign,* with the initial letters standing for these different hip joint movements. Hip joint pain is often referred in the anterior femoral triangle, whereas sacroiliac pain is referred over the sacroiliac joint.
3. The Thomas test to assess hip flexion or contracture can be done in this position.
4. In the supine position, the Hoover test can be done. In this test the patient pushes against resistance to elevate one leg while the examiner evaluates the pressure on the other heel. When a patient is genuinely trying to raise his leg, he puts pressure on the calcaneous of his opposite leg to gain leverage and the examiner can feel this downward pres-

sure on his hand. If the patient does not bear down as he attempts to raise his leg, this may indicate noncompliance.

The supine position is an excellent opportunity to examine the knee joint, the ankle joint, and the hip joint more specifically. In addition, the hip and sacroiliac joint can be examined in this position.

C. Patient in the Prone Position

In the prone position, the spinous processes throughout the cervical through lumbosacral regions can be palpated for tenderness over the spinous process versus the paravertebral muscles.

The hip extension test can be done, which may be positive in reproducing anterior thigh pain seen in L_4 radiculopathy.

D. Patient in the Standing Position

Observe the patient moving from the supine to the standing position. Is it done with exaggerated behaviors or is it smooth? In a standing position the following could be assessed.

1. Pelvic crest heights to see pelvic tilt, pelvic obliquity, or leg length discrepancy.

2. Lumbosacral and thoracolumbar mobility can be assessed by having the patient bend over and then measuring the distance between fingertips to ground.

3. A more accurate assessment of thoracolumbar mobility can be done by using the Schober's test. In this position, a 15-cm line is drawn over the spine and the spinal excursion is measured. A 4- to 5-cm excursion would be expected. In addition, interspinous mobility can be assessed by placing the fingertips on the spinous processes when possible.

4. This position provides for palpation of the greater trochanter, ischial tuberosity, sciatic notch, and the scapular, cervical, and thoracolumbar sacral paraspinal muscles.

5. The standing position provides an excellent opportunity to assess Romberg's sign for posterior column stability.

6. Posture should be observed from the front, back, and side. Normal spinal curvature should be assessed to see if the normal lordosis is flattened and to see whether thoracic kyphosis is accentuated.

7. Chest expansion at nipple level can be done to assess for rigidity of the spine and chest wall. Asymmetries and balance should be noted.

RECOMMENDED READING

Hoppenfeld S. *Physical Examination of Spine and Extremities.* Norwalk, CT: Appleton-Century-Crofts, 1976.

Mayo Clinic and Mayo Foundation. *Clinical Examination in Neurology.* Philadelphia: WB Saunders, 1981.

Polley H, Hunder G. *Physical Examination of Joints.* Philadelphia: WB Saunders, 1978.

The Pain Clinic Manual, Second Edition,
edited by Stephen E. Abram and J. David Haddox.
Lippincott Williams & Wilkins,
Philadelphia, © 2000

6

Psychological Assessment of Patients Experiencing Chronic Pain

Mary Lou Taylor

M. L. Taylor: Department of Anesthesiology, Medical College of Wisconsin, Milwaukee, Wisconsin 53226.

Most patients referred for treatment of chronic pain and all patients being considered for multidisciplinary pain treatment, spinal cord stimulator, or pump implantation need to be scheduled for a psychological evaluation. Evaluation includes a clinical interview and completion of questionnaires.

I. PURPOSES OF PSYCHOLOGICAL ASSESSMENT
  Purposes of psychological assessment include the following:
  A. To determine whether the patient is a good candidate for a particular treatment
  B. To tailor a treatment program to a patient's individual needs
  C. To identify psychological factors that may need to be addressed before pain treatment begins or that may need referral to psychiatry
  D. To establish a baseline from which to judge treatment effectiveness

II. SUBJECTS COVERED
  Subjects covered in the psychological assessment include the following:
  A. Pain
    1. Patient's understanding of current pain condition
    2. Patient's understanding of acute versus chronic pain and goals for treatment
    3. History of pain since it began, from patient's point of view, including past treatments
  B. Effects of Pain Experience
    1. Activity limitations
    2. Changes in work, finances
    3. Secondary gain (financial gain, decrease in responsibility, increase in support and attention due to pain, etc.)
    4. Role changes

47

        5. Perception of blame (Is pain a result of another person's actions? Is anger/injustice an issue?)

        6. Role of fear, guarding

   C. Family Functioning

        1. Level of support

        2. Possible sources of reinforcement of pain

        3. Stressors that may influence pain level and management of pain

        4. Identification of family members who may need to be a part of treatment

   D. Educational and Work History

   Current work status, including any compensation issues, disability applications, and lawsuits

   E. History of Psychological Functioning and Past Treatment

   F. Current Psychological Functioning

        1. Screen for major psychological disorders. Active schizophrenia, paranoid ideation, dissociative identity disorder (multiple personality), or factitious disorder make any invasive treatment of pain very risky or contraindicated.

        2. Assess levels of depression and anxiety.

        3. Identify any cognitive deficits (may be secondary to preinjury intellectual level, injury, or medications/drug use), which may impact on treatment.

        4. Screen for past or current drug/alcohol abuse or addiction.

        5. Assess levels of learned helplessness, external locus of control, or anger management issues that may impact on treatment.

        6. Assess motivation and likelihood of compliance with treatment.

III. ASSESSMENT INSTRUMENTS

   A. Clinical Interview

   The clinical interview allows for a behavioral sampling of pain behaviors, interpersonal skills, and certain functional abilities (grooming, sitting tolerance, etc.) as well as a gathering of information.

   B. Tests

   Many tests exist for evaluating pain experience and general and specific psychological functioning. Normally, only selected tests are administered for an initial assessment. Others are administered on an as-needed basis or as ongoing assessment of treatment efficacy.

        1. Pain Clinic Questionnaire. Most pain clinics administer a version of the International Association for the Study of Pain Data Base questionnaire, adapted to its population. Items cover the nature of the pain; how it began; previous treatments and outcomes; family, social, vocational, and legal issues; and tobacco, alcohol, and medication use.

        2. Multidimensional Pain Inventory. This is a short, standardized questionnaire for chronic pain patients, designed to assess current psycho-

social functioning in relation to pain, responses to pain by a significant other, and activity levels. Patients' responses are rated on 12 individual scales and are classified into one of three profiles, including "Adaptive Coper," "Dysfunctional," and "Interpersonally Distressed."

3. Symptom Checklist 90—Revised. This 90-item self-report instrument provides quantification of patient functioning on nine scales, including somatization, obsessiveness, interpersonal sensitivity, depression, anxiety, hostility, phobic anxiety, paranoid ideation, and psychoticism. It is a good screen for psychological characteristics that may need to be a focus of treatment.

4. Other tests commonly used in treatment or research with chronic pain patients include the following:

  a. Psychological instruments

    (1) Minnesota Multiphasic Personality Inventory. The MMPI is a 567-item comprehensive assessment of psychopathology. Though some clinics use the MMPI routinely, its length and the content of questions make it unpalatable to many patients. Shorter instruments may provide adequate information with greater efficiency. It is often used in pain research.

    (2) Millon Behavioral Health Inventory. The MBHI is a 150-item true/false instrument developed and normed for a general medical population, which yields eight basic coping styles, psychogenic attitudes, psychosomatic correlates, and prognostic indices.

    (3) Beck Depression Inventory. The BDI is a 21-item questionnaire that is easy to administer and can be used repeatedly to track depression over time. Its inclusion of multiple somatic symptoms (sleep disturbance, fatigue, decreased interest in sex) may overinflate scores for chronic pain patients.

    (4) Spielberger State/Trait Anxiety Inventory. The STAI is a 40-item questionnaire that measures anxiety levels as a character trait (how you generally feel) and as a measure of current functioning (how you feel at this moment).

  b. Pain and coping instruments

    (1) McGill Pain Questionnaire. The MPQ is a short instrument that assesses sensory, affective, and evaluative components of pain. Its sensitivity to treatment effects makes it useful for evaluations of outcome.

    (2) Coping Strategies Questionnaire. The CSQ is a 50-item self-report questionnaire that assesses six cognitive coping responses (catastrophizing, diverting attention), and 2 behavioral responses. It can be useful in measuring changes in coping as a result of treatment.

IV. RECOMMENDATIONS BASED ON INITIAL PSYCHOLOGICAL ASSESSMENT
    A. For evaluations for implanted stimulators or pumps:
        1. Recommendation for implantation
        2. Recommendation for psychological pain management treatment prior to implantation
        3. Referral for treatment of depression, addictive behaviors, or other psychological issues; then reevaluation for procedure
        4. Advice against implantation due to psychological factors that would interfere with motivation, compliance, or efficacy of treatment
    B. For general pain management patients:
        1. Recommendation for multidisciplinary pain management program to address physical and psychological aspect of chronic pain
        2. Recommendation for individual pain management counseling to ready the patient for a more demanding multidisciplinary program
        3. Recommendation for individual psychotherapy
        4. Referral to psychiatry
        5. Referral to vocational counseling / training
        6. Recommendation for further acute pain management, without need for further psychological treatment
        7. No further psychological treatment indicated

RECOMMENDED READING

Jamison RN. *Mastering Chronic Pain: A Professional Guide to Behavioral Treatment.* Sarasota, FL: Professional Resource Press, 1995.

Main CJ, Spanswick CC. Personality assessment and the Minnesota Multiphasic Personality Inventory: 50 years on: Do we still need our security blanket? *Pain Forum* 1995;4(2):90–97.

Nelson DV, Kennington M, Novy DM, Squitieri P. Psychological selection criteria for implantable spinal cord stimulators. *Pain Forum* 1996;5(2):93–103.

Turner JA, Romano JM. Psychologic and psychosocial evaluation. In: Bonica JJ, ed. *The Management of Pain,* 2nd ed. Philadelphia: Lea & Febiger, 1990.

The Pain Clinic Manual, Second Edition,
edited by Stephen E. Abram and J. David Haddox.
Lippincott Williams & Wilkins,
Philadelphia, © 2000

7

The Pain-Focused Psychologic Evaluation

Stanley L. Chapman

*S. L. Chapman: Department of Anesthesiology, Division of Pain Medicine,
Emory University School of Medicine; Center for Pain Medicine,
Section of Anesthesiology, The Emory Clinic, Inc.,
Atlanta, Georgia 30322.*

I. SCREENING FOR COMPREHENSIVE PSYCHOLOGIC INTERVIEW
   A. The purpose is to evaluate the need for a more comprehensive psychologic interview.
   B. A psychologic interview is recommended for all patients with significant chronic pain.
   C. The following factors, identified from a medical interview and examination, suggest the need of a more in-depth psychologic interview:
      1. High level of pain severity on a chronic basis
      2. Evidence of significant depression or anxiety
      3. Vague, dramatized, or diffuse complaints that do not fit with expectations based on medical evidence
      4. Substance abuse or chemical dependency (may require addictionology input)
      5. Very low level of activity or unemployment not clearly necessitated by medical problem
      6. Major concurrent or recent stresses in the patient's life
      7. Family alienation, discord, or overprotection
      8. Patterns of significant emotional or behavioral disturbances in the patient's past, including poor coping with previous stresses, multiple health problems not clearly linked with medical findings, school and work failures, interpersonal distress, and/or previous significant difficulty with depression, anxiety, or excessive substance use.
   D. Useful Tests for Screening
      1. Beck Depression Inventory (Beck et al., 1961)
         a. Consists of 21 items, each of which measures a symptom of depression. For each item, patients choose among four statements that range in severity from 0 to 3.

    b. Only requires about 10 minutes for patient to fill out.

    c. Screens for depression, including measures of

        (1) Affect (such as sadness, dissatisfaction, irritability)

        (2) Negative cognition (such as pessimism, feelings of being a failure, guilt)

        (3) Somatic changes (such as poor sleep, appetite, low energy, difficulty getting started)

        (4) Suicide potential (ranging from wishing one were dead to having a definite plan for suicide)

    d. Has short form of 13 items, which correlates highly with score on longer form.

    e. Referral is indicated to psychology if patient scores 8 or above on long form or 5 or above on short form (moderate depression range), and/or if patient endorses item wishing he/she were dead or expressing suicidal planning.

2. Multidimensional Pain Inventory (Kerns et al., 1985)

    a. Consists of 61 items, with a score of 0 to 6 for each item.

    b. Requires about 15 to 20 minutes for patient to fill out.

    c. Devised specifically for patients with chronic pain to measure relevant parameters associated with behaviors and attitudes associated with pain.

    d. Scores are expressed in relation to a normative group of chronic back pain patients.

    e. Scores are presented in two sections.

        (1) Psychosocial section presents scores (relative to normative group of chronic back pain patients) on pain severity, degree to which pain interferes with activities, perceived overall control over life, overall level of emotional distress, and perceived level of interpersonal support related to pain.

        (2) Behavioral section presents scores on:

            (a) How patient sees spouse or significant other responding to pain and related problems, including:

                (i) Number of angry or irritated responses

                (ii) Number of responses designed to help

                (iii) Number of responses designed to distract patient from pain

            (b) Activity level, reflecting degree of participation in

                (i) Household chores

                (ii) Outdoor work

                (iii) Activities away from home

                (iv) Social activities

    f. From their overall pattern of scores, patients can be divided into one of several categories:

        (1) Adaptive copers—cope well with pain and related problems, have high likelihood of responding well to appropriate targeted

interventions for pain, are unlikely to need interdisciplinary comprehensive pain treatment; may not be candidates for psychologic evaluation.

(2) Dysfunctional—multiple problems in coping with pain and related problems, unlikely to respond favorably to simple interventions, often are candidates for interdisciplinary comprehensive pain rehabilitation programs; need psychologic interview.

(3) Interpersonally distressed—report a loss or lack of social and emotional support in the context of pain and related problems—likely to need a psychologic interview to include evaluation of family and other relationships.

(4) Hybrid—contains significant features of at least two of the preceding clusters but lacks statistical power to place in any one cluster.

II. PSYCHOLOGIC INTERVIEWING
   A. Should be performed if indicated from screening described above
   B. It often is helpful to interview the patient and significant other(s) separately.
      1. Significant others may include family members, important friends, previous treating professionals, and case managers or rehabilitation providers.
      2. Significant others often can identify important observable behaviors that the patient may not report, including observations of verbal complaints, activity levels, substance use, compliance with treatment, attitudes expressed toward treatment, and social and medical history.
      3. Interviewing significant others allows comparison of their observations with those of the patient and gives the interviewer some clues regarding the veracity of patient self-report data. Because treatment decisions are likely to be based on such self-report data, this assessment can be critical.
      4. Significant others' responses can affect the patient's behaviors significantly. Frequently observed responses include
         a. Providing attention, sympathy, and support contingent on pain behaviors, which can serve to increase the likelihood of those behaviors
         b. Increased withdrawal of the family in response to pain, which can heighten depression and isolation
         c. Anger and resentment of the family in response to loss of income or function on the part of the patient, and the stress that those losses bring to the family
         d. Family members' advice and opinions regarding the nature and reality of the pain, and treatments and strategies for coping with pain, can either enhance or detract from treatment goals. Commonly observed areas of family input and advice include
            (1) Searching for the cause of the pain versus working on managing it more effectively

          (2) Staying active despite pain versus withdrawing from activities

          (3) Working or not

          (4) Taking medications of various kinds

          (5) Focusing on acceptance and management of pain versus finding the cure

          (6) Complying with recommendations of physicians, psychologists, physical therapists, and other health practitioners

          (7) Applying for disability benefits or not

C. Significant Areas of Inquiry

   1. Pain complaints

      a. Location, description, and patterns of occurrence

         (1) Pain complaints that are diverse and diffuse, vague and poorly described, and/or presented with highly dramatized language suggest the possible importance of emotional, behavioral, and environmental factors.

         (2) Relationship of pain occurrence or intensity should be considered in relation to such factors as stress, reactions of others, activities, weather, time of day, sleep, and medications.

      b. Circumstances surrounding pain onset: relationship to accident, injury, or disease; stressful events; and major life changes

      c. Presence of multiple pain complaints or health problems: possibly suggesting poor coping, susceptibility to stress, hypochondriasis (i.e., focusing on physical complaints), and/or other underlying psychologic condition

      d. Nonverbal pain behavior (i.e., bracing, guarding, rubbing painful areas, verbal complaints, sighing, wincing, changes in posture, etc.). Should be evaluated for

         (1) Consistency of observations with verbal reports. (For example, it is common for patients to say they are unable to sit for more than a brief period of time but to sit for a 60-minute interview without overt signs of increasing pain. Doing so does not necessarily represent malingering and can be related to factors of distraction or mental focusing, loss of perspective regarding abilities, desire to please the interviewer, etc.).

         (2) Consistency with expectations from medical evaluation. Research reveals a positive correlation between severity of medical condition and the presence of such behaviors.

         (3) Demand characteristics (i.e., intended effect on observer). High intensity pain behavior can represent a "crying out" for treatment or for understanding of the intensity or reality of the problem.

         (4) Direct discussion with the patient about his or her awareness of these behaviors, tendency to hide or demonstrate them, and intended effects can be helpful in interpreting them.

2. Physical, social, and recreational activities
   a. Evaluation is often improved by asking the patient to describe a typical day or week.
   b. It is important to assess multiple factors regarding activities.
      (1) Nature of activities restricted
          (a) Consistency with expectations based on medical findings
          (b) General versus specific. Restriction of almost all activities, particularly if inconsistent with clear medical findings, may suggest the importance of psychologic and environmental factors. Restriction of social activities may relate to low self-esteem, self-consciousness, poor communication patterns, lack of assertiveness, and/or depression.
      (2) Efforts to engage in previously enjoyed activities. If patient has not made significant efforts to engage in these activities, suspect significant psychologic or environmental factors.
      (3) Pacing and consistency. Many patients make pain and dysfunction worse by failing to pace activities within the day and by engaging in much more activity on some days than on others.
      (4) Knowledge of body mechanics and posture
3. Work
   a. Poor supervisor rating of work performance was found in the Boeing study (Bigos et al., 1986) to be a precursor of work-related injury and failure to return to work. Ask about work history and performance, relationships with supervisors and employers, reasons for changing jobs, job satisfaction, and patient perceptions of how well he or she was treated.
   b. Evaluate the patient's attempts to return to work and perceived job abilities.
      (1) Ask the details about what the nature of the patient's previous work was, what efforts the patient has made to return to that job, what other jobs the patient has sought, what vocational tasks the patient believes he or she can do, and what the nature of the patient's efforts to find work within those restrictions has been.
      (2) Evaluate how consistent these efforts are with the patient's perceived job abilities, work possibilities, and likely functional restrictions. Patients who have made few efforts to return to some kind of work within such restrictions may be depressed, have low confidence in their ability to be successful, and/or have major secondary gain issues.
   c. Assess employer's and supervisor's attitude and response toward the patient's pain.
   d. Assess financial incentives—patient's and family's income, salary from work, disability considerations, hiring of attorney.

4. Sleep
   a. Nature, history, and frequency of sleep patterns and difficulties
      (1) Diurnal cycle—sleeping during the day may be an avoidance behavior and likely precludes adaptive sleep at night.
      (2) Difficulty getting to sleep frequently is related to anxiety, inactivity or excessive sleeping during the day, caffeine use, and/or failure to distract oneself from pain.
      (3) Early-morning awakening can occur because of dependence on medication and increased pain during sleep (often related to sleep posture); it is also a frequent symptom of depression.
   b. Effects of loss of sleep on pain level, cognitive abilities, irritability, and ability to perform activities of daily living.
5. Social relationships and history
   a. Social responses to pain behaviors
   b. Quality and quantity of social support, historically and presently
      (1) Marital and family
      (2) Friendships
      (3) Relationships with treatment professionals, insurance representatives, employers and supervisors, attorney
   c. Social responses to interview: relationship with interviewer, appropriateness of responses, listening, humor, eye contact
   d. Sexual responses, historically and presently: quality and nature of sexual interactions, interference of pain, attitude and response to any sexual difficulties, communication, and compensatory adjustments
   e. Presence of pain and health problems in members of the patient's family
      (1) Responses of patient and family to problem
      (2) Influences on patient's view of pain and its treatment
   f. Expectations from significant others regarding pain and how it should be handled
6. Emotional status
   a. History of emotional function
      (1) Previous depression, anxiety, psychiatric illness, ability to adjust to previous stresses
      (2) Behavioral problems, including substance abuse, impulsive behavior, anger problems, trouble with the law
      (3) History of physical, sexual, and/or emotional abuse
      (4) History of other major trauma, losses
   b. Current emotional function
      (1) Emotional strengths and weaknesses
      (2) Contributing factors to emotional difficulties, including behaviors, attitudes, beliefs, and environmental stressors and reinforcers

        (3) Nature of emotional problems, such as depression, anxiety, and anger; frequently result from losses and health problems, and contribute to pain and affect treatment outcome.

    c. Depressive symptoms include sadness, pessimism, guilt, dissatisfaction, feelings of failure, hopelessness, social withdrawal, suicidal ideation or planning, sleep loss, appetite disturbance, difficulty getting started, low energy, poor concentration, and loss of libido.

    d. Anxiety symptoms include irritability, worry, poor concentration and memory, distractibility, panic reactions, obsessive thinking, compulsive behaviors, and many types of physical symptoms (muscle tension, heart racing, sweating, tremors, shortness of breath, headaches, ulcers, etc.).

    e. Symptoms of anger include acting-out behaviors, impulsivity and irritability, temper outbursts and interpersonal conflicts, and difficulties.

7. Cognitive-attitudinal factors (thoughts, beliefs, and expectations)

    a. Beliefs regarding the nature of pain

        (1) Causes

        (2) Contributing factors

    b. Beliefs regarding treatment

        (1) Perceived reasons for success and failure of previous treatments

        (2) Perceived current treatment needs

    c. Needed role of treatment staff: educators/guiders versus agents of cure

    d. Needed patient role: active treatment collaborator versus passive recipient of care

8. Expectations of success or failure with treatment options.

    a. Health locus of control—belief that health depends on: one's own behaviors; the skill and behaviors of physicians or other providers; luck, chance, or fate.

        (1) Can be measured by the Multidimensional Health Locus of Control Scale (Wallston and Wallston, 1978), which includes three scales measuring degree of belief that health depends on each of these factors.

        (2) Also can be ascertained less formally during interview.

        (3) Has been found to be an important predictor of compliance and outcome of treatment for chronic problems.

        (4) Related to psychologic construct of self-efficacy (degree of belief that one has the skills and the means to effect rewarding outcomes), which correlates significantly with emotional adjustment and with success of treatments whose outcome depends on behavior.

  b. Attitude toward pain and its role in life.
   (1) Catastrophe versus inconvenience
   (2) Requiring cure versus acceptance and management
  c. Goals for treatment

III. MENTAL STATUS EXAMINATION

 A. Affect: nature, range of expression, appropriateness, relationship to content, stability

  1. Depression: detectable through observations of facial expression, eye contact, spontaneity and responsiveness to interviewer, voice intonation, psychomotor speed, initiative to ask for information or help, laughter/humor, and report of symptoms listed earlier)

  2. Anxiety

   a. Detectable through observed muscle tension, perspiration, tics or tremors, psychomotor agitation (such as pacing or inability to sit still), shortness of breath, poor concentration and memory, distractibility, anxious voice intonation, and report of symptoms listed earlier).

   b. Psychophysiologic evaluation described in Section IV can provide objective measures of anxiety-related symptoms.

  3. Anger: detectable through language, voice tone, facial expression, content of statements

 B. Cognitive abilities: ability to think, attend, concentrate, and remember

  1. Orientation to person, time, place

  2. Distractibility

  3. Quality of associations and responsiveness to interview questions: logical and cohesive versus tangential, rambling

  4. Ability to analyze, draw inferences, understand questions

  5. General fund of information, including knowledge and understanding of medical condition

  6. Memory: can be evaluated from ability to give history and remember content of interview

  7. Processing of information: one means of evaluation is "serial sevens" task: asking patient to count backward from a given number in increments of seven

  8. Consistency of cognitive abilities with history and educational level (to evaluate possible loss)

 C. Social Skills

  1. Quality of relationship to interviewer: sociability, friendliness, cheerfulness, hostility, detachment, responsiveness

  2. Social appropriateness of responses

  3. Appearance and hygiene.

IV. PSYCHOPHYSIOLOGIC EVALUATION

 A. Biofeedback measures can be helpful to measure physiologic correlates of pain and anxiety and can help determine whether biofeedback may be a helpful treatment.

B. Physiologic measurement is useful under a variety of situations.
   1. Resting state, with no instructions
   2. While patient is trying to relax
   3. During simulated or actual stress, which can include imagining a personally relevant stressful situation or being placed in such a situation, such as being asked to do difficult mental arithmetic
C. Repeated measures should be taken to evaluate the consistency of responses across time periods.
D. Several types of measures can be relevant.
   1. EMG (electromyographic) biofeedback measures muscle tightness from electrodes placed on the surface of the skin.
      a. Tightness can relate to medical problems (such as scoliosis), anxiety and bracing, guarding and other postural effects, and usually can be controlled (at least partially) through improved body mechanics and application of relaxation methods.
      b. Multiple muscle groups can affect any given painful area and should be evaluated.
      c. The absolute level of tightness of any muscle can be compared with normative values.
      d. Significant problems also are detectable through asymmetries [i.e., when a muscle on one side (not necessarily the side with pain) reads significantly higher than the corresponding muscle on the other side].
      e. A comprehensive evaluation assesses muscle activity during movement (dynamic EMG) and while the patient is stationary (static EMG) in a variety of postures.
      f. Evaluation during activities or situations common in the patient's day is particularly relevant (e.g., while a patient who is an office worker is speaking on the phone or working at a computer keyboard).
   2. Thermal biofeedback
      a. Measures skin temperature from placement of a temperature-sensitive sensor. Sensor most commonly is placed on a finger or hand (occasionally a foot), as anxiety tends to reduce peripheral blood flow.
      b. Skin temperature correlates closely with blood circulation to the area evaluated, but also can vary significantly, depending on many factors, including room temperature, recent activity, and recent caffeine or nicotine use.
      c. An adaptation period of about 10 minutes after placement of the sensor is necessary for meaningful evaluation.
      d. Thermal biofeedback is particularly relevant for anxiety problems (as hand warming often occurs with relaxation), Raynaud's disease, complex regional pain syndromes, and other prob-

lems associated with sympathetic overactivity or circulatory difficulty.

3. Skin conductance or electrodermal biofeedback
   a. Measures sweat gland activity, another correlate of anxiety and sympathetic activity.
   b. Sensors typically are placed at the tips of two fingers of a hand.
4. Other physiologic measures that can be used for evaluation and training include heart rate, blood pressure, photoplethysmograph (measures dilation of blood vessels and has been used for migraine headache and erectile dysfunctions), and electroencephalogram (varies with state of consciousness and alertness and has been used in treatment of seizures), among others.

RECOMMENDED READING

Beck AT, Ward CH, Mendelson M, et al. An inventory for measuring depression. *Arch Gen Psychiatry* 1961;4:561–571.

Bigos SJ, Spengler DM, Martin NA, et al. Back injuries in industry: A retrospective study. III. Employee-related factors. *Spine* 1986;11:252–256.

Kerns RD, Turk DC, Rudy TE. The West Haven–Yale Multidimensional Pain Inventory (WHYMPI). *Pain* 1985;23:345–356.

Wallston KA, Wallston BS. Development of the Multidimensional Health Locus of Control (MHLC) scales. *Health Educ Monogr* 1978;6:160–170.

The Pain Clinic Manual, Second Edition,
edited by Stephen E. Abram and J. David Haddox.
Lippincott Williams & Wilkins,
Philadelphia, © 2000

8

Diagnostic and Prognostic Nerve Blocks

Quinn H. Hogan

Q. H. Hogan: Department of Anesthesiology, Pain Management Center, Medical College of Wisconsin, Milwaukee, Wisconsin 53226.

Chronic painful conditions often have few distinguishing features to aid in certain diagnosis. Moreover, the subjective nature of pain makes exact communication difficult. In this setting the performance of diagnostic neural blockade offers the possibility of defining the nature and route of nociceptive signals. The general format is that if analgesia follows injection into a tissue or around a nerve supplying a tissue, that is the site of the pain generator. Additionally, a temporary prognostic block allows the patient and physician to determine the desirability of attempting longer-lasting relief with decompressive or neurodestructive techniques.

I. IDENTIFYING PAIN PATHWAY
   A. Tissue Infiltration
      1. Determine depth of pain-generating site by injection at various depths.
         a. Skin or scar infiltration can identify origin from neuromas in incision site.
         b. Muscle infiltration into trigger points identifies myofascial pain.
         c. Pain that persists is from deeper sites such as visceral, deep somatic (joints, bursae, bones), or deep neural structures.
   B. Somatic Peripheral Nerve Block
      1. Identify a site of nerve injury such as neuroma (e.g. Morton's) or entrapment (e.g., carpal tunnel).
      2. Identify a pathway for nociceptive signals (e.g., genitofemoral after inguinal hernia repair).
      3. Determine the contribution of peripheral input to a painful condition, such as greater occipital pathway for chronic headache.
      4. Differentiate between peripheral and central components of pain. If pain persists after successful peripheral nerve block, a central mechanism may be dominant. Pain relief does not exclude a central pathology contribution.

C. Visceral Nerve Block
1. Distinguishes nociceptive signals traveling by visceral pathways
   a. Pain relieved by celiac or hypogastric plexus block but not relieved by intercostal block has origin in viscera and not abdominal wall.
   b. Thoracic pain relieved by stellate ganglion block may have visceral origin, while intercostal block relieves chest wall pain.
2. Local anesthetic celiac block should precede neurolytic injection of alcohol or phenol.
D. Sympathetic Blocks
1. Determine the extent to which sympathetic innervation contributes to generating pain in neuropathic pain, central pain, and RSD (CRPS I).
2. Identifies the contribution of sympathetic activity and reversibility of other nonpainful conditions such as hyperhidrosis, sensorineural hearing loss, long QT syndrome, and peripheral vascular disease.
3. Technique must include
   a. Confirmation that sympathetic interruption occurred (warming, eye signs, loss of sweating, loss of sympathogalvanic response)
   b. Confirmation that there is no somatic blockade by careful evaluation of sensory and motor function
4. If sympathetic block fails to provide relief, comparison with somatic block is helpful: No relief following somatic block may indicate central pain or psychologic mechanism.
5. Alternatives to local anesthetic injection at the paravertebral sympathetic chain include
   a. Intravenous regional guanethedine or bretylium.
   b. Intravenous phentolamine (see Chapter 21, p. 181)
E. Differential Neuraxial Blockade
1. The intention is to inject local anesthetic into the subarachnoid or epidural space in a sequence of concentrations that block sympathetic but not somatic pathways.
   a. Spinal, 5 ml saline—placebo
      10 ml 0.25% procaine—sympathetic block
      10 ml 0.5% procaine—somatic block
   b. Epidural, 5 ml saline—placebo
      10 ml 0. 5% lidocaine—sympathetic block
      10 ml 1% lidocaine—somatic block
   c. Pain relief after placebo indicates psychologic mechanism.
   d. Pain relief after sympathetic (but not placebo) block indicates sympathetic mechanism.
   e. Pain relief after somatic block (but not either other block) indicates somatic mechanism.
   f. Failure to produce relief by any of the injections indicates central pain or psychologic mechanism.

F. Compression/Ischemia Block
1. C fibers (slow pain and sympathetic efferents) continue to conduct after tourniquet application while Aα (motor), Aβ (soft touch), and Aδ (sharp, fast pain) fail in that order.
2. Technique
    a. Perform careful sensory exam.
    b. Elevate arm to exsanguinate.
    c. Inflate tourniquet to 100 mmHg above systolic blood pressure.
    d. Monitor loss of sensory modalities and point at which pain subsides.

II. DIAGNOSTIC PROCEDURES FOR BACK PAIN
A. Sacroiliac Injection
1. Well innervated so probably a possible pain source, but diagnostic maneuvers are unreliable. No diagnostic imaging.
2. Two ways to inject the area
    a. Starting at the midline, direct the needle under the posterior edge of the iliac crest inferior to the posterior superior iliac spine. The needle is unlikely to enter the actual joint space, so drug will be injected into the sacroiliac ligament.
    b. Using imaging (fluoroscopy or CT), a 22-g spinal needle can be directed into the actual joint at its most inferior extent, where there is no overhanging iliac bone.
B. Facet Injection
1. Facet arthropathy is a likely cause of cervical or lumbar back pain, but distinguishing this etiology from other sources of back pain is unreliable by history and exam.
2. Injection into the joint requires careful imaging and meticulous needle placement.
    a. Contact with the joint may re-create pain that resembles the patient's usual pain.
    b. Injection of contrast confirms intraarticular placement.
    c. Use no more than 1 ml of local anesthetic solution since larger volumes may spread to adjacent structures and especially the epidural space.
3. Alternatively, the medial branch of the posterior primary ramus of the spinal nerve can be blocked to denervate the joint. Injection of 1 ml of local anesthetic is made at the upper edge of the transverse process where the superior articular process joins.
    a. Each joint has two nerves innervating it (e.g., the $L_{4/5}$ joint receives innervation from the L_3 and L_4 nerves), so two blocks are necessary to fully denervate (in this example, on the transverse processes of L_4 and L_5).
    b. It is impossible to completely block one joint without partially denervating the adjacent joints.

        4. After injection, inquire about pain at rest, and repeat postures or movements that had previously resulted in pain to identify change in pain.

  C. Intervertebral Disc Injection

      1. Performed with fluoroscopic or CT imaging, and ideally in conjunction with a radiologist

      2. As up to 3 ml of contrast is injected, the patient is asked to compare the sensation created with their usual pain.

      3. Examination of the images following contrast injection can identify disruption of the annulus of the disc.

      4. Typically, several adjacent discs are examined.

      5. The proper indications for the procedure are still debated. It is probably necessary only when MR is indeterminant.

  D. Selective Spinal Nerve Injection

      1. Also known as *foraminal injection,* the intent is to deliver anesthetic only to that segmental nerve.

      2. May be used to identify level of radiculopathy and to plan level of surgical procedure.

      3. The needle is passed by paravertebral puncture and is placed just within the intervertebral foramen.

         a. The S_1 nerve can be reached by needle passage through the posterior sacral foramina.

         b. Gentle needle contact with the nerve may produce a pain that radiates in the fashion of the patient's typical pain, confirming the diagnosis.

         c. Local anesthetic should not exceed about 1 ml to limit spread into the epidural space.

      4. Examination after anesthetic injection confirms decrease of pain and decreased provocation of pain (e.g., straight leg lift, bending).

      5. Be cautious not to inject if pain ensues. Imaging is necessary to confirm placement and level, as well as to avoid injection too medially into the subarachnoid space or cord.

      6. Pain relief following spinal nerve block poorly predicts outcome from ganglionectomy or rhizotomy.

III. LIMITATIONS OF DIAGNOSTIC BLOCKADE

There are several problems with the concept of using neural blockade for diagnosis and prognosis

  A. The model that pain originates from a single site and transmitted by a single pathway is not always accurate.

      1. Following injury, spinal cord function is changed, so low-intensity stimuli may produce pain.

      2. Signals from multiple sites converge on individual dorsal horn neurons, a phenomenon enhanced by high-intensity sensory input.

3. Injured nerves become sensitized at the site of trauma and in the dorsal root ganglion so pain may follow minimal stimuli, mechanical irritation of these sites, and may occur spontaneously.
4. These observations mean that block of the injured nerve may not relieve pain, and block of nerves innervating uninjured tissue may provide relief.
5. Block of the nerve to the site of original injury may not end pain if dorsal horn sensitization has caused a large area of allodynia. Alternately, normalization of dorsal horn function following block may produce unexpected prolonged relief.

B. Dorsal horn response to peripheral stimuli depends on descending signals from the brain.
   1. Analgesia may result from stress or pain during a block, which enhances descending pain inhibition, creating the impression that the block produced relief.

C. Local anesthetic application does not produce a simple temporary neural transection.
   1. Afferent signals, possibly enough to produce pain, especially during sensitization, persist after even intense neural blockade.
   2. When checking for somatic block after sympathetic nerve blockade, despite a lack of motor change or loss of sensation to touch, analgesia could be due to loss of somatic pain sensation.
   3. The size concept (small fibers are more sensitive to local anesthetic) is not reliable. The exact pattern of differential blockade of various sensory modalities is a complicated mix of physical and pharmacologic factors, and cannot be produced in a predictable, stable way.

D. Local anesthetics have systemic effects.
   1. Minimal effect on afferent signals from high-intensity stimulation
   2. Substantial effect on sensitized states
      a. Spontaneous signals from neuromas and dorsal root ganglia are sensitive to low circulating concentrations of local anesthetic.
      b. Sensitized dorsal horn is less responsive with systemic local anesthetic.
   3. Large-dose blocks (e.g., lumbar sympathetic block) most likely to create adequate circulating levels.

E. Assumptions about anatomy may be misleading.
   1. Segmentation, dermatomes, and landmarks are highly variable between subjects.
   2. Injected solution spread is highly variable.
   3. Imaging may eliminate some of the uncertainty that variability produces.
   4. Patterns of visceral sensory innervation, deep somatic sensation, and sympathetic motor innervation are not fully confirmed and do not match somatic sensory patterns.

    F. Psychosocial influences affect reliability of diagnostic block.
        1. Physician is looking for pathophysiologic data, but the patient's agenda may be to document illness, identify a source of hope, or please the doctor.
        2. Placebo response is always a large factor.
            a. All patients may respond to placebos.
            b. Placebo effect especially prominent in chronic pain and with injections.
            c. Physicians expectations are a component in placebo responses.
            d. Suspect a placebo response if the analgesia is incomplete, is inconsistently repeatable, or lacks the appropriate time course for the onset or duration of the active agent.
            e. Response to a placebo does not mean the pain is imagined or contrived.

IV. RECOMMENDATIONS FOR DIAGNOSTIC AND PROGNOSTIC BLOCKS
    A. Confirm that the block worked. No conclusion can be derived if there is not evidence for an effective block.
        1. Identify evidence of sympathetic blockade with temperature, sweating, or sympathogalvanic response changes in the area of interest. Eye signs are only fully adequate if the face is the area of interest.
        2. Document sensory changes in the area innervated by a blocked somatic nerve.
        3. Confirm that no undesired blockade occurred (sensory/motor changes after sympathetic block; effects on adjacent nerves after somatic block).
    B. Carefully evaluate the response to a block.
        1. A thorough preblock exam is necessary.
        2. Measure pain (e.g., visual analog scale) before and after block. Measure pain during activity that has provoked the pain before block.
    C. Consider a placebo injection.
        1. This is particularly important if the block is used to plan surgery or neurodestructive procedure.
        2. Blind both the patient and the physician. An assistant can prepare and keep track of active or saline injectate.
        3. Placebo response means the results from active agent are suspect, but does not mean the patient is lying.
        4. Interpret all responses to diagnostic neural blockade with caution.

RECOMMENDED READING

Abram SE. Pain mechanisms in lumbar radiculopathy. *Anesth Analg* 1988;67:1135–1137.

Hogan Q, Abram S. Neural blockade for diagnosis and prognosis: A review. *Anesthesiology* 1997; 86:216–241.

Hogan Q, Taylor ML, Goldstein M, Stevens R, Kettler R. Success rates in producing sympathetic blockade by paratracheal injection. *Clin J Pain* 1994;10:139–145.

Ness T, Gebhart GF. Visceral pain: A review of experimental studies. *Pain* 1990;41:167–234.

Raja SN, Treede R-D, Davis KD, Campbell JN. Systemic alpha-adrenergic blockade with phentolamine: A diagnostic test for sympathetically maintained pain. *Anesthesiology* 1991;74:691–698.

Raymond S, Gissen AJ. Mechanisms of differential nerve block. In: Strichartz G, ed. *Local Anesthetics.* New York: Springer-Verlag, 1987:95–164.

Turner JA, Deyo R A, Loeser JD, von Korff M, Fordyce WE. The importance of placebo effects in pain treatment and research. *JAMA* 1994;271:1609–1614.

PART III

Treatment Methods

The Pain Clinic Manual, Second Edition,
edited by Stephen E. Abram and J. David Haddox.
Lippincott Williams & Wilkins,
Philadelphia, © 2000

9

Pain Rehabilitation Programs

Stanley L. Chapman

*S. L. Chapman: Department of Anesthesiology, Division of Pain Medicine,
Emory University School of Medicine; Center for Pain Medicine,
Section of Anesthesiology, The Emory Clinic, Inc., Atlanta, Georgia 30322.*

Pain rehabilitation programs became widespread starting in the 1960s to treat patients with chronic pain whose problems had remained refractory to conventional medical approaches. These programs encompass comprehensive interdisciplinary interventions designed to help patients increase their physical and emotional function despite the presence of a condition associated with chronic pain.

I. GOALS OF REHABILITATION PROGRAMS
  A. Maximize physical function and activity level within physical limitations.
  B. Minimize medications to include only those necessary to enhance or maintain function.
  C. Improve self-management of pain and related problems so as to reduce reliance on health care system.
  D. Improve emotional function so as to reduce depression, anxiety, chronic anger, and other harmful emotional states associated with pain.
  E. Find suitable employment, if possible.
  F. Help in the fair and just settlement of disability issues.
  G. Reduce subjective pain intensity.
II. STRUCTURES OF PROGRAMS
  A. Comprehensive Interdisciplinary Evaluation: medical, psychological, and physical. The following are criteria for inclusion of patients in rehabilitation:
    1. Pain problem is chronic (i.e., it has extended past the healing period of 3 to 6 months following an injury or illness).
    2. Pain problem has significantly affected physical and psychosocial function. Patient has significant number of "the D's": disuse, dysfunction (physical, emotional, familial), drug dependency, many dollars of previous health care costs, depression, demoralization, dependence on doctors, disability/employment issues, distress.

3. Patient does not have a pain problem in which function can be restored through easier and less costly means, such as simple advice, medications, etc.
4. Patient is not a clear surgical candidate.
5. Patient has ability to communicate and learn basic information.
6. Patient does not have an acute health problem or outside stress that would keep him or her from participating fully in rehabilitation.
7. Patient's goals are compatible with those of the program.
   a. Patient understands that the primary goal is to increase function (physical, psychosocial, often vocational) and demands active participation in treatment.
   b. Patient agrees to attend treatment regularly, comply with treatment recommendations, and keep diaries and other records as prescribed.
   c. Patient agrees not to receive treatment elsewhere while attending the program.
   d. Patient signs treatment contract, which specifies his or her role in treatment.
B. Program is goal-oriented, coordinated, interdisciplinary, and inclusive.
   1. Goals and decisions regarding treatment are made by patient and treatment team together.
   2. A program manager is designated to ensure coordination of all aspects of treatment among professionals and between professionals and patient.
   3. All professionals actively treating the patient meet regularly at specified intervals (usually weekly) in a team conference to discuss and coordinate treatment.
      a. Patient's input always is discussed as part of this conference.
         (1) Patient may be present for some or all conferences.
         (2) Patient's goals, perception of progress, satisfaction, attitude, and compliance are discussed.
         (3) Program manager communicates results of team conference to patient.
      b. Professionals reevaluate goals and treatment needs at each team conference.
         (1) Ensure consistent treatment.
         (2) Evaluate need for additional assessment or referrals.
         (3) Discuss optimal handling of observed patient problems.
         (4) Reevaluate plan, including intensity and length of treatment.
         (5) Reevaluate follow-up plan.
      c. Team conferences are documented and summarized as part of the patient's record.
C. Programs need to have an intensity sufficient to help patients reach their goals step by step. Initially, most patients' treatment days include at least 5 hours of activity and instruction.

1. Inpatient programs are becoming less common because of reduced insurance reimbursement or approval. Potential advantages of such programs include the following:
   a. Ability to structure a "therapeutic community," in which the patient's environment is controlled throughout the day so as to reinforce function continually, consistently, and intensively.
   b. Staff observation of patient behaviors, which reduces reliance on patient self-report.
   c. Removal of patient from environment that may have conditioned pain behaviors.
   d. Ability to supervise medication use and observe effects of medications or their withdrawal immediately and continually.
   e. Avoidance of dependency on transportation to facility, which may interrupt treatment or aggravate pain.
2. Outpatient programs can include intensive all-day treatment in which patients return home or to a local motel, or can be structured so that patients attend treatment on a less intense basis. The potential advantages include the following:
   a. Opportunity for patients to practice recommended exercises and skills in their naturalistic environment and report back to staff on results.
   b. Opportunity for family report of observations of patient responses to treatment.
   c. Elimination of stress of taking patient away from home environment while undergoing treatment.
   d. More flexible scheduling is possible and may allow some patients to continue working while undergoing treatment.
   e. Opportunity to observe effects of treatment interventions over longer periods of time.
   f. Reduced problems with maintenance of behaviors as patient moves from hospital to home.
   g. Reduced cost in comparison to inpatient programs.
3. Programs often are most effective when treatment is gradually tapered from greater to lesser levels of intensity.
   a. Patients then can have intense supervision while they are acquiring new skills, behaviors, and attitudes, and an opportunity to practice them in the home environment.
   b. Follow-up needs to be planned carefully to enhance independence and control cost while preventing relapse. Relapse prevention may include the following:
      (1) Education of support system (family, significant others, employer, rehabilitation provider or case manager, outside treating professionals, etc.) in their roles in maintaining and extending treatment gains

(2) Preplanning and/or rehearsal in handling problems which may occur, including pain flare-ups and problems with maintaining function

(3) Maintenance of communication with treatment facility
  (a) Planned follow-up visits
  (b) When and whom to call if problems develop

(4) Planning of daily schedule and self-monitoring of patient behavior through patient record-keeping and diaries

III. TREATMENT PARAMETERS NECESSARY FOR REHABILITATION
  A. Patient must be involved and communicate actively with staff rather than be a passive recipient of care.
  B. Professionals are teachers and facilitators who actively listen and communicate with patients.
  C. Focus is on improved management of pain and related problems, not on curing a disease.
  D. Treatments must contribute to improved management of pain and related problems by patient.
     1. Treatments that relieve pain in the short term and have to be repeated over and over again are contraindicated.
     2. Treatments should help increase function.
        a. Medications that help patients function better by relieving pain are consistent with rehabilitation.
        b. The patient must use pain relief provided by medical treatments to increase levels of physical, social, and/or vocational functioning.

IV. MAJOR ROLES OF DISCIPLINES
  A. Physician's Role
     1. Educate patient in medical aspects of pain.
        Medical education often is provided in group settings. The following are examples of common topics:
        a. Chronic pain versus acute pain
           (1) Nature and definitions
           (2) Different treatment approaches needed
           (3) Different patient roles required.
        b. Physiologic/medical rationale for rehabilitation, reactivation, and multidisciplinary treatment
        c. Role of medical testing
        d. Body/mind and body/behavior relationships
        e. Medications—types, indications and contraindications, side effects, and proper patient compliance
     2. Explain results of comprehensive medical evaluation to patient and family.
     3. Provide medical interventions that enhance function, such as medications, injections, and other modalities for relief of pain and related problems, such as sleep loss, depression, and anxiety.

    4. Reinforce importance of rehabilitation and patient compliance with interdisciplinary treatment.

    5. Provide information to other professionals about how medical and physical function can be enhanced.

B. Psychologist's Role

    1. Evaluate behaviors and cognitions of patient and relationships as they affect pain and related problems. (See Chapter 7.)

    2. Conduct group therapies to enhance adaptive coping.

       a. Group education topics often include the following:

          (1) Relationship of pain to emotions, such as depression, anxiety, and anger

             (a) Stages of dealing with grief and loss (from Kubler-Ross, 1969): denial, anger, bargaining, depression, acceptance

             (b) Vicious cycles (reciprocal influences) of pain and depression, anxiety and/or tension

             (c) Gate theory of pain (Melzack and Wall, 1965)

          (2) Role of beliefs, attitudes, and cognitions in pain and its rehabilitation (i.e., positive thinking and focus, development of self-efficacy, and avoidance of catastrophization and of focus on pain and misery)

          (3) Stress management skills, including relaxation (described later), balanced activity, pacing, energy conservation, planning, and humor

          (4) Pain and relationships: communication, assertiveness, handling social situations, and sexual issues and problems

          (5) Behavioral self-control methods, including self-monitoring, goal setting, and self-reward

          (6) Behavioral methods for improved sleep

       b. Besides didactic groups, patients can benefit from groups that encourage active discussion of their behaviors, feelings, and reactions to such issues as the presence of pain, changes in function and relationships, and response to treatment. Benefits of such groups can include

          (1) Modeling of adaptive coping of better-functioning patients, leading to increased hope and recognition that pain and related problems can be managed successfully.

          (2) Recognition of commonality of problems associated with chronic pain, leading to increased self-esteem

          (3) Reduced isolation through sharing of feelings with a supportive group

          (4) Feedback and suggestions from other group members regarding management of pain and related problems

          (5) Opportunity to be helpful to others and appreciated by them, reducing feelings of worthlessness

    c. Groups including family members or significant others can focus on relationship issues and/or improving others' understanding and handling of pain and related problems.

    d. Long-term support groups can help reinforce and maintain improved coping and help patients deal with problems as they occur following the termination of treatment.

3. Provide individual and family therapies to work more intensively on emotions, behaviors, cognitions, and relationships.

4. Teach relaxation methods.

    a. Commonly employed methods include progressive muscle relaxation (sequentially tensing and letting go of muscles throughout the body), deep (diaphragmatic) breathing, imagery, focusing intensively on positive images or memories, and meditation methods.

    b. Patients generally are given tapes with instructions to practice such methods daily.

    c. Goal is to learn to relax deeply through application of brief relaxation methods throughout each day.

    d. Success in developing relaxation skills has been found to reduce pain and improve management of stress and pain, as well as sleep.

    e. Relaxation skills can be enhanced with biofeedback, which measures physiologic parameters.

        (1) EMG (electromyographic) biofeedback can be used to reduce muscle tightness, which leads to pain. It generally is the most commonly employed biofeedback method at pain centers.

        (2) Thermal biofeedback is used to reduce anxiety and improve peripheral blood circulation through measurement of temperature, generally taken from a finger or toe.

        (3) Electrodermal biofeedback measures skin conductance/resistance and is highly correlated with anxiety in some patients.

        (4) Other types of biofeedback include heart rate, blood pressure, and photoplethysmograph (measuring dilation of blood vessels), among others.

        (5) Biofeedback increases the credibility of relaxation by allowing patients to see its physiologic effects.

        (6) In most research studies, pain levels are only modestly correlated with physiologic parameters measured from biofeedback.

        (7) Biofeedback may be most effective in contributing to an improved patient perception of control and self-efficacy, which helps to reduce the commonly observed helplessness and depression.

    f. Self-hypnosis training, which involves the use of selective attention processes to change perceptions, can reduce pain levels in those patients with hypnotic susceptibility.

5. Set up behavior modification plans and reward contingencies so as to increase patients' functional behaviors. Successful behavior change is more likely to occur with:
   a. Specific goal-setting and behavioral contracts with active patient involvement.
   b. Teaching others in the patient's environment (including other professional staff inside and outside the center and family members/significant others) how to be consistent in reinforcing and encouraging needed change.
C. Physical Therapist's Role
   1. Teach and demonstrate exercises to increase strength and range of motion so as to enhance physical function. These exercises generally need to be practiced daily for optimum benefit.
   2. Teach proper body mechanics and posture.
   3. Teach proper conditioning and engage patients in appropriate aerobic activity.
      a. Exercise may help stimulate endorphin release, increase blood circulation to painful areas, and improve the balance and availability of neurotransmitter substances important in controlling pain and depression.
      b. Exercise can be critical for managing stress, distracting a person from pain, and helping that person achieve a greater sense of well-being.
      c. Different forms of exercise are appropriate for different patients, depending on the nature of their pain and limitations.
         (1) Establishing limits, through medical and physical evaluation and patient input and experience, is important.
         (2) Patients need to work to maximize function within these limits.
         (3) Parameters to consider in designing an exercise plan include general medical condition and fitness, patient goals and enjoyment of activity, the current level of exercise, the specific nature of the pain problem, the setting of exercise (e.g., flatness and slope of surface, land versus water), duration of activity, number of times activity needs to be repeated per day, and so on. Many patients with musculoskeletal pain can be much more active in a well-heated pool, as the warmth can help with blood circulation and pain and the buoyancy of the water protects joints from stress.
         (4) The following are general principles for activity programs:
            (a) Stay within assigned limitations.
            (b) Work on increasing activity level gradually from current level.

(c) Pace activities by taking numerous breaks when necessary.

(d) Be consistent day by day. If too much pain follows an activity, scale that activity back and gradually increase from lower level. If necessary, find an alternative activity so as to maintain an increased fitness and activity level.

(e) Avoid spending days in bed or being totally inactive.

(f) Recognize the difference between "hurt" and "harm." Increased pain from an activity does not mean medical harm.

4. Educate patients about modalities for pain relief and use them as appropriate. Examples include the use of heat and cold, transcutaneous electrical nerve stimulation, massage, and so on.

   a. Like medications, modalities must contribute to enhance function.

   b. Whenever possible, teaching patients to use and apply these modalities is preferable to having them applied by a professional, to reduce dependency and passivity, and to reduce the cost of professional time.

   c. Teaching family members to apply certain modalities (such as massage) may be appropriate if doing so helps restore function and does not create an unhealthy dependency.

5. Aid in the return to work process.

   a. Establishment of functional capacity through standardized testing to determine abilities and restrictions in doing physical tasks

   b. Ergonomic analysis of workplace

   c. Work with prospective employer to set up physical demands of workplace to fit patients' needs

D. Vocational Counselor's/Specialist's Role

1. Analysis of education and work history, including evaluation of work abilities, skills, and problems

2. Assessment of interests through interview and standardized testing

3. Work with physical therapist to establish functional capacity, with particular reference to cognitive skills, including intelligence and knowledge, and psychomotor and interpersonal skills.

4. Evaluate reemployment potential.

   a. Comparison of skills with available work

   b. Attitude toward work

   c. Motivation to work

   d. Role of disability status, current or pending

5. If potential for employment is present, coordinate with patient, professional team, perspective employer(s), and case manager/rehabilitation provider to expedite return to work.

a. Identify and work on obstacles, including physical, financial, social, psychologic, and attitudinal.
(1) Work with patient to improve employment skills, job-seeking skills, including knowledge of work possibilities, assertiveness, interview presentation, resume writing, and so on.
(2) Discuss with employer how work can be set up to enhance possibility of success (physical demands, hours, scheduling, etc.) and how the treatment team can aid the employer.
(3) Discuss needs and possibilities of further assistance with the case manager or rehabilitation provider (further training, work hardening, etc.).
(4) Attend team conferences to discuss patient needs with professional team members.
b. Provide needed documentation.
E. Role of Other Disciplines Critical in Pain Rehabilitation
1. Nursing—for patient education, program management, quality review, assistance to physician
2. Occupational therapist—for adaptive devices, work simplification, energy conservation methods, use of leisure time, proper activity management
3. Nutritionist—for proper diet and weight loss
4. Disability evaluation specialist—for impairment and disability ratings, to help settle disability issues by providing information important for case settlement or closure
5. Multiple medical specialists—for medical evaluation, consultation, and treatment
6. Specialists from other disciplines—including, as examples, recreational therapist, kinesiologist, massage therapist, social worker, pharmacologist, and/or chaplain—may need to be involved for optimal outcome.
F. Accreditation
The Commission on Accreditation of Rehabilitation Facilities (CARF) has devised standards with which chronic pain programs must comply to receive accreditation. These standards have been adapted from recommendations of committees consisting of experts in the field. Some states mandate accreditation by CARF for reimbursement for patients evaluated and treated through their Workers' Compensation system. The following are major areas addressed by the accreditation standards:
1. Promoting organizational quality, including philosophy, governance, organizational structure and management, fiscal management and planning, personnel and personnel development, health, physical plant, and transportation

2. Promoting program quality, including patient rights, intake management, orientation, individual program planning, discharge planning and implementation, and records of persons served

3. Promoting outcome measurement and management, including program evaluation, assessing the quality of services provided to the persons served, and analysis and utilization of information

4. Specific program standards for comprehensive pain management programs, defined as providing "coordinated, goal-oriented, interdisciplinary team services to improve functioning and decrease the dependence on health care systems by persons with pain. The program is applicable to those persons who have limitations that interfere with their physical, psychologic, social, and/or vocational functioning" (CARF, 1996). Examples of key standards for all such programs include

   a. Services provided by a coordinated team, which meets regularly in conference

   b. Conferences with patient's family

   c. Medical director who is Board certified within his or her specialty, with at least 2 years of experience in an interdisciplinary chronic pain management program, with membership in a national or regional pain society, who receives ongoing annual continuing medical education in pain management

   d. Physicians other than the medical director need to have 1 year's such experience and the same membership and continuing medical education requirements listed earlier for the medical director.

   e. Program evaluation regularly conducted and reviewed to measure functional and medical outcomes, including appropriate use of medication and effective management of pain, as well as discharge disposition and status of postdischarge functional abilities. (See the following section for a description of some measures that can be used for evaluation of chronic pain rehabilitation programs.)

   f. Team to consist of person served, physician, psychologist, and at least three other disciplines (among 13 listed)

   g. Psychologists must be members of a local, regional, or national pain society; have 1 year's experience in an interdisciplinary comprehensive pain management program; and participate at least once per year in a continuing education activity in pain management.

   h. Weekly interdisciplinary team conference unless needs of person served indicate once every other week is sufficient

   i. If patient has a moderate to severe impairment of physical/functional status, moderate to severe pain behaviors, or at least moderate impairment of cognitive and/or emotional status, services must be provided by pain team members for a minimum of 5 hours per day, 5 days per week.

V. OUTCOME MEASURES
   A. Important to evaluate at pretreatment and at follow-up intervals after treatment in order to evaluate program effectiveness
   B. Careful measures must be taken to avoid biased or inaccurate responding.
   C. Outcome should be evaluated in comparison with cost and outcomes from other centers and from other treatments designed for the same types of patients.
   D. Outcome measures must be reliable and valid.
   E. Standardized measures that are also used at other centers allow comparability of findings.
   F. Examples of major outcome measures include
      1. Subjective pain intensity
         a. Usually measured by a visual analog scale
            (1) Patient marks current level of pain or average level of pain over a period of time on a horizontal line.
            (2) Endpoints of scale usually range from "no pain" to "pain as bad as it could be" or "excruciating, worst pain imaginable."
            (3) Scored from 0 to 10 or from 0 to 100, depending on placement of mark along the line. If the line is 10 cm long (as is common), the scorer can represent distance from "no pain" endpoint.
            (4) Many forms of such scaling exist, including movement of a slide rule to designate pain level, and different labeling of endpoints to measure pain relief or maximum or minimum pain levels.
         b. Measurement is also possible by words chosen from the McGill Pain Questionnaire (Melzack, 1975).
            (1) Contains 20 lists of words reflecting different categories of pain experience, including sensory, affective, and evaluative dimensions.
            (2) Three to six words within each category are listed in order, representing progressively more intense levels of pain perception.
            (3) Subject chooses most applicable word if one or more apply within each category.
            (4) Number of words chosen and mean rank of words chosen help evaluate the dimensions and intensity of pain level.
      2. Activity—often measured from a daily diary reflecting "uptime," or time spent on one's feet during the day
      3. Medications
         a. Complex to measure through a single number

b. One attempt to quantify the detriment potential of medications used is the Medication Quantification Scale (Steedman et al., 1992).
   (1) Each medication is placed in a category with a given "detriment potential," ranging from 1 (aspirin/acetaminophen) to 6 (strong narcotics).
   (2) For each category of medication taken, dose level ranges from 1 (subtherapeutic dose) to 4 (supertherapeutic dose).
   (3) Score for each medication taken is product of dose level and category designation.
   (4) Score for each medication category used is added to derive total MQS score.
   (5) MQS is controversial, in that it assumes linear progression of detriment potential for categories of medications and dose levels of medications, and an absence of interaction between the two. It also ranks opioids as the most detrimental medication class.

4. Work status
   a. Important parameters may include full-time versus part-time employment, hours, income level, changes from prior work status, participation in school or training, and/or work satisfaction.
   b. Outcome may depend on definition of "work," subject selection, and disability incentives, as well as effectiveness of program.
   c. Requires evaluation at least 3 to 6 months after treatment for data to be meaningful.
5. Posttreatment utilization of health care system and cost of health care
6. Emotional status/coping with pain and related problems
   a. Patients can rate overall coping on a visual analog scale or can rate degree of improvement among choices (e.g., "significantly improved," "slightly improved," "not improved," "slightly worse," "significantly worse.")
   b. Many questionnaires, including (as examples) the Multidimensional Pain Inventory and Beck Depression Inventory (described in chapter entitled, "The Pain-Focused Psychologic Evaluation") can evaluate dimensions of status and function.
7. General health status questionnaires
   a. Sickness Impact Profile (Bergner et al., 1981) measures overall degree of interference of illness on medical, psychosocial, and other (sleep, work, etc.) dimensions of functioning.
   b. The Medical Outcomes Study Short Form 36 (SF-36; Ware & Sherbourne, 1992) is a 36-item questionnaire that measures health status along eight scales, including Physical Function, Role Function—Physical, Bodily Pain, General Health, Vitality, Social Function, Role Function—Emotional, and Mental Health.

8. Patient satisfaction questionnaires measure patient perceptions of treatments received and can be helpful in improving program outcomes. Patient satisfaction measurement is required for accreditation through CARF.
   a. Patient satisfaction generally is modestly correlated with treatment outcome.
   b. The Treatment Helpfulness Questionnaire (Chapman, Jamison & Sanders, 1996) is a standardized way of measuring patient perceptions of the degree of helpfulness of treatment modalities experienced in pain centers.
9. The American Academy of Pain Medicine has commissioned the Committee on Uniform Outcome Measures, which currently is working to establish a program evaluation system that can be utilized to allow comparable data collection by pain rehabilitation programs.

VI. OUTCOMES FROM REHABILITATION PROGRAMS FOR CHRONIC PAIN MANAGEMENT

Numerous studies have evaluated major outcomes of pain management programs. Outcome data depend greatly on patient selection and measures used. Flor, Fydrich, and Turk (1992) reported on a metaanalysis of 65 outcome studies, encompassing 176,850 patients receiving treatment for chronic pain at multidisciplinary pain centers. Major findings from this analysis include

A. Mean cost of professional expenses of $8,100 for such multidisciplinary pain centers (versus about $15,000 for lumbar surgery).
B. Mean reduction in subjective pain intensity of about 25% following pain rehabilitation, which was maintained at 5 years' follow-up.
C. Sixty-five percent of patients discontinue use of opioid medications at posttreatment and at 1-year follow-up (versus 6% who do not receive rehabilitation but receive various other treatments for pain).
D. Reduction in hospital rate after treatment of three to six times versus those not treated, with significant reduction in likelihood of surgery.
E. Very variable return-to-work statistics, with average of about 40% to 50% of patients working following pain rehabilitation, significantly more than in its absence or following lumbar surgery.

RECOMMENDED READINGS

Bergner M, Bobbitt RA, Carter WB, et al. The Sickness Impact Profile: Development and final revision of a health status measure. *Med Care* 1981;19:787–805.

Chapman SL, Jamison RN, Sanders SH. Treatment Helpfulness Questionnaire: A measure of patient satisfaction with treatment modalities provided in chronic pain management programs. *Pain* 1996; 68:349–361.

Commission on Accreditation of Rehabilitation Facilities: 1996 Standards Manual and Interpretive Guidelines for Medical Rehabilitation, Tucson, 1996.

Flor H, Fydrich T, Turk DC. Efficacy of multidisciplinary pain centers: a meta-analytic review. *Pain* 1992;49:221–230.

Kubler-Ross E. *On Death and Dying.* New York: Macmillan; 1969.

Melzack R. The McGill Pain Questionnaire: Major properties and scoring methods. *Pain* 1975;1:277–299.

Steedman SM, Middaugh SJ, Kee WG, et al. Chronic pain medications: Equivalence doses and method of quantifying usage. *Clin J Pain* 1992;8:204–214.

Ware JE, Sherbourne CD. The MOS 36-item short-form health survey (SF-36): I. Conceptual framework and item selection. *Med Care* 1992;30:473–483.

The Pain Clinic Manual, Second Edition,
edited by Stephen E. Abram and J. David Haddox.
Lippincott Williams & Wilkins,
Philadelphia, © 2000

10

Physical Therapy in the Pain Clinic Setting

Donna Marie Schramm-Bloodworth

*D. M. Schramm-Bloodworth: Department of Physical Medicine and Rehabilitation,
Baylor College of Medicine, Houston, Texas 77030.*

Physical therapy is one of many modalities available to the physician treating patients with chronic pain. Other modalities include parenteral and injected medications, psychological evaluation and treatment, biofeedback, and vocational and social services. Each modality provides a different benefit to the patient with chronic pain, including, respectively, modulating the transmission of noxious stimuli; instructing the patient about his pain syndrome and coping with its presence; sensitizing the patient to autonomic effects of stress and instructing the patient in conscious relaxation; and assisting the patient in vocational placement or in accessing federal or contractual entitlements. Physical therapy benefits the patient by improving the patient's personal function and fitness.

Physical therapeutics include sustained stretch, strength training, endurance training, training in the use of assistive devices or adaptive techniques, and thermal and electrical modalities. A patient will benefit from physical therapy when deficits exist in flexibility, strength, endurance, or personal mobility. Patients also learn back and joint mechanics and the prevention of injury in physical therapy. A limited effect of physical therapy prescription is decreasing pain. Thermal and electrical modalities may modulate the perceptions of pain, and some studies have shown stretching to decrease reports of pain. However, direct results of physical therapy prescription are improved flexibility, increased strength and endurance, and correct use of assistive devices or body mechanics.

I. PHYSICAL THERAPEUTICS

    A. Sustained Stretch Exercises

        1. Sustained stretch is the most basic of exercises. When range of motion is lost and contracture of a joint capsule or muscle has developed, sustained stretch is beneficial to restore normal muscle length and the joint's full range of motion. Examples of patients who benefit from sustained stretch are patients with adhesive capsulitis of the shoulder and

patients with painful knee osteoarthritis and knee flexion contracture. In the chronic pain setting patients with diagnoses of reflex sympathetic dystrophy and with low back pain with hip flexion and hamstring contracture benefit from sustained stretch.

a. Benefits

(1) Sustained stretch returns a contracted muscle to its "normal" resting length and allows the contracted or restricted joint to move through its entire range of motion. Some studies have found that the stretched muscle is less painful and that stretching, along with a strengthening program, improves the strength of the muscle more than strengthening alone. Relief of contracture also allows the patient to perform personal care and mobility tasks. Using the example of adhesive capsulitis, the patient who may not have been able to perform grooming and hygiene tasks regains this ability when sustained stretch restores range of motion about the shoulder.

(2) The therapist should normalize the resting lengths of muscles and the range of motion around a joint prior to beginning strengthening exercises so that muscles will be strengthened through the entire range of motion, including extremes of lengthening and shortening contraction.

(3) Other benefits of sustained stretch include the relief of pain and the potentiation of strength in low-back-pain patients, the possible prevention of injury with vigorous activity, the reduction of periarticular edema, and increased oxidation capacity of muscle tissue.

b. Indications

(1) To maintain flexibility, most persons should stretch regularly. In the setting of the chronic pain clinic, physicians prescribe sustained stretch for three groups of patients:

(a) Patient with intact motor systems in whom contracture limits self-care or personal mobility

(b) Patient with intact motor systems in whom contracture is painful

(c) Neurologically impaired patients with spasticity. Examples of contracted neurologically intact patients include patients with adhesive capsulitis of the shoulder, and patients with knee osteoarthritis and knee flexion contracture. The population of patients with adhesive capsulitis have difficulty with hair care, upper body dressing, and perineal hygiene. Patients with knee arthritis and flexion contracture experience abnormal loading forces on the flexed knee during ambulation that increase pain and decrease the efficiency of movement. For patients with reflex sympathetic dystrophy, sustained stretch combined with thermal or cooling modalities may improve range of motion of contracted joints.

(2) Physicians also prescribe sustained stretch for the neurologically impaired patient, with diagnoses like spinal cord injury, brain injury, and stroke, as an initial treatment of spasticity.

(3) Patients with diagnoses of primary fibromyalgia, patients with low back pain and hip flexion, hamstrings, or hip adductor contracture, or patients with piriformis syndrome should also participate in sustained stretch.

c. Technique

(1) To apply sustained stretch the therapist stabilizes the bone proximal to the contracted joint and slowly applies steady pressure to the bone distal to the contracted joint. The therapist only stretches the joint in its natural arc of motion. The therapist stretches to the end range achievable in the contracted joint and holds that end-range position for 30 seconds to a few minutes. The patient and the therapist then release the stretch, rest briefly, and repeat the stretch. On subsequent stretches a few more degrees of motion should be attainable. During this therapeutic intervention, the therapist works actively while the patient is fairly passive. The therapist may have the patient assist the stretch by having the patient vigorously contract the shortened muscle group in order to fatigue it, and then relax for the stretch that the therapist applies.

(2) In a joint that moves in several planes, sustained stretch to restore the normal range of motion in each plane should occur. "Frozen shoulder," or adhesive capsulitis, provides an example. In this condition, range of motion of the joint in flexion, abduction, internal and external rotation is limited. The therapist begins sustained stretch of the joint in flexion and then abduction, and later applies stretch to internal and external rotators. By contrast, flexion contractures of the knees, common in patients with osteoarthritis, require the application of sustained stretch of the hamstring muscles.

d. Frequency

(1) Sustained stretch is most effective when performed daily. A patient may perform sustained stretch independent of the therapist, once the therapist has instructed the patient in the correct technique.

(2) The patient or therapist holds the stretch for at least 30 seconds.

  e. Risks and complications

   (1) To prevent injury and to apply stretch correctly, the therapist must isolate the contracted joint from the joints proximal and distal to it. The joint should only be stretched in its natural plane of motion.

   (2) Injuries that may occur as a result of improper stretching include the fracture of osteopenic bones and joint subluxation.

B. Thermal and Electrical Methods

 Physicians and therapists elect to use thermal or electrical methods before, during, or after stretch and exercise to reduce swelling, pain or soreness, or spasm resulting from the painful disorder or from stretch and exercise. The patient, therapist, or physician may use heat or cold in a number of chronically painful conditions. Whether cold or heat is used depends largely on the person's preference. However, in acute injuries and those with swelling, practitioners tend to use cold; heat is used in the absence of swelling or suture lines, and in some chronic conditions.

  1. Thermal methods. Commonly used thermal modalities include hot packs, paraffin baths, K-pads, and ultrasound, a form of deep heat. Hot packs are a form of superficial heat, as are K-pads and paraffin dips.

   a. Benefits. The benefits of thermal modalities include local vasodilatation and increased blood flow, decreased muscle spasm and improved soft-tissue distensibility, and decreased pain. The patient may also perceive psychological relaxation.

   b. Indications. Superficial heat and even deep heat, as in adhesive capsulitis of the shoulder and moderate to severe hamstring contracture, may be used during or just before stretch to promote tissue distensibility, to help local and psychological relaxation, and to decrease pain.

   c. Techniques.

    (1) Hot packs are a form of superficial heat. They come in many forms: microwaved moist towels, gel-filled hydrocollator packs, K-pads that circulate warm water, and electric heating pads.

    (2) The therapist, physician, or patient using heat methods must take caution to avoid burns. Gel-filled hydrocollator packs steep in a 140-degree water bath. Therapists handle the pack with tongs and wrap the pack in at least six layers of toweling before placing it on the patient.

    (3) Microwaved towels, while a useful homemade heat source, may be extremely hot. Tongs for handling and extra toweling to wrap the moist towels are recommended.

    (4) K-pads, often used in hospital settings, circulate heated water. They have a thermostat adjustable from 92° to 104°, changed

by a hex key. In our hospital, thermostats are set at 94° to minimize the possibility of burns.

(5) Physicians should caution patients against the use of electric heating pads. Hydrocollator packs and microwave towels eventually cool. An electrical heating pad can continue to heat. Unfortunately, many reports exist of persons being burned by heating pads after falling asleep on them. Diabetic patients with poor vasculature and sensory deficits, and spinal cord-injured persons with sensory levels are at risk, even if they do not fall asleep, if the heating element settles on an insensate area.

(6) Ultrasound provides heat to deep structures, up to several centimeters, whereas hot packs and other superficial heat sources heat to a tissue depth of less than 1 cm. Physical therapists apply the deep-heating modality of ultrasound in conjunction with sustained stretch to relieve contracture around osteoarthritic joints and adhesive capsulitis. Ultrasound preferentially heats bony surfaces, reflecting heat to contiguous structures.

d. Risks and contraindications
   (1) Absolute contraindications to thermal modalities include anesthetic areas, obtunded patients, and areas of poor venous or arterial flow. Also hemorrhage, malignancy, and acute inflammatory states preclude the use of heat.
   (2) Physicians are advised against applying heat to patients with spinal cord injury, diabetes, sensory neuropathies, angiopathies, and other peripheral vascular disease.

2. Cryotherapy
   a. Cryotherapy, or cold methods, include vapocoolants, ice massage, ice packs, and ice baths. Cryotherapy generally decreases inflammation and swelling. Its ability to decrease muscle spasm is claimed but not proven. Cryotherapy may modulate pain by direct cooling of superficial nerves.
   b. Cold packs applied over a painful joint or area while the patient is attempting range of motion of a painful joint is a common technique to improve patient performance. In the setting of postoperative total knee replacement, the therapist often applies an ice pack to the operated knee during or after stretch to relieve muscle spasm and joint pain.
   c. Avoid cryotherapy in patients with cryoprecipitate diseases, Raynaud's phenomena, angiopathy, and atherosclerotic vascular disease.

3. Transcutaneous electrical stimulation
   a. Transcutaneous electrical nerve stimulation, or TENS, is an electrically powered pain-modulating modality developed in the 1960s.

Originally developed as a transcutaneous screening tool to determine which patients would benefit from implanted technology, TENS emerged as an effective pain-modulating modality.

b. Indications

   (1) Physicians prescribe TENS for acute, postoperative, and chronic pain syndromes.

   (2) However, in the realm of chronic pain, patients with diagnoses of various arthritides, postherpetic neuralgia, arachnoiditis, neuritis, radiculopathy, and plexus and peripheral nerve injuries may benefit from TENS.

c. Technique and technology

   (1) TENS units, about the size of a deck of playing cards, consist of three parts: a pulse generator, an amplifier, and one or two sets of electrodes.

   (2) TENS units generate an electrical impulse that may vary in waveform shape, frequency, pulse width, and amplitude. Applied TENS impulses feel like vibration.

   (3) With conventional applications of TENS (i.e., high frequency and narrow pulse width), dorsal column stimulation occurs and modulates and dampens the transmission of noxious stimuli. Other forms of TENS, like "burst" and "brief, intense" and "acupuncture-like" TENS, which utilize wide pulse width with fast or slow frequencies and which induce muscle contractions, may also stimulate areas of the brain stem that modulate pain.

   (4) During an adequate TENS trial, the therapist adjusts pulse width and frequency to achieve deeper and broader perceptions of stimulation. The therapist also places electrodes cutaneously along the nerve trunk that innervates the painful area. Distal-most placement occurs first and then the therapist migrates the electrodes proximally along the nerve trunk to optimize stimulation. Placebo responders fall out quickly as the efficacy of TENS diminishes with repeated applications. Literature suggests that a 1-month trial of TENS varying lead placement, frequency, and pulse width of impulses will identify the one-third of patients who will benefit from TENS for at least 1 year.

d. Risks and contraindications

   (1) Patients with demand pacemakers should not use TENS.

   (2) TENS is not used over the eyes or the carotid sinus, and its use is generally not recommended for pregnant women, unless used for labor pain, where it has occasional benefit in early stages.

C. Strengthening and Endurance Exercises

Strengthening and endurance exercises form two large distinct classes of exercise. Strengthening exercises consist of three to ten repetitions, moving a muscle-fatiguing load through full range of motion of a joint. *Weight training* is another term for *strengthening exercise.* Endurance exercises, by contrast, are low-load or resistance activities that rapidly and repetitively move large muscle groups to drive heart rate. This class of exercise, also called *cardiovascular fitness exercise,* develops endurance or stamina for activity, as opposed to strength.

   1. Strengthening exercises. Strengthening exercises, or weight training, increase the strength and bulk of the muscle groups exercised. Three types of strength training exist: isometric, isotonic, and isokinetic.

      a. Isometric strengthening. Isometric exercises involve no movement of the load, or weight; the exercise is static, and the length of the muscle does not change. When one "sets a muscle" or locks a joint firmly in one position, a muscle contracts isometrically.

      b. Isotonic strengthening. Isotonic contractions move a fixed weight, or load, through the full range of motion of a joint. This exercise is dynamic, but the speed of the movement may vary at different points along the arc of motion. Weight training with dumbbells and barbells, or "free weights," is the familiar form of isotonic strengthening.

         (1) In physical therapy, instead of weights, therapists often substitute "Therabands," or large elastic bands that offer resistance to motion. Therabands are convenient, inexpensive, and lightweight; moreover, the patient can use them at home to continue an exercise program. The resistance of Therabands varies with the color: Yellow has the lowest resistance and is the easiest to stretch; black is the stiffest and hardest to stretch. In between yellow and black, from easiest to hardest, are red, green, and blue. (For a mnemonic, the order, from hardest to easiest, is alphabetical.)

      c. Isokinetic exercises. Isokinetic exercises are also dynamic but must be done with a special cammed machine, which controls the speed of contraction as the muscle group moves the load. Through the arc of motion against a fixed speed, the load resisted may actually vary.

         (1) A common example of isometric loads in the environment are doors on a hydraulic controller. Regardless of how hard one pushes or pulls the door, it closes at only one speed.

      d. Indications. In practice, isometric exercises are helpful when a patient has pain with range of motion of a joint (e.g., acute arthritis). Isometric exercises, or setting the muscle against gravity or against a load, allow the patient to strengthen the muscle without moving the painful joint. Patients with weakness in gravity, or paresis, due to upper (stroke) or lower motor neuron dysfunction, start with isometric strengthening, contracting the muscle at progressive points along the arc of motion. This activity increases strength while minimizing joint and tendon injury in the weakened limb. The limitation of isometric exercise is that the muscle is only strengthened at the length at which it is contracted.

(1) Physical therapists commonly use isotonic exercises to strengthen patients. Patients use the Theraband in the gym as well as at home as part of a strength-building program. Isotonic strengthening has obvious and empiric utility because humans perform isotonic contractions throughout the day during the completion of activities of daily living and mobility.

(2) Range-of-motion exercises are a special type of isotonic exercise. With weakened patients who have improved from isometric exercise and can move their limbs through a full range of motion against gravity, do not add additional weight until they can comfortably move the weakened limb through five to 10 repetitions of full range of motion. Unweighted movement of a limb for the purposes of strengthening is called range-of-motion exercise.

(3) Persons encounter isokinetic exercise in commercial gyms with cammed isokinetic equipment. Isokinetic equipment has safety advantages for the general and unsupervised public. With free weights, the user must control the motion of the weight. Isokinetic equipment moves a load on a fixed axis of rotation, decreasing the user's need to stabilize the load.

e. Risks and contraindications

(1) Patients with unstable medical and surgical conditions—including unhealed fractures, second- and third-degree sprains, unstable angina, and uncompensated cardiac, pulmonary, endocrine, hypertensive, thrombotic, and hematologic disorders—may not participate in strengthening, endurance, or flexibility exercises.

(2) Risks of strengthening exercises include sprains and strains, as well as more serious injuries from improper use of equipment, improper technique, or unstable medical conditions. Fractures in patients with osteoporosis can occur rarely.

2. Endurance exercise. Endurance exercise refers to aerobic exercise or cardiovascular fitness exercise. Endurance exercises involve the repetitive, rapid use of large muscle groups to increase the heart rate. Examples of endurance exercises include speed walking, jogging, running, swimming, stair stepping, and cycling.

a. Benefits

    (1) The benefits of endurance exercise include reduced resting heart rate, reduced heart rate during submaximal activities, increased stroke volume, improved muscle enzyme metabolism, and more efficient shunting of blood to working muscle. Cardiovascular conditioning improves the efficiency of oxygen delivery and energy metabolism in the body.

    (2) The concept of reduced heart rate during submaximal activity is complex but relates directly to personal mobility and to personal and community activities of daily living. At rest, a lower baseline heart rate indicates efficiency. For example, a person prior to beginning a jogging program has a resting heart rate of 88; after participating in a jogging program for 6 weeks the person may have a resting heart rate in the 70s. During mild to moderate activity, or submaximal activity, this efficiency is apparent. For example, a person prior to beginning a jogging program increased her heart rate from 88 to 106 when vacuuming the house; after 6 to 8 weeks of a jogging program, when the person vacuumed the same house, the her heart rate changed from a new resting baseline of 72 to 84. A different, more strenuous example is provided by running to catch a bus: The unconditioned person might increase heart rate from resting level of 90 beats per minute (BPM) to 150 BPM after running 100 feet to catch a bus; after 6 to 8 weeks of regular conditioning, the heart rate after running the same 100 feet at the same speed might be only 110 beats per minute. In each example the same submaximal workload is done but the lower heart rate required to complete the activity indicates improved oxygen and energy utilization efficiency.

    (3) Like isotonic strengthening exercises, endurance exercise has daily and practical applications because, throughout the day, individuals perform isotonic and endurance activities. In the setting of chronic pain, patients adopt sedentary lifestyles that lead to generalized weakness and deconditioning. Isotonic strengthening and endurance exercise improves strength and stamina for common activities, and these exercises form the basis of most therapy scripts.

b. Technique

    (1) Aerobic exercise specifically improves the endurance of the muscle groups exercised, and generally improves endurance and "fitness" of the cardiovascular system. Exercise must be of adequate intensity to raise the heart rate to 70% to 85% of the person's maximum heart rate for 20 to 30 minutes. Maximum

heart rate is determined approximately by age (maximum heart rate = 220 − age in years) or exactly by a maximal exercise treadmill test.

(2) For patients with stable cardiac disease, 60% of maximum heart rate for 15 minutes is the initial intensity of exercise. Patients more than 40 years of age or with cardiac risk factors should receive medical clearance to participate in an exercise program prior to its initiation. Patients with cardiac disease should be monitored for exercise-induced hypotension and signs of cardiac disease (pallor, angina, diaphoresis, etc.) during exercise. Patients with chronic obstructive pulmonary disease should also be monitored. Aggressive aerobic exercise may exacerbate heart failure or peripheral arterial insufficiency and cause claudication.

c. Risks and contraindications

(1) As with strengthening exercise, patients with unstable medical and surgical conditions—including unhealed fractures, second- and third-degree sprains, unstable angina, and uncompensated cardiac, pulmonary, endocrine, hypertensive, thrombotic, or hematologic disorders—may not participate in strengthening or in endurance or flexibility exercises.

(2) Risks of endurance exercises include sprains and strains, as well as more serious injuries from improper use of equipment or from improper technique or unstable medical conditions. Fractures of osteoporotic bones can also occur with endurance exercises.

D. Adaptive Equipment and Adaptive Techniques

1. Adaptive techniques and adaptive equipment exist to facilitate completion of activities of daily living and personal mobility when a person is limited by pain or by another impairment, such as paresis or contracture.

2. In the chronic pain setting, physicians prescribe mobility aids, such as canes and walkers, to unweight painful spines or painful lower limbs.

3. Patients with complex regional pain syndrome type I, arthritis, or radicular pain may improve mobility when prescribed a cane or walker. Physicians may prescribe wheelchairs for expedient personal mobility in severe cases of CRPS-I that preclude weight bearing. Orthotics, or braces, stabilize lower limbs with permanent weakness. Patients may develop permanent foot drop or ankle weakness as sequelae to lumbar stenosis, arachnoiditis, severe radiculopathy, or peroneal neuropathy.

4. Occupational therapists, who rehabilitate persons for activities of daily living, provide equipment with long handles to facilitate reaching during bathing, dressing, and other activities.

5. Physical therapists can instruct the patient with arthritis in joint conservation techniques or the patient with low back pain in back conservation techniques. Also, occupational therapists teach work simplification and energy conservation techniques to patients with low endurance due to heart or lung disease, or chronic pain.

II. PHYSICAL THERAPY PRESCRIPTION

A. The Basic Components

The components of a physical therapy prescription include the patient's name, the patient's referral diagnosis, precautions or activities to avoid, the frequency and duration of treatment, the goals for the therapy referral, and the date of the patient's return visit to the referring physician.

1. The referral diagnosis

a. The patient's referral diagnosis may be *chronic pain;* however, a review of the benefits that physical therapy offers reveals few modalities that relieve pain. The physician's careful musculoskeletal examination of the patient will reveal areas of contracture or regional weakness or generalized poor condition and mobility; physicians should list these musculoskeletal deficits as impairments along with the referral diagnosis.

b. For example, a patient with chronic lumbar radiculopathy may have hip flexor and hamstring contracture, abdominal and gluteal weakness, slumped posture, and pectoralis contracture. If the physician includes these areas of weakness and contracture on the physical therapy referral along with the more general diagnosis of lumbar radiculopathy, the specificity and quality of the order improves.

c. Another example is provided by the CRPS-I patient. Physical findings may include allodynia and hyperesthesia of the hand, contracted range of motion for finger and wrist flexion and extension, limited supination and pronation at the wrist, and adhesive capsulitis of the ipsilateral shoulder, as well as myofascial trigger points in ipsilateral cervical paraspinal muscles. If the physician includes these impairments along with the referral diagnosis, the physician alerts the therapist to other deficits and allows for more specific and directed treatment of the patient beyond desensitization techniques and edema control most often applied to patients with CRPS-I.

2. Precautions (Table 10–1).

a. The physician may list the patient's significant medical history as the precautions on the physical therapy script. The notation "Precaution: seizures, diabetes, hypertension" provides the therapist and emergency personnel with baseline data in the case of an emergency during therapy.

TABLE 10-1. *Precautions for common concomitant diagnoses*

CAD:	Keep heart rate below 60% of maximal heart rate. Avoid SBP over 170 and DBP over 98. Contact MD if there is cyanosis, hypotension, pallor, or angina.
Hypertension:	Similar to CAD. Postpone therapies if SBP < 100 because of medication.
Seizures:	In the event of seizure, lie patient on the floor on his or her side and contact MD.
Diabetes:	Rest patient and offer snack if there is diaphoresis or confusion.
Spinal fusion:	Wear back/cervical orthotic for all standing and sitting activity. No sitting longer than 15 minutes.
Fractures:	Generally non-weight-bearing.
Total hip precautions:	Do not cross legs or flex hip > 90°. Weight-bearing as allowed by orthopedic surgeon.
Osteoporosis:	Fracture risk with minimal or no trauma. Do not force stretch and do not manipulate.
Spinal cord stimulators:	Avoid overhead lifting and bending of > 90° at the waist.

      b. The physician may also list more specific limitations.
  3. Therapy goals (Table 10–2)
      a. Therapy goals describe the intended result from the therapy referral.
      b. Goals include the reduction or elimination of the impairments associated with the referral diagnosis.
      c. Using the example of the patient with chronic radiculopathy, goals include reduction of hip flexion contracture and improved flexibility of the hamstrings, increased strength of the abdominal and gluteal muscles, and observance of back conservation techniques during household activities.
  4. Frequency
      a. The frequency with which the patient attends therapy depends on the exercise. Stretching should be done daily. For therapy to remain cost-effective, the patient should participate in a home program for daily stretching.

TABLE 10-2. *Example of therapy goals*

Reduce contracture of _____.
Improve flexibility of _____.
Improve strength of _____.
Increase endurance _____.
Maintain proper body mechanics during _____.
Reduce edema in _____.
Unweight painful motion of _____.

   b. To gain strength, the patient must perform strengthening exercises three to four times per week. Six to 8 weeks is required to improve strength 20% to 40%.

   c. Endurance exercises improve the cardiovascular fitness when the patient performs them three to five times per week.

   d. The patient requires the supervision of the therapist to master new exercises and to correct exercise technique to avoid injury. The therapist also requires frequent visits with the patient while the patient is learning posture and conservation techniques. Attention to posture must be reinforced during activity.

B. Other Components (Table 10–3).

When prescribing therapy, the physician may prescribe stretching, strengthening, or endurance exercises, as well as instruction or assistive devices the patient is to receive. However, for physicians who are not rehabilitation specialists, standard practice does not generally include these specifics.

III. CONCLUSIONS

A. Physical therapy primarily benefits the pain patient by restoring flexibility, range of motion, strength, and endurance for exercise as well as activities of daily living. Some modalities, such as cold, TENS, and stretch, may directly impact perceptions of pain.

B. Physical therapy modalities include stretch, strengthening, and endurance exercises; thermal and electrical modalities; and instructional and adaptive applications.

C. Examination of the patient for contracture, weakness, and poor endurance, as evidenced by high resting heart rate or shortness of breath during routine physical exam, indicate impairments and diagnoses that physical therapy prescription can help. Physicians should include the referral diagnosis, other diagnoses that may indicate activity limitations, or precautions on the therapy script. Familiarity with stretching, strengthening, and endurance activity is helpful but not requisite.

TABLE 10-3. *Obligatory and optional components of the physical therapy prescription*

Obligatory	Optional
Name of patient	Stretching exercise
Referral diagnosis	Strengthening exercise
Precautions	Endurance exercise
Goals of referral	Instruction
Date of MD follow-up	Adaptive devices
	Heat, cold, TENS

Appendix. Therapy Prescription for Selected Diagnoses

The literature reveals therapy regimens for some specific musculoskeletal diagnoses but the treatment of many conditions is empiric.

A. Axial Musculoskeletal Low Back Pain
1. Stretches to the hip flexors and hamstrings and lumbar paraspinals, and to the hip adductors and lateral lumbar flexors (quadratus lumborum) if tight
2. Strengthening of the abdominals with pelvis tilts, crunches and knee to chest exercises and prone press-ups
3. Progressive endurance to 30 minutes of aerobic activity
4. Assistive devices: lumbar roll while sitting
5. Thermal or cold or electrical modalities as needed before or after therapy
6. Education about back conservation and biomechanics
7. The patient's diagnosis, other significant medical diagnoses, specific precautions and goals
8. Duration—8 weeks

B. Chronic Low Back Pain After Laminectomy
1. Stretching of identified contracture
2. Strengthening via prone press-ups, spinal stabilization, and latissimus pull-downs
3. Low-impact endurance activity (rapid walking or stationary cycling) starting at 10 minutes duration
4. Superficial heat prior to therapies for 20 minutes
5. Education about posture and lifting techniques
6. Duration three times per week for 8 weeks
7. The patient's diagnosis, other significant medical diagnoses, specific precautions, and goals

C. Lumbar Spondylolisthesis
1. Stretch the lumbar paraspinals
2. Strengthen the lumbar flexors—namely, the abdominals; limit lumbar extension to isometric activity only.
3. Assistive devices include braces that promote lumbar flexion or that block lumbar extension.
4. Modalities include superficial heat.
5. Education includes posture and lifting techniques.
6. The patient's diagnosis, other significant medical diagnoses, specific precautions, and goals

D. Lumbar Radiculopathy
1. Stretch of the hamstrings and generalized flexibility
2. Strengthening of the abdominals and gluteals, pelvic tilts; arm and leg extensor strengthening
3. Endurance exercise with progressive lumbar stabilization and progress to sustain lumbar posture on treadmill
4. Modalities include ice massage of spasm in lumbar paraspinals and trial of TENS.
5. Assistive devices include a cane if ambulation is painful or unsteady due to motor weakness or sensory loss.
6. Education includes back conservation and body mechanics.
7. The patient's diagnosis, other significant medical diagnoses, specific precautions, and goals

E. Complex Regional Pain Syndrome of the Upper Extremity
1. Sustained stretch of contracted joints, including shoulder flexion, abduction, and internal and external rotation; elbow flexion and extension; and wrist flexion, extension, supination, and pronation, and finger flexion and extension. Gentle but progressive range of motion, even of painful joints, should occur. Stretch must be gentle as osteoporosis and the risk of fracture accompany the diagnosis of RSD.
2. Strengthen markedly weakened and painful joints first isometrically or isotonically out of gravity to restore normal range of motion. Strengthen moderately weakened joints with active and active assisted range of motion and progress to weighted exercise. Strengthening in a water medium (pool therapy) may allow for antigravity buoyancy, for gentle constant resistance, and for a desensitization medium. Strengthening activities will require modifications if hand pain prevents adequately grasping a weight. Pool therapy with air-filled "water wings" that can be worn on the wrist or arm creates resistance under water and allows strengthening exercises without the patient holding a weight.
3. Endurance activity if the patient has become sedentary. Walking in a pool or on land will minimize jarring; a patient with significant hand pain may not safely grasp a bicycle.
4. Modalities may include modulating devices like TENS and desensitization techniques like stroking, pool therapy, and fluidotherapy (a heated modality in which air is bubbled through sawdust-like material, creating movement of the material over the extremity). The physician may prescribe ultrasound over some areas of contracture, but the physician and therapist should monitor for worsening edema.
5. Assistive devices include edema control gloves, resting, and supportive hand splints.

6. The patient may benefit from instruction about work simplification and one-handed techniques for ADLs or change of the dominant hand if hand pain is severe.
7. The patient's diagnosis, other significant medical diagnoses, specific precautions, and goals

F. Complex Regional Pain Syndrome of the Lower Extremity
1. Stretch of the foot and ankle if primarily involved may be facilitated by having the patient work in a pool, starting in deeper water (clavicle) height, touching the toe to the bottom. The patient can increase stretch to the foot and ankle by increasing weight bearing and contact of the foot to the pool bottom while decreasing water depth (xyphoid height, waist height, etc.). The foot and ankle can also be manually stretched on land.
2. Strengthening or bracing of the painful joint or structure occurs after normal range of motion is restored.
3. Strengthening of the musculature proximal to the painful area will be necessary if the patient has been off the extremity for more than 2 weeks. For example, patients with foot and ankle CRPS who use crutches and do not weight-bear on the extremity will have ipsilateral weakness of hip and knee extensors.
4. Endurance activity if the patient has become sedentary; walking in a pool or swimming may be the only aerobic activity that the patient can tolerate.
5. Modalities may include modulating devices like TENS and desensitization techniques like stroking, pool therapy, and fluidotherapy. The physician may prescribe ultrasound over some areas of contracture, but the physician and therapist should monitor for worsening edema.
6. Adaptive devices include canes, walkers, or wheelchairs to promote pain-free mobility.
7. The patient's diagnosis, other significant medical diagnoses, specific precautions, and goals.

RECOMMENDED READING

De Lateur B. Therapeutic Exercise. In: Braddom RL, ed. *Physical Medicine and Rehabilitation.* Philadelphia: WB Saunders, 1996:401–420.

Detorri JR. The effects of spinal flexion and extension exercises and their associated postures in patients with acute low back pain. *Spine* 1995;20 (21):2303–2312.

Khalil TM, Asfour S, Martinez SM, et al. Stretching in the rehabilitation of the low back pain patient. *Spine* 1992;17(3): 311–317.

Lewit K, Simons DG. Myofascial pain relief by post-isometric relaxation. *Arch Phys Med Rehab* 1984; 65:452–56.

Lindstrom I. Mobility, strength and fitness after a graded activity program for patient with subacute low back pain. *Spine* 1992;17(6):641–652.

Munning F. Does stretching really help performance and prevent injury? *Your Patient and Fitness* 1990;4(6):12–16.

Owens MK, Ehrenreich D. Literature review of non-pharmacologic methods for the treatment of chronic pain. *Holistic Nursing Pract* 1991;6(1):24–31.

Reitman C, Esses S. Conservative options in the management of spinal disorders, Part 1. *Am J Orthop* 1995;24(2):109–116.

Rodriquez AA. Therapeutic exercise in chronic neck and back pain. *Arch Phys Med Rehab* 1992;73: 870–875.

Saal JA, Saal JS. Nonoperative treatment of herniated lumbar intervertebral disc with radiculopathy. *Spine* 1989;14(4):431–435.

Takemasa R. Trunk muscle strength in and effect of trunk muscle exercises for patients with chronic low back pain. *Spine* 1995;20(23):2522–2530.

The Pain Clinic Manual, Second Edition,
edited by Stephen E. Abram and J. David Haddox.
Lippincott Williams & Wilkins,
Philadelphia, © 2000

11

Psychological Strategies for Managing Chronic Pain

Mary Lou Taylor

M. L. Taylor: Department of Anesthesiology, Medical College of Wisconsin, Milwaukee, Wisconsin 53226.

Pain clinics generally treat patients who have had pain for a lengthy period and for whom seeking a cure is no longer a reasonable option. Often such patients feel helpless. A major goal of psychological pain management strategies is to provide the patient with tools for controlling the effects of pain in their lives. By replacing maladaptive responses and behaviors with effective coping strategies, patients can increase their sense of control and decrease functional disability.

Treatment can be provided individually, in groups, or with a combination of both, according to the patient's needs.

I. MAJOR TREATMENT COMPONENTS
A. Patient Education
1. Goals are to eliminate misperceptions or misunderstandings regarding chronic pain, to decrease anxiety, and to increase the patient's motivation to take an active role in pain management. Pain management treatment will fail if the patient really believes that a brain tumor is the cause of his/her headache, or does not understand the relationship between stress, muscle tension, and headaches, for example.
2. Topics include
   a. Differences between acute and chronic pain
   b. Gate Control Theory of pain
   c. Hurt versus harm
   d. Circular relationship between pain, anxiety, and depression
   e. Relationship between stress and autonomic nervous system arousal
   f. Learning and reinforcement of pain behaviors
   g. Need for exercise and physical conditioning

B. Cognitive/Behavioral Therapy
1. The goals of cognitive/behavioral therapy (CBT) are focused on changing maladaptive behaviors and the thoughts, attitudes, or beliefs that precede those behaviors. Results of successful therapy include increased functional ability and decreased pain-related anxiety and depression.
2. Topics include
   a. Problem exploration
      Patients are assisted in identifying thoughts, beliefs, or attitudes that may increase their distress in painful situations (e.g., "This is never going to end").
   b. Cognitive restructuring
      Techniques such as thought records, thought stopping, and thought switching help the patient recognize maladaptive cognitions early and substitute more balanced, productive, and adaptive ones. These techniques may also be applied to the treatment of anxiety and depression.
   c. Environmental factors/reinforcement theory
      Patients learn to identify factors in their environment that may be reinforcing pain behaviors. Getting away from a stressful work situation may be an obvious reinforcer, but increased family cooperation or decreased home responsibilities when showing pain behaviors may be just as strongly, though more subtly, reinforcing.
   d. Sleep management
      Relaxation training and behavioral techniques improve sleep quality in most patients
   e. Stress and anger management
      Patients are taught to identify stressors or anger triggers that increase arousal and pain levels. Interventions may include assertiveness training and communication skills.
   f. Distraction
      Patients are taught to identify times when focusing on pain actually increases pain perception. Distraction techniques, either active (getting involved in an activity) or passive (relaxation or meditation), can give the patient more control over pain perception.
   g. Increasing self-efficacy
      Helping the patient set appropriate goals and break goals down into smaller steps increases the patient's belief that goals are attainable. Research has shown that increasing a person's belief that he can achieve a goal actually increases the likelihood of success.
C. Relaxation/Biofeedback
1. Goals
   Both relaxation and biofeedback for chronic pain are used to enable the patient to identify and modify muscle tension in the body. They decrease

autonomic arousal in general and decrease emotional distress as well. Relaxation techniques are generally as effective as or more effective than biofeedback and are less costly and more generalizable. However, biofeedback is recommended in certain situations (i.e., thermal biofeedback for migraines or Raynaud's).

2. Relaxation techniques include
   a. Progressive muscle relaxation
      By systematically tensing and relaxing separate muscle groups, patients learn to be aware of the difference between tension and relaxation and get control over muscle tightness. It is not recommended for headaches, which may be exacerbated by the tensing/relaxing cycle.
   b. Focused breathing
      Patients are taught to focus on their breathing while silently repeating a soothing word or phrase with each exhalation. Research indicates that even one 10-minute practice daily can produce long-term decreases in autonomic arousal.
   c. Autogenic relaxation
      Patients use self-instruction to systematically relax each body part with suggestions of warmth and heaviness (e.g., "My right foot is warm and heavy"). This provides good generalization and gives patients control.
   d. Imagery
      Once relaxed, patients can use imagery in several ways:
      (1) General relaxation can be increased by imagining oneself in a safe, comfortable place.
      (2) Temperature rises in extremities can be induced by images of warmth (e.g., sunbathing, warm water).
      (3) Pain-coping skills can be increased through systematic desensitization, guiding the patient through a series of progressively stressful images, while maintaining relaxation and imagining successful coping responses.
      (4) Pain perception can be changed by imaging changes in body parts, such as picturing a tight muscle unwinding.
   e. Hypnosis or self-hypnosis
      In a deeply relaxed state, the patient experiences a heightened sensitivity and susceptibility to suggestion. Hypnosis is effective in pain control for hypnotically susceptible patients, though the underlying mechanisms are unclear. In pain management the suggestions are often discussed beforehand, and patients are taught self-hypnosis techniques to increase internal control.
3. Biofeedback techniques include
   a. EMG biofeedback

EMG biofeedback reads electrical activity in the muscle between two surface electrodes and transforms it into an analog signal. A tone decreases in pitch and frequency as the muscle relaxes. By using the auditory feedback, the patient is aware of tension decreases that may be too small to feel. It is useful for targeting specific muscles.

b. Thermal biofeedback

By listening to auditory feedback, the patient can learn to increase the temperature of hands or feet. This technique is a treatment of choice for migraine headaches and Raynaud's phenomenon and is useful in general relaxation and decreasing temperature extremes in reflex sympathetic dystrophy.

II. OTHER PSYCHOLOGICAL FACTORS AFFECTING PHYSICAL CONDITIONS

A. Evaluation

As with all other medical disorders, some patients will present with pre-existing psychological disorders that will impact on their ability to cope with chronic pain. Psychotic disorders, dissociative identity disorder, severe obsessive-compulsive disorder, dementia, cognitive dysfunction due to traumatic brain injury, and severe personality disorders may make chronic pain management therapy difficult or may require specialized treatment. Anxiety, depression, and posttraumatic stress disorder are commonly treated as part of the pain management program.

B. Treatment Options

1. Referral to psychiatry or long-term psychological treatment, with no pain management therapy
2. Coordination between outside therapists/psychiatrists and pain management therapists
3. Individualized pain management therapy
4. Group therapy is not usually appropriate for patients with significantly disruptive psychological disorders.

III. GROUP THERAPY

A. Rationale

Chronic pain patients often feel very isolated and misunderstood. It can be very helpful to learn pain management techniques in a group, to see that others experience similar feelings, and to help group members to encourage each other.

B. Patient Selection

The patient needs

1. To have basic interactional skills and at least a low-average level of intelligence
2. To be free of psychotic symptoms and severe personality disorders
3. To demonstrate at least moderate motivation and compliance

    4. To have reliable transportation to assure regular attendance

C. Group Formats

    1. In an outpatient pain management center, group therapy usually includes 2 hours of psychotherapy and 1 hour of didactic physical therapy weekly. The format may be two hourly sessions or one 2-hour session, and usually runs for 5 to 8 weeks.

    2. Intensive rehabilitation-focused clinics include daily physical therapy, occupational therapy, and psychotherapy groups in a structured program lasting 3 to 6 weeks.

    3. If the patient is being weaned from a high level of pain medication, intensive inpatient pain management programs are useful.

D. Topics in Group.

Group therapy covers all the topics outlined above, including pain education and cognitive behavioral coping techniques.

RECOMMENDED READING

Integration of behavioral and relaxation approaches into the treatment of chronic pain and insomnia. *NIH Technol Assess Statement* 1995, Oct. 16–18, pp. 1–34.

Lipchik GL, Milles K, Covington EC. The effects of multidisciplinary pain management treatment on locus of control and pain beliefs in chronic non-terminal pain. *Clin J Pain* 1993;9 (1): 49–57.

Slater MA, Doctor JN, Pruitt SD, Atkinson JH. The clinical significance of behavioral treatment for chronic low back pain: An evaluation of effectiveness. *Pain* 1997;1 (3):257–263.

Turk DC, Meichenbaum D. A cognitive-behavioral approach to pain management. In: Wall PD, Melzack R, eds. *Textbook of Pain,* 3rd ed. London: Churchill Livingstone, 1994:1337–1348.

The Pain Clinic Manual, Second Edition,
edited by Stephen E. Abram and J. David Haddox.
Lippincott Williams & Wilkins,
Philadelphia, © 2000

12

Electrical Stimulation of the Nervous System

Arun Rajagopal and Stephen E. Abram

A. Rajagopal: Departments of Anesthesiology and Symptom Control and Palliatative Care, The University of Texas M.D. Anderson Cancer Center,Houston, Texas 77030.
S. E. Abram: Department of Anesthesiology and Critical Care Medicine, University of New Mexico, Health Sciences Center—School of Medicine, Albuquerque, New Mexico 87131.

I. INTRODUCTION

Interest in the therapeutic use of electrical stimulation for pain management increased greatly following publication of Melzack and Wall's gate control theory of pain in 1965. The theory proposed that activation of large (A-beta) afferent fibers could interfere with the transmission of noxious stimulation at the dorsal horn level. Since high-frequency square wave electrical stimulation activates large fibers at a lower current than that required for activation of small nociceptive afferents, it was postulated that it should be possible to provide analgesia with certain types of electrical stimuli. The dorsal columns seemed a logical site to stimulate since these structures contain the central projections of large afferent axons.

Transcutaneous electrical stimulation has widespread acceptance for the treatment of a variety of chronic and cancer pain syndromes and is used as an adjunctive treatment for acute postoperative pain and labor pain in some centers. The most common indication for spinal cord stimulation is for unilateral extremity pain, with radiculopathy and reflex sympathetic dystrophy (CRPS type I) being the principal causes. More recently, there has been considerable interest in the use of this modality for patients with angina and ischemic peripheral vascular disease. Peripheral nerve stimulation is used in a few centers for posttraumatic or compression neuropathies where pain is confined to a single peripheral nerve distribution. Deep brain stimulation has not achieved extensive use but is currently being used in a few centers for patients unresponsive to less invasive measures.

II. TRANSCUTANEOUS ELECTRICAL NERVE STIMULATION (TENS)

A. History

1. The application of electrical signals of low voltage to cutaneous sites for analgesia began in the early 1970s. Initially used prognostically to determine response to spinal cord stimulation.

2. Found to be useful therapeutically; of little benefit in predicting response to spinal stimulation.

B. Modes of Action

1. General description: TENS delivers an electrical stimulus that can be varied with respect to pulse width, amplitude, and pulse rate (frequency).

   a. Pulse width is the duration of each pulse.
      (1) Usually measured in microseconds.
      (2) The longer the duration of the pulse, the more power delivered to the skin and the wider the radiation of electrical stimulation and cutaneous sensation.

   b. Amplitude is the intensity of current.
      (1) Sensation with increasing amplitude varies from a light tingling to painful sensation and muscle contractions.
      (2) Usually measured in milliamperes (mA).

   c. Frequency is the number of pulses delivered per second.
      (1) Measured in hertz (Hz).
      (2) The frequency selected determines what type of nerve fiber is stimulated.

2. Specific modes of stimulation

   a. High-frequency stimulation
      (1) Selectively stimulates large-diameter, myelinated A fibers.
      (2) Produces increased latency and, at high currents, block of C fibers.
      (3) Is used for 30 minutes or more per session.
      (4) If analgesia is transient, may be worn continuously.

   b. Modulated settings
      (1) The frequency, the amplitude, or both can be varied during stimulation.
      (2) Patients may tolerate higher amplitudes and experience more effective levels of stimulation with modulated settings.
      (3) Used in a fashion similar to high-frequency TENS.

   c. Low-frequency, high-intensity stimulation
      (1) "Acupuncture-like" stimulation.
      (2) Activates C and A-delta fibers.
      (3) Intensity increased to provide uncomfortable or mildly painful sensation.
      (4) Used for short periods of time.

   d. Burst mode
      (1) Short bursts (e.g., 5 to 10 pulses) of high-frequency stimulation delivered at low rates (e.g., 1 to 2 Hz).
      (2) Similar to low-frequency stimulation in effect and utilization.

3. Method of use

   a. After the patient has been evaluated, the physician or other health care provider determines optimum sites for placement of electrodes.

      b. The areas of pain are usually discrete (e.g., "trigger points") and localized to a specific area on the body.

      c. After placement of electrodes, the patient narrates to the provider the degree of relief, the location of the stimulation, and the degree of discomfort experienced while the settings on the unit are adjusted.

      d. After an optimal setting is reached, the patient is allowed to control the intensity of the stimulus as needed for relief.

C. Use in Cancer Patients

  1. With careful selection of the proper patient, TENS can be a useful adjunct in therapy for cancer pain. It is particularly useful in the patient with

      a. Discrete musculoskeletal involvement.

      b. Peripheral nerve irritation.

      c. Bone pain (e.g., metastasis to a rib or vertebral body).

  2. Works best in early cancer pain before the pain is too widespread or too severe.

  3. Effective in a wide variety of conditions, including patients on opioids

D. Contraindications

Caution should be exercised in placing a TENS unit in the following situations:

  1. In patients who have implanted pacemakers—possible cause of programming changes in certain types of pacemakers.

  2. Placement of the unit over the neck, specifically the carotid sinus.

  3. Relatively contraindicated across the heart or with the electrodes placed in an anteroposterior fashion across the chest.

  4. In incompetent patients.

  5. Near the eyes.

E. Side Effects

  1. Localized skin irritation or breakdown under the electrodes

      a. Most likely to occur when used in areas of reduced sensation.

      b. Most likely with prolonged, high-intensity use.

  2. Contact dermatitis from electrodes, gel, or adhesive tape

III. SPINAL CORD STIMULATION (DORSAL COLUMN STIMULATION, DCS)

A. Mechanism of Action

  1. Activation of axons in the dorsal columns

      a. These fibers consist of ascending branches of large peripheral sensory axons.

      b. Antidromic activation of dorsal column fibers activates interneurons in the dorsal horn.

  2. Direct blockade of nociceptive input

      a. There is evidence that spinal cord stimulation blocks ascending pain transmission directly.

         (1) In some patients, reduced sensation below the level of spinal stimulation is achieved as analgesia occurs.

(2) Electrodes placed anterior/posterior produce analgesia at lower currents than electrodes placed over the dorsal columns only.

   3. Sympathetic inhibition

      a. Patients with peripheral vascular disease show improved blood flow.

      b. Patients with angina show analgesia and improved cardiac function.

B. Patient Selection

   1. Conditions associated with fairly high success rates:

      a. Lumbar and cervical radiculopathy.

      b. Reflex sympathetic dystrophy (CRPS type I).

      c. Pain associated with peripheral vascular disease.

      d. Intractable angina pectoris.

   2. Conditions with lower success rates, with some patients responding:

      a. Pain and spasticity associated with spinal cord injury.

      b. Peripheral neuropathy.

      c. Nonradicular low back pain.

      d. Postamputation pain.

   3. Conditions unlikely to respond:

      a. Postherpetic neuralgia.

      b. Brachial plexus avulsion.

      c. Poststroke pain.

C. Technique

   1. Percutaneous trial/permanent implantation procedure

      a. The lead is advanced through the epidural needle and is positioned posteriorly close to the midline on the affected side using fluoroscopic guidance.

      b. Lead wires tunneled subcutaneously laterally; externalized and external pulse generator is attached.

      c. If analgesia is achieved, the external wires are removed, a subcutaneous pocket is excavated in a suitable location for the implanted pulse generator, and a new set of lead wires is tunneled from the epidural lead to the implanted pulse generator.

   2. Percutaneous trial only

      a. Following epidural electrode placement the electrode is left as a strictly percutaneous lead.

      b. An external pulse generator is used to test analgesic efficacy, usually for 24 to 48 hours.

      c. The electrode is removed and, if analgesia is achieved, a permanent electrode and pulse generator are placed at a later time.

      d. Permanent electrode may be percutaneous or placed via limited laminotomy.

D. Disadvantages of DCS

   1. Placement of the lead in the exact location can be difficult.

        a. Patient must experience paresthesias to painful area—needs to be awake during placement.

        b. Lead migration may cause loss of efficacy.

        c. Anterior placement or anterior migration of the leads can lead to uncomfortable motor stimulation.

    2. Analgesia in low lumbar and sacral areas can be difficult to achieve.

    3. Fibrosis around the lead can reduce efficacy, particularly with percutaneous leads.

  E. Contraindications

    1. Failure to achieve satisfactory analgesia with the external trial.

    2. Presence of a cardiac demand pacemaker or implanted defibrillator.

    3. Patients who require magnetic resonance imaging (MRI) scan.

IV. PERIPHERAL NERVE STIMULATION

  A. History and General Description

    1. A single peripheral nerve is directly stimulated using a totally implanted system.

    2. Is indicated for peripheral mononeuropathy.

    3. May be helpful in sympathetically maintained pain if pain distribution follows a peripheral nerve.

  B. Technique

    1. Screening

        a. Percutaneous high-frequency stimulation of the affected nerve is used for 30 to 60 minutes.

        b. No studies to indicate prognostic benefit, but it would make sense not to proceed if percutaneous trials are totally unsuccessful.

    2. Operative procedure

        a. Patient is anesthetized and the affected nerve is carefully isolated at a site proximal to the nerve damage.

        b. A lead similar to that used for operative placement of spinal cord stimulator is secured against nerve with fascial flap interposed.

        c. Lead wire is tunneled subcutaneously to an appropriate site for placement of the pulse generator (same as used for DCS).

V. DEEP BRAIN STIMULATION

  A. History

    1. "Deep brain stimulation," the placing of electrodes in certain areas of the brain for subsequent electrical stimulation, began approximately 20 years ago.

    2. Subsequent studies utilizing a rat model demonstrated that abdominal surgery could be easily performed using only deep brain stimulation.

    3. Although the procedure has been an accepted modality in pain management practice for many years, there is still considerable controversy regarding its efficacy.

4. Much of this controversy stems from the fact that there is still a paucity of literature that definitely establishes which areas of the brain provide the best analgesia and for which types of pain.

B. Rationale
   1. Electrical stimulation of three areas of the brain have been studied using various animal and human models:
      a. The somatosensory areas of the ventrobasal thalamus.
      b. Periventricular gray matter (PVG) and adjoining nuclei.
      c. Rostral ventral periaqueductal gray (PAG) and caudal ventral PVG.
   2. There is some evidence to suggest that certain types of pain respond to stimulation at certain sites, although there is no consistency of response.
      a. Somatogenic pain, the pain caused by nociceptive input from damaged peripheral nerves, seems to respond to PVG/PAG stimulation.
      b. Neurogenic pain arising from central nervous system destruction or deafferentation seems to respond to stimulation of the somatosensory thalamus.
   3. Although many studies corroborate these findings, a number of studies also suggest exactly the opposite. This may be due in part to the extreme degree of precision needed to place the electrodes.

C. Stimulation Parameters
   1. In addition to the placement of electrodes, different patterns of analgesia can be experienced by varying the parameters of stimulation.
   2. Typically, high-frequency stimulation is used (100 to 333 Hz) with a short pulse width (about 0.1 msec).
   3. Stimulation is also achieved by using either unipolar or bipolar leads.
   4. As can be seen, the range of frequencies used is large, and this could account for the discrepancies in studies assessing efficacy.

VI. CONCLUSION

Electrical stimulation by one of the means discussed in this chapter can be a useful adjunct in the field of pain management. The only noninvasive technique discussed, TENS, is a useful modality in patients with specific, discrete areas of pain. It is safe, has relatively few contraindications, and has a proven record of providing analgesia in specific types of pain. As advances in technology make implantable devices smaller and less traumatic to place and as the field of pain management continues to expand in new areas, the role of implanted devices will undoubtedly continue to grow.

RECOMMENDED READING

Dubuisson D. Neurosurgical treatment of pain. In: Warfield CA, ed. *Principles and Practice of Pain Management.* New York: McGraw-Hill; 1993:467–480.

Duncan GH, Bushnell MC, Marchand S. Deep brain stimulation: A review of basic research and clinical studies [Review]. *Pain* 1991;45:49–59.

Jessurun GAJ, DeJongste MJL, Blanksma PK. Current view on neurostimulation in the treatment of cardiac ischemic syndromes [Review]. *Pain* 1996;66:109–116.

McLean B, Fives HE. Stimulation-induced analgesia. In: Warfield CA, ed. *Principles and Practice of Pain Management.* New York: McGraw-Hill; 1993:413–426.

North RB. The role of spinal cord stimulation in contemporary pain management. APS J 1993;2(2):91–99.

Strege DW, Cooney WP, Wood MB, Johnson SJ, Metcalf BJ. Chronic peripheral nerve pain treated with direct electrical nerve stimulation. *J Hand Surg* 1994;19A:931–939.

The Pain Clinic Manual, Second Edition,
edited by Stephen E. Abram and J. David Haddox.
Lippincott Williams & Wilkins,
Philadelphia, © 2000

13

Principles of Clinical Pharmacology

James E. Heavner

J. E. Heavner: Departments of Anesthesiology and Physiology,
Texas Tech University Health Sciences Center, Lubbock, Texas 79430.

I. GENERAL CONCEPTS

A. Following drug administration, the drug is acted upon by the body (the pharmacokinetic phase) and acts on the body (the pharmacodynamic phase). Drug interactions can occur in either phase.

1. Pharmacodynamics. Generally refers to the biochemical and physiologic effects of drugs and their mechanisms of action.

   a. Drug receptors. A term coined to denote the component of the organism with which a drug is presumed to interact. The receptor can be any functional macromolecular component of the organism.

   b. Agonist. A drug that binds to physiologic receptors and mimics the effects of endogenous regulatory ligands (e.g., hormones, neurotransmitters).

   c. Antagonist. A drug that binds to receptors and does not mimic, but interferes with, the binding of the endogenous agonist.

   d. Partial agonist. A drug that is only partially effective as an agonist.

   e. Negative antagonists or inverse agonists. Drugs that stabilize the receptor from undergoing productive agonist-independent conformational changes.

   f. G protein–coupled receptors. Receptors in the plasma membrane that regulate distinct effector proteins through the mediation of a group of GTP-binding proteins known as G proteins.

   g. Desensitization (also referred to as refractoriness or down-regulation). Diminished effect of the same concentration of a drug often follows continued or subsequent administration of the drug.

   h. Affinity. Refers to the strength of attraction between a drug and its receptor.

   i. Intrinsic activity. A term (α) that describes the relationship between the effect (E) elicited by a drug (D), and the concentration of drug/receptor (R) complexes $E = \alpha(DR)$. The concept addresses the fact that a factor or factors in addition to DR determines magnitude of response. The terms *intrinsic activity* and *efficacy* are commonly used interchangeably.

It is important to remember that not all drug effects are mediated via receptors. Examples would be bulk cathartics and antacids.

2. Pharmacokinetics. Refers to the time course of changes in drug and metabolite concentrations in fluids, tissues, and excreta of the body, and the mathematical relationships developed to describe the time course.
    a. Predict whether effective concentrations of drugs are reached and maintained at the site of action.
    b. Determine whether drug concentrations exceed safe levels (i.e., produce unacceptable toxicity).
    c. Establish dosage regimens for different routes of administration— for example, transcutaneous, oral, intrathecal, epidural, intravenous, subcutaneous, cutaneous patches, drug-laced lollipops, patient-controlled analgesia devices (epidural, intravenous), constant-infusion devices (subcutaneous, intravenous, intrathecal, epidural).

II. MAJOR PHARMACOKINETIC BUILDING BLOCKS

The major pharmacokinetic building blocks are diagrammatically represented in Fig. 13-1.

A. Absorption

Drugs administered by an extravascular route must be absorbed. No absorption is required when a drug is injected intravascularly or at the target site (Fig. 13-2).

1. Intravascular injection of a given dose of drug produces plasma concentration of drug that is dependent on the method of injection (bolus, incremental dosing, constant infusion) and on speed of injection (Fig. 13-3).
2. Administration of the same dose of drug by a nonvascular route produces plasma concentration that is dependent upon formulation of medication (sustained release or not) as well as other factors (e.g., pH at absorption site and pKa of the drug).

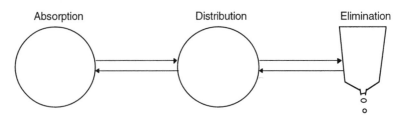

FIG. 13-1. Major pharmacokinetic building blocks.

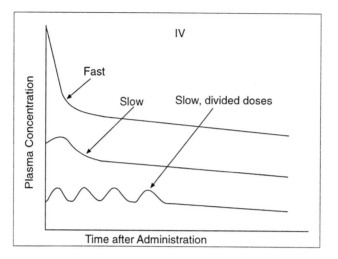

FIG. 13-2. Hypothetical plasma concentration of drug versus time plot following rapid, slow, or slow, divided IV administration.

B. Distribution

Once a drug enters systemic circulation, it is distributed to the various organs of the body.

1. Distribution is influenced by how well each organ is perfused with blood, organ size, binding of drug within blood and in tissues, and permeability of tissue membranes.

2. Changes in distribution of cardiac output (e.g., peripheral vasodilation) will alter drug distribution.

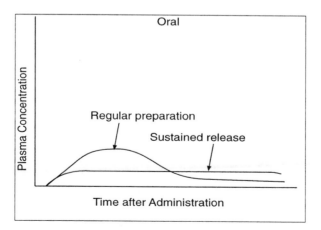

FIG. 13-3. Hypothetical plasma concentration of drug versus time plot following oral administration of a standard formulation versus a sustained-release formulation.

   3. Intrathecal injection of drug represents a special case wherein spread
      of the drug within the cerebrospinal fluid represents distribution.
C. Elimination
   The liver and kidneys are the two principal organs of elimination of most
   pain medications.
   1. The kidneys are the primary site for excretion of the chemically unal-
      tered drug.
   2. The liver is the usual organ for drug metabolism; however, the kidneys
      and other organs can also play an important metabolic role for certain
      drugs.
D. Kinetics of Absorption, Distribution, and Elimination
   As indicated by the double arrows in Fig. 13-1, drug may move out of and
   back into the absorption, distribution, or elimination site.
   1. The rate of movement in each direction is usually assigned a parame-
      ter, k, a rate constant that represents rate of movement.
   2. If the rate of removal exceeds the rate of return, drug will ultimately be
      removed from a site (Fig. 13-4).
E. Zero-Order and First-Order Kinetics
   Fig. 13-5 illustrates a hypothetical representation of zero- and first-order
   kinetics.
   1. Zero-order kinetics are those in which rate of change of drug concen-
      tration is independent of drug concentration. Usually the initial decrease

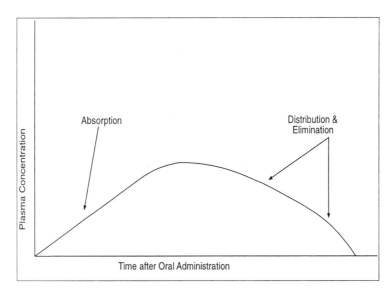

FIG. 13-4. Hypothetical plasma drug concentration versus time plot following oral drug administration, illustrating the simultaneous absorption, distribution, and elimination of the drug.

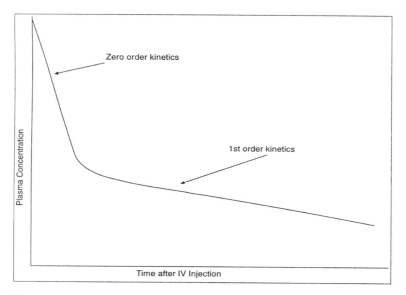

FIG. 13-5. Hypothetical plasma drug concentration versus time plot following iv drug administration, illustrating the portions of that plot representing zero and first-order kinetics.

in plasma concentration of a drug following intravenous injection of drug is zero order, but following parenteral administration, it usually is first order.

   2. First-order kinetics are those in which rate of change of drug concentration is dependent on drug concentration.
   F. Compartments
   1. Pharmacokinetic models may include single-compartment models or models with several ($n = 2 \rightarrow \infty$) compartments.
   2. Usually compartments do not correspond to anatomically identifiable parts of the body.
   3. Inflection points on a plasma concentration-versus-time plot are considered to indicate distribution of drug into different "compartments."
III. INFORMATION DERIVED FROM PHARMACOKINETIC CONCEPTS
   A. Volume of Distribution (Vd)

V_d = amount of drug injected ÷ plasma concentration of drug

(e.g., $V_d = 200$ L in the following situation: 10 mg morphine intravenous (iv) ÷ [0.05 mg/L morphine/ml plasma])

   B. Volume of Distribution Under Steady-State Conditions (V_{dss})
   This is a multicompartment term that represents the volume in which a drug

appears to be distributed during steady state if the drug existed throughout that volume at the same concentration in the measured fluid (plasma or blood).

This is more complicated to calculate than V_d. The equation will be given, but a sample calculation will not be done.

$$V_{dss} = (\text{Dose} * \div \text{AUC*}) \cdot (\text{AUMC} * \div \text{AUC*})$$

(See "Recommended Reading")

C. Mean Resonance Time (MRT). This is the average time the number of molecules introduced reside in the body. MRT is used to calculate V_{ss}.

$$\text{MRT} = (\text{AUMC} * \div \text{AUC*})$$

(Simplest of two methods to calculate MRT)

D. Half-life
Half-life is the time it takes for the plasma concentration, or the amount of drug in the body, to be reduced by 50%.

E. Context-Sensitive Half-life
This is the time to halving of the blood concentration after termination of drug administration by an infusion designed to maintain a constant concentration.

F. Clearance (CL)
At the simplest level, clearance of a drug is the rate of elimination by all routes, normalized to the concentration of drug (C) in some biologic fluid. It is important to note that clearance does not indicate how much drug is being removed, but rather the volume of biologic fluid (e.g., blood or plasma) that would have to be completely freed of drug to account for the elimination.

$$\text{CL} = \text{rate of elimination} \div C$$

At steady state

$$\text{CL} = \text{Dosing rate} \div C_{ss}$$

(C_{ss} = steady-state concentration of drug)
(or Dosing rate $= \text{CL} \cdot C_{ss}$)
For a single dose

$$\text{CL} = \text{Dose} \div \text{Area Under the Curve (AUC)}$$

G. Area Under the Curve
This value is obtained by integrating the area under the drug concentration versus the time curve.

H. Bioavailability
The amount of drug that actually reaches the systemic circulation after administration by a nonvascular route expressed as a fraction of the dose F_1.

---

*Refers to a tracer label of a drug, for example.

I. Bioequivalency

Two products are considered to be bioequivalent if the time/concentration profiles of the active ingredient are so similar that they are unlikely to produce clinically relevant differences in either therapeutic or adverse effects. The common measures used to assess bioequivalence are AUC, C_{max}, C_{min}, and t_{max}. (C_{max} = the maximum concentration [e.g., in plasma]; C_{min} = the minimum concentration of drug required to obtain a predetermined intensity of response; t_{max} = the time to maximum concentration.)

J. Maintenance dose (Dosing Rate; DR)

The dose and dosing interval required to maintain the desired concentration of drug in the plasma.

$$DR = (\text{target concentration}) \cdot (CL/F)$$

(F = bioavailability)

This equation is in its simplest form. A more complex equation is required to determine dosing interval for intermittent dosage.

K. Loading Dose

The "loading dose" is one or a series of doses that may be given at the onset of therapy with the aim of achieving the target concentration rapidly.

$$\text{Loading dose} = \text{target } C_p \cdot V_{ss}/F$$

IV. DRUG INTERACTIONS

A. Drug Interactions

Drug interactions may be pharmacodynamic or pharmacokinetic in nature.

1. Pharmacodynamic interactions

    a. Competitive or surmountable antagonists—commonly observed with antagonists that bind reversibly at the receptor site of the agonist. Competitive antagonists shift the log dose/effect curve for the agonist to the right. The maximal effect is unaltered, but the agonist appears to be less potent.

    b. Noncompetitive antagonist—prevents the agonist at any concentration from producing a maximum effect.

    c. Reversible and irreversible antagonists—if an antagonist binds at the active site for the agonist, reversible antagonists will be competitive and irreversible antagonists will be noncompetitive.

2. Pharmacokinetic interactions (see Fig. 13-6)

    a. Pharmaceutic incompatibility. One drug or vehicle reacts chemically or physically with another when two or more drug formulations are mixed.

    b. Alteration in absorption. One drug (e.g., epinephrine) alters the absorption of another (e.g., local anesthetic).

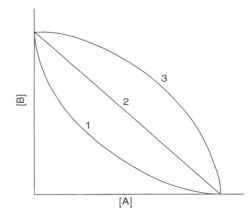

FIG. 13-6. Isobolograms for the response to mixtures of drugs. The sets of concentrations of drugs A and B, which as a mixture produce an effect (e.g., 50% of a maximal response), are plotted. Strict additivity, which means [A] + [B] = a constant results in a curve of slope −1 (**2**). If the curve is concave (**3**), some antagonism is present; if the curve is convex (**1**), synergism is present.

   c. Alterations of drug biotransformation enzymes. Possibilities include enzyme induction by one drug that alters the biotransformation of another drug, or inhibition by one drug of an enzyme that biotransforms another. Alterations may either shorten or prolong the duration of action of a drug, depending upon (a) the importance of biotransformation in terminating the action of a drug; (b) whether or not an active product is formed; and (c) whether biotransformation is increased or decreased.

   d. Alterations in protein binding. Drugs that bind to the same protein can displace each other, resulting in higher free fraction of one or both drugs.

   e. Changes in renal or hepatic clearance. Generally, these are a consequence of changes in renal or hepatic blood flow, although other actions (e.g., effects on active reuptake by the kidney) can result from one drug influencing the disposition kinetics of another. Blood flow changes are most noted when the liver or kidney extracts a high fraction of drug from the blood presented to it. Lidocaine, meperidine, and morphine are examples of drugs that have high hepatic extractions.

   f. Changes in excretion through the lungs. These may be important in anesthesia, as pulmonary excretion is a major pathway for elimination of gaseous and volatile inhalation anesthetic agents. Drugs that depress ventilation, such as opioids, may delay pulmonary excretion of inhalation agents.

g. Changes in distribution. These can affect the onset and duration of action of many drugs administered intravenously more profoundly than do changes in excretion and metabolism. Any drug that affects either cardiac output or flow distribution will affect the rate of drug delivery and the total amount delivered, especially to the brain and heart.

h. Addition. This refers to simple additivity of fractional doses of two or more drugs, the fraction being expressed relative to the dose of each drug required to produce the same magnitude of response. That is, response to X amount of drug A = response to Y amount of drug B = response to $\frac{1}{2}X_A + \frac{1}{2}Y_B$ = response to $\frac{1}{4}X_A + \frac{3}{4}Y_B$, and so on.

i. Synergism. This refers to the situation where the response to fractional doses as described previously is greater than the response to the sum of the fractional doses (e.g., $\frac{1}{2}X_A + \frac{1}{2}Y_B$ produces more than the response to X_A or Y_B).

j. Potentiation. Refers to the enhancement of action of one drug by a second drug that has no detectable action of its own.

RECOMMENDED READING

Benet LZ, Kroetz DL, Sheiner LB. Pharmacokinetics. The dynamics of drug absorption, distribution, and elimination. In: Hardman JE, et al., eds. *The Pharmacological Basis of Therapeutics*, 9th ed. New York: McGraw-Hill; 1996:3–27.

Hughes MA, Glass PSA, Jacobs JR. Context-sensitive half-time in multicompartment pharmacokinetic models for intravenous anesthetic drugs. *Anesthesiology* 1992;76:334–341.

Ross EM. Pharmacodynamics. Mechanisms of drug action and the relationship between drug concentration and effect. In: Hardman JE, et al., eds. *The Pharmacological Basis of Therapeutics*, 9th ed. New York: McGraw-Hill; 1996:29–41.

Rowland M. *Clinical Pharmacokinetics: Concepts and Applications*. Baltimore: Williams & Wilkins; 1995.

The Pain Clinic Manual, Second Edition,
edited by Stephen E. Abram and J. David Haddox.
Lippincott Williams & Wilkins,
Philadelphia, © 2000

14

Local Anesthetic Pharmacology

Christian R. Schlicht

C. R. Schlicht: Department of Anesthesiology, University of New Mexico, Health Sciences Center—School of Medicine, Albuquerque, New Mexico 87131.

In 1860, Nieman isolated the alkaloid cocaine from cocoa leaves. Topical cocaine became the first local anesthetic (LA) used clinically. Since that time many LAs have entered into clinical use. This discussion focuses on amino amide and amino ester LAs used for infiltrative anesthesia.

I. MECHANISM OF ACTION

LAs block conduction of impulses in excitable tissues such as peripheral and central nerves, through sodium channel deactivation. By binding to and blocking transmembrane sodium channels, the ordinary inward flux of sodium ions during depolarization is negated. Resting and threshold potentials are not altered. However, the rate of depolarization is markedly slowed, thereby preventing the initiation of action potentials. Several theories for specific mechanisms of action have been proposed:

A. Calcium-Mediated LA Inhibition of Sodium Flux
B. Interference of Membrane Permeability Through LA Expansion of the Membrane Volume
C. LA-Induced Surface Changes of the Axolemma
D. LA Interaction with a Specific Receptor on the Neuronal Membrane

II. STRUCTURE/ACTIVITY RELATIONSHIP

A. Basic Concepts
1. LAs consist of a lipophilic unsaturated benzene-ring head and a hydrophilic tertiary amine tail, separated by a hydrocarbon chain.
2. The linkage between the hydrocarbon chain and the lipophilic portion can be an amide or an ester bond; this results in vastly different LA properties, and the general division of LAs into amino ester and amino amide agents.
3. Some antihistamine and anticholinergic drugs share the general chemical structure of LAs but offer only weak LA properties.

B. Potency
    1. Potency generally correlates with lipid solubility.
    2. Potency increases with the total number of carbon atoms in the molecule.
    3. The minimum blocking concentration (C_m) of LAs is the lowest concentration that blocks impulse propagation; it is a direct indication of potency analogous to the minimum alveolar concentration (MAC) of inhalational anesthetics.
C. Ionization
    1. The degree of ionization determines the lipid solubility and consequently potency of LAs.
    2. The unchanged, free-base form of the drug is the most lipid-soluble form and has the best membrane penetration.
    3. The portion of the drug available in the cation or base form is governed by the pKa and the ambient pH.
III. PHARMACOKINETICS
Pharmacokinetics describes how a drug moves through the body. The use of LAs for infiltrative anesthesia depends on local physical factors as well as on systemic pharmacokinetic properties. The latter determines the absorption, distribution, and elimination of LAs.
A. Absorption
    1. Absorption depends primarily on the local vascularity and the local concentration of the LA.
    2. Variables include
        a. Site of injection
        b. Presence of vasoconstrictors. These can enhance neuronal uptake, prolong duration of action, and limit systemic toxicity.
        c. Degree of tissue binding
B. Distribution
    1. Distribution is determined by tissue blood flow and the relative blood and tissue solubilities of LAs.
    2. Variables include
        a. Tissue perfusion. The vessel-rich group (brain, lung, liver, kidney, heart) is responsible for the initial uptake (alpha phase); redistribution (beta phase) then occurs to lesser perfused tissues.
        b. Tissue mass. Most LAs will stay in the largest tissue mass (i.e., muscle tissue).
C. Elimination
    1. Ester metabolism
        a. Amino esters are metabolized by plasma cholinesterases, predominantly pseudocholinesterase.
        b. Ester hydrolysis is rapid and extensive, yielding water soluble metabolites, which are excreted in the urine.

2. Amide metabolism
   a. Amino amides are metabolized by microsomal liver enzymes through biotransformation; hepatic compromise may predispose to toxicity.
   b. Amide metabolism is far slower than ester hydrolysis.
   c. Very little drug is excreted unchanged.

IV. AMINO ESTER LOCAL ANESTHETICS
   A. Cocaine
      1. Is first known LA.
      2. Is used as topical anesthetic agent primarily.
      3. Possesses vasoconstrictive properties specifically useful for ENT surgery.
   B. Procaine
      1. First synthetic LA
      2. Weak LA, slow onset, and short duration of action
      3. Low systemic toxicity
   C. Chloroprocaine
      1. Rapid onset, short duration, low systemic toxicity
      2. Hydrolyzed some four times faster than procaine
      3. Rapid fetal metabolism
      4. Used almost exclusively in obstetric epidural anesthesia
      5. Myelotoxicity and neurotoxicity reports are probably due to the preservative sodium metabisulfite.
   D. Tetracaine
      1. Ten times as potent but hydrolyzed four times slower than procaine
      2. Slow onset of action
      3. Produces a profound motor block
      4. Almost exclusively used in spinal anesthesia
   E. Benzocaine
      1. Poorly water soluble; therefore not injectable
      2. Used extensively as topical anesthetic

V. AMINO AMIDE LOCAL ANESTHETICS
   A. Lidocaine
      1. First available amino amide agent
      2. Most versatile and most frequently used LA
      3. High potency, rapid onset, moderate duration of action
      4. Available for topical, infiltrative, spinal, and epidural use
      5. Drug absorption can be slowed by as much as 50% with the addition of vasoconstrictors.
      6. Only agent approved for intravenous regional anesthesia
      7. Capable of producing systemic analgesia in central pain states

B. Mepivacaine
1. Similar overall properties to lidocaine.
2. Less versatile than lidocaine; not available topically
3. Particularly useful for brachial plexus blockage
4. Prolonged fetal hepatic degradation
C. Bupivacaine
1. Moderately fast onset, long duration of action, profound conduction blockage
2. High potency, albeit high potential for systemic toxicity (i.e., cardiotoxicity)
3. Offers significant separation of sensory and motor blockage.
4. Drug of choice for labor epidural analgesia and postoperative analgesia in combination with opioids
D. Ropivacaine
1. Newest amide LA
2. Similar properties to bupivacaine with slightly lower potency and shorter duration in terms of motor blockage
3. Only local anesthetic prepared as a pure s-isomer rather than a racemic mixture
E. Prilocaine
1. Similar chemical properties to lidocaine
2. Least toxic LA
3. Capable of causing methemoglobinemia
F. Etidocaine
1. Derivative of lidocaine
2. More intense motor blockage than sensory blockage with early cardiotoxicity

RECOMMENDED READING

Arthur GR. Pharmacokinetics of local anesthetics. In: Strichartz FR, ed. *Local Anesthetics.* Berlin: Springer-Verlag, 1987: 165–186.

Butterworth JF IV, Trichartz GR. Molecular mechanisms of local anesthesia: A review. *Anesthesiology* 1990;72:711–734.

De Jong RH. *Local Anesthetics.* St. Louis: Mosby-Year Book, 1994.

Denson DD, Mazoit JX. Physiology, pharmacology, and toxicity of local anesthetics: adult and pediatric considerations. In: Raj PP, ed. *Clinical Practice of Regional Anesthesia.* New York: Churchill Livingstone, 1991: 73–105.

Scott DB, Lee A, Fagan D, et al. Acute toxicity of ropivacaine compared with that of bupivacaine. *Anesth Analg* 1989;69:563–569.

Tucker GT, Mather LE. Properties, absorption, and disposition of local anesthetics. In: Cousins MJ, Bridenbaugh PO, eds. *Neural Blockage in Clinical Anesthesia and Management of Pain,* 2nd ed. Philadelphia: JB Lippincott, 1988.

The Pain Clinic Manual, Second Edition,
edited by Stephen E. Abram and J. David Haddox.
Lippincott Williams & Wilkins,
Philadelphia, © 2000

15

Local Anesthetic Toxicity

Christian R. Schlicht

C. R. Schlicht: Department of Anesthesiology, University of New Mexico, Health Sciences Center—School of Medicine, Albuquerque, New Mexico 87131.

Generally, local anesthetic (LA) drugs are void of side effects if they are administered in the proper anatomic location and in the proper dosage. However, unrecognized intravascular or intrathecal injections can lead to potentially life-threatening systemic reactions primarily of the central nervous and cardiovascular systems. Other specific adverse reactions can include local tissue toxicity, allergic reactions, and methemoglobinemia.

I. SYSTEMIC TOXICITY
    A. Cardiovascular Toxicity

The cardiac toxicity of LAs parallels their potency, with the exception of bupivacaine and etidocaine, which are more cardiotoxic than predicted. Manifestations of toxicity may vary from initial mild hypertension to conduction abnormalities and circulatory arrest.

        1. Mechanism

           a. LAs decrease the rate of conduction of cardiac electrical impulses through their action on cardiac sodium channels. Lidocaine is a fast-in, fast-out blocker, whereas bupivacaine has fast-in, slow-out properties. Subsequently, bupivacaine accumulates, especially when given in high concentrations or rapid administration rates. This results in reentry-type arrhythmias.

           b. There is a dose-dependent decrease in myocardial contractility through inhibition of intracellular calcium release.

           c. Cardiovascular depression also results from LA action on medullary autonomic sites.

           d. LAs act on vascular smooth muscle directly; they vasoconstrict in low doses and vasodilate at higher concentrations.

        2. Treatment

The cardiovascular toxicity of LAs is markedly increased by concomitant hypoxia, acidosis, hyperkalemia, and hypercarbia. Much of the treatment focuses on reversing these processes to prevent ongoing toxicity.

    a. High doses of epinephrine intravenously may be necessary for a prolonged period of time to support heart rate and blood pressure.

    b. Atropine may be useful in bradycardia states.

    c. DC cardioversion may be successful.

    d. Ventricular arrhythmias are more responsive to bretylium than lidocaine.

    e. Magnesium sulfate may be useful intravenously for reentry-type arrhythmias.

B. Central Nervous System Toxicity

Frequently, central nervous system (CNS) alterations are the first evidence of an inappropriate or unrecognized intravascular injection of LAs. This tends to occur at significantly lower doses than necessary to produce symptoms of cardiac toxicity.

    1. Mechanism

        a. Convulsant activity results from selective depression of inhibitory fibers in the brain.

        b. Generation of global convulsions from focal excitation probably occurs in the amygdala.

    2. Basic principles

        a. A direct correlation exists between anesthetic potency and CNS toxicity of various LAs.

        b. CNS toxicity is increased by hypercarbia, acidosis, and prior administration of drugs that slow metabolism (i.e., cimetidine).

        c. A high rate of administration or high concentration of LAs will result in toxicity at a lower dose than otherwise predicted.

        d. More potent agents (i.e., bupivacaine, etidocaine) are absorbed into the circulation slower than less potent ones (i.e., lidocaine, mepivacaine).

    3. Signs and symptoms

        a. Premonitory symptoms are lightheadedness and dizziness, followed by auditory, olfactory, and visual disturbances such as tinnitus, a metallic taste, and difficulty in focusing.

        b. Objective signs are usually excitatory, including shivering, facial muscle twitching, tremors, and nystagmus.

        c. Eventually, generalized tonic/clonic seizures occur, followed by respiratory distress and cardiovascular collapse.

    4. Treatment

        a. For mild symptoms, supplementary oxygen and assistance with ventilation are recommended to prevent hypoxemia and hypercarbia.

        b. With significant ventilatory problems the airway may need to be secured with the help of succinylcholine; this also prevents further metabolic acidosis as a result of increased muscular activity during the convulsion.

   c. For control of the central electrical activity of the convulsion, benzodiazepines (i.e., diazepam) or barbiturates (i.e., thiopental) are indicated.

II. LOCAL TISSUE TOXICITY

Local anesthetic agents in the concentrations and volumes typically used in regional anesthesia are relatively free of significant local tissue irritation. However, preservatives of local anesthetic solutions as well as contamination of the LA may result in local tissue toxicity.

  A. Neurotoxicity

    1. Neurotoxicity is rare but may occur under special circumstances.

      a. Injection of inappropriate large volumes or high concentrations of agents

      b. Chemical contamination of LAs

      c. Neural ischemia secondary to local pressure

      d. Direct trauma from the injection needle

    2. The margin between median blocking concentrations and neurotoxic concentrations is very high, perhaps more than fifty-fold.

    3. Intrathecal or epidural chloroprocaine has been implicated in neurotoxicity due to the preservative sodium bisulfite and the low pH of the solution.

    4. Intrathecal administration of concentrated lidocaine (5%) has been shown to cause neurotoxicity, particularly when injected through spinal microcatheters.

    5. A syndrome of transient nerve root irritation has been described following spinal anesthesia with several local anesthetics, particularly lidocaine.

  B. Muscle Tissue

    1. Skeletal muscle changes with histopathologic significance have been observed following intramuscular injections of LAs.

    2. More potent, longer-acting agents cause a higher degree of tissue damage.

    3. Generally, these changes reverse spontaneously within several weeks.

III. ALLERGIC REACTIONS

True allergic reactions to LAs are rare, whereas adverse reactions are relatively common. Discriminating between the two can be difficult.

  A. Basic Principles

    1. Allergic reactions to amino ester agents occur due to the parent compound para-aminobenzoic acid, a known allergenic agent; these are far more common than reactions to amino amides.

    2. Amino amide agents contain the preservative methylparaben, which is generally the allergenic agent.

    3. There is no known cross-reactivity between amide and ester agents.

   4. A thorough history will often discriminate between symptoms of allergy (e.g., urticaria, bronchospasm) and those of adverse reactions (e.g., fainting, tinnitus).
   5. Prior documented allergic reactions to amino esters can be avoided by switching to an amino amide.
   B. Testing
      1. Provocative skin testing is possible, but the reliability and the scientific basis of the testing have been challenged.
      2. A negative skin test still necessitates switching classes of local anesthetics.
   C. Treatment
      The treatment is identical to that of any allergic reaction and may include volume resuscitation, epinephrine, histamine receptor blockage, and steroids, depending on severity.
IV. METHEMOGLOBINEMIA
   A. Basic Principles
      1. This is a unique systemic effect associated with prilocaine and benzocaine.
      2. This is generally seen only with doses of prilocaine exceeding 500 mg.
      3. The metabolism of prilocaine yields o-toluidine, which is responsible for the oxidation of hemoglobin to methemoglobin.
      4. This may result in clinically significant cyanosis.
   B. Treatment
      1. This phenomenon usually reverses spontaneously.
      2. Intravenous methylene blue will reverse the process.

RECOMMENDED READING

De Jong RH. *Local Anesthetics.* St. Louis: Mosby-Year Book, 1994.
Incaudo G, Schatz M, Patterson R, et al. Administration of local anesthetics to patients with a history of prior adverse reaction. *J Allergy Clin Immunol* 1978;61:339.
Kasten GW, Martin ST. Bupivacaine cardiovascular toxicity: Comparison of treatment with bretylium and lidocaine. *Anesth Analg* 1985;64:911.
Reiz S, Nath S. Cardiotoxicity of local anesthetic agents. *Br J Anesth* 1986;58:736.
Spiegel DA, Dexter F, Warner DS, et al. Central nervous system toxicity of local anesthetic mixtures in the rat. *Anesth Analg* 1992;75:922.

The Pain Clinic Manual, Second Edition,
edited by Stephen E. Abram and J. David Haddox.
Lippincott Williams & Wilkins,
Philadelphia, © 2000

16

Systemic Opioid Therapy for Noncancer Pain

Stephen E. Abram

S. E. Abram: Department of Anesthesiology and Critical Care Medicine, University of New Mexico, Health Sciences Center—School of Medicine, Albuquerque, New Mexico 87131.

There has been considerable resistance within the medical community to the long-term use of opioids for noncancer pain. There are multiple reasons for this:

1. Likelihood of tolerance development with eventual loss of efficacy
2. Dose escalation that will lead to mental clouding
3. Development of addiction
4. Fear of action against prescribing physician by drug regulatory agencies
5. Concern that patients may be selling drugs

Experience from the cancer pain population has caused many pain management practitioners to reassess some of the conventional thinking on this subject. Many cancer patients experience excellent analgesia for prolonged periods with minimal dose escalation and minimal side effects.

I. OPIOID EFFICACY
   A. Responsiveness to Opioids: Great Variability
   B. Factors Associated with Lower Response
      1. Neuropathic pain
      2. Incident pain
      3. Cognitive impairment
      4. Psychological distress
   C. Some patients with the preceding factors may have excellent responsiveness—presence does not contraindicate opioid use.
II. TOLERANCE
   A. Rapid dose escalation occurs occasionally.
   B. Rapid development of tolerance to analgesic effect is relatively uncommon.
   C. Intense noxious input (e.g., from fracture, osteomyelitis, pancreatitis, sickle cell crisis) may be the cause of escalating drug dose.

    D. Highly potent drugs with high intrinsic activity such as fentanyl, Sufentanil may be more effective in patient needing high opioid doses because of tolerance or intense nociception.

III. DECISION TO PRESCRIBE OPIOIDS LONG-TERM
    A. Good Therapeutic Efficacy
        1. Selected medication produces complete or substantial analgesia.
        2. No rapid dose escalation
        3. Improvement in functional activity
    B. No History of Substance Abuse
    C. Minimal or Tolerable Side Effects

IV. SIDE EFFECTS
Tolerance to most side effects occurs, but persistence of some adverse effects may limit usefulness.
    A. Cognitive Impairment
        1. May not be evident to patient during opioid use.
        2. Becomes obvious after medication discontinued.
    B. Sedation
    C. Nausea
    D. Constipation
    E. Insomnia
    F. Sexual impairment

V. OPIOID-INDUCED HYPERALGESIA
    A. Mechanisms of neuronal plasticity involved in development of hyperalgesia following persistent noxious stimulation or neuropathic pain
        1. Cascade of intracellular events initiated by release of excitatory amino acids (EAAs)
        2. Involvement of translocation of protein kinase C (PKC)
    B. Similar mechanisms implicated in the development of opioid tolerance
        1. Thermal hyperalgesia demonstrated in animals made tolerant to morphine
        2. Increased intracellular PKC results from prolonged exposure of opiate receptor to exogenous opioids—increases responsiveness of NMDA receptor to EAAs
        3. Increased PKC, induced by neuropathic pain or by exogenous opioid exposure, reduces opiate receptor responsiveness, leading to tolerance
    C. Possible mechanism of central hyperalgesia among patients on long-term opioids
        1. Discontinuation of opioids may actually lead to reduction in pain levels.
        2. Requires prolonged abstinence before beneficial effects are seen.

VI. RISK OF ADDICTION AND ABUSE
Continues to be a major concern of prescribing physicians, patients, law enforcement personnel.

A. Physical Dependence
  1. Physiologic condition characterized by abstinence syndrome following abrupt cessation
  2. Not an indicator for addiction—patients abusing opioids not necessarily physically dependent; patients taking opioids for pain control often physically dependent, but not addicted
  3. Most pain patients no longer needing opioids can taper and discontinue medications with minimal adverse effects.
B. Addiction
  1. Defined as compulsive use of a substance resulting in physical, psychologic, or social harm to the user and continued use despite that harm.
  2. Three components
     a. Loss of control over drug use
     b. Compulsive drug use
     c. Continued use despite harm
  3. Possibly difficult to recognize addiction in patients with chronic pain. Signs may include
     a. Intense desire for drug; inappropriate concern over continued availability
     b. Unsanctioned dose escalation
     c. Use of drug to treat symptoms not targeted by therapy or unapproved use when asymptomatic
     d. Aberrant drug-related behaviors
C. Therapeutic dependence
  1. In patients with drug-induced benefit, threat of discontinuation produces anxiety and drug-seeking behavior.
D. Pseudoaddiction
  1. When pain is undertreated, patients may exhibit drug-seeking behaviors similar to those seen with addiction.
  2. Symptoms subside when pain is adequately treated.

VII. DRUG DIVERSION
A. Term used to describe use of prescription drugs for untended purposes (e.g., sale of drugs for street use)
  1. Difficult to document
  2. Possibly determined on the basis of negative drug screen
     a. Have patient document most recent dose of opioid.
     b. If recent enough to be detectable, obtain drug screen; make sure screen detects prescribed drug.
     c. If drug screen is negative for prescribed drug, there is likelihood of drug diversion.

VIII. OPIOID CONTRACT
A. Agreement with patient based on decision to provide long-term opioid prescription

B. Definition of terms under which physician will continue to prescribe, expectations of patient behavior

C. Permission for random drug screening to ensure patient is taking prescribed drugs and is not using nonsanctioned controlled substances or illegal drugs

D. Opioid contract—example

IX. GUIDELINES FOR OPIOID TREATMENT OF NONCANCER PAIN

A. Exhaust other conservative treatment options before considering long-term opioid use.

B. Rule out contraindications to opioid use.

C. Single practitioner prescribes all opioids and other analgesics.

D. Provide informed consent regarding side effects, complications, physical dependence, risks for pregnant, lactating women, etc.

E. Establish rules of behavior for patient (opioid contract) and responsibility of physician for ongoing care; patient should agree to discontinuation of therapy if analgesic effect is minimal, there are significant side effects, or there is failure to achieve improvement in activity or function.

F. Prescribe medications by the clock; agree to several-week period of dose titration; provide several additional rescue doses while titrating regular dose.

G. Assess degree of pain relief, functional improvement, side effects.

H. Patients should return to clinic at least monthly during dose titration; may wish to continue monthly visits for patients on schedule II drugs.

I. Consider tapering and discontinuing opioids in response to repeated violations of contract; patient should understand that this is the consequence of aberrant behavior; may consider referral to addiction medicine.

RECOMMENDED READING

Abram SE, Mampilly GA, Milosavljevic D. Assessment of the potency and intrinsic activity of systemic versus intrathecal opioids in rats. *Anesthesiology* 1997;87:127–134.

Buckley FP, Sizemore WA, Charlton JE. Medication management in patients with chronic non-malignant pain. A review of the use of a drug withdrawal program. *Pain* 1986;26:153–266.

Clark HW, Sees KL. Opioids, chronic pain and the law. *J Pain Symptom Manage* 1993;8:297–305.

Mao J, Price DD, Mayer DJ. Mechanisms of hyperalgesia and morphine tolerance: A current view of their possible interactions. *Pain* 1995;62:259–274.

Portenoy RK. Opioid therapy for chronic non-malignant pain: Current status. In: Fields HL, Liebeskind JS, eds. *Progress in Pain Research and Management,* vol 1. Seattle: IASP Press, 1994:247–287.

Weissman DE, Haddox JD. Opioid pseudoaddiction—an iatrogenic syndrome. *Pain* 1989;36:363–366.

CONTROLLED SUBSTANCE CONTRACT

For most patients with chronic noncancer pain the problems and side effects of narcotics far outweigh the benefits. However, there are some patients who benefit from the use of these drugs. The patients who do well are those who experience profound pain relief (most or all of their pain is relieved), who continue to get good relief over time without needing higher narcotic doses, and who are able to increase their daily activities as a result of the reduced pain. In addition, the patients who do well do not show signs of addiction. Signs of addiction include calling between appointments for more narcotics; asking the pharmacy for early refills; asking many different doctors, clinics, or the emergency room for pain medications; taking medications in higher doses or more frequently than prescribed; or using alcohol, marijuana, or other non-prescribed mind-altering substances.

Taking narcotics may interfere with your ability to concentrate and think clearly. Side effects may also include constipation, dizziness, itching, drowsiness, nausea, and difficulty urinating. If you already have or develop any of these problems, please tell your doctor.

Taking narcotics regularly for a long period of time usually causes physical dependence. This means that if you stop taking the medications suddenly, you could experience withdrawal symptoms, such as watering eyes, runny nose, sweating, tremors, difficulty sleeping, agitation, diarrhea, and abdominal pain. Taking narcotics over a long period of time may put you at risk for developing an addiction. This means that you could become preoccupied with taking narcotics or other drugs to the point that other important aspects of your life—such as family, friends, work, and health—could suffer.

Individuals who are addicted are often unaware of their addictions. Therefore it is very important that your doctor follow you closely to assess whether you are developing an addiction. To conduct this ongoing assessment your doctor may need to check your blood or urine for narcotics and other drugs. Your doctor may also need to be in contact with your family members and friends, because the symptoms of addiction may be recognized by others before you recognize them.

The prescribing of narcotics is closely regulated by state and federal regulatory agencies. If your use of controlled substances is not in compliance with governmental regulations or if you are using additional controlled substances or illegal drugs, your doctor could be at risk of losing the right to prescribe controlled substances or could even lose his or her medical license. Therefore we are unwilling to continue prescribing narcotics if you violate this agreement, both because of the potential harm to you and because of the risk to our livelihood.

Taking narcotics during pregnancy may be harmful to developing babies. Women must be certain that they are not pregnant now and that they do not get pregnant while taking narcotics.

I understand what is written above. As a condition of receiving regular doses of narcotics from my doctor, I agree to the following:

1. I will take my medication as prescribed by my doctor. I will not take more than is prescribed, I will not allow other individuals to take my medications, and I will not take narcotics prescribed by other doctors.
2. I will avoid alcohol and all illegal drugs while I am taking narcotics.
3. If I feel tired or mentally foggy, I will not drive, operate heavy machinery, or serve in any capacity related to public safety.
4. I will submit a urine or blood test for narcotics and other drugs whenever my doctor requests. My doctor may ask that a clinic staff member observe me as I produce the urine specimen.
5. I will allow my doctor to receive information from any health care provider or pharmacist about use or possible misuse of alcohol and other drugs. This permission shall expire only upon my written cancellation of this agreement.
6. I will allow my doctor to contact my family and friends to help monitor my conditions. If my doctor recommends, I will see a specialist to help determine whether I am developing an addiction. I will allow the pain clinic doctors to send a copy of this agreement to my other doctors or to the pharmacy where I obtain my prescriptions.
7. I understand that my doctor will not be available to prescribe medication during evenings and weekends. It is my responsibility to call my doctor at least three business days in advance of running out of medications. **Under no circumstances will allowances be made for lost or stolen prescriptions or drugs.**
8. I will not obtain pain medications from any doctors outside of this clinic. In the event of an **EMERGENCY,** I will alert the emergency room doctor of my special arrangement (medication contract). The doctor should provide me with only enough medication to last until I can be seen in the pain clinic.
9. I will keep all my clinic appointments, and if I must reschedule I will notify the clinic prior to my scheduled time.
10. If asked, I will bring all of my unused pain medication to each clinic visit.
11. I will have all of my pain medications filled at one pharmacy, to be agreed upon by me and my pain clinic physician.
12. I understand that narcotic therapy will be stopped if:
    a. My doctor feels the medication is harming me, is not providing adequate pain control, or is not improving my activity or functioning.
    b. I sell, abuse or misuse my medication.
    c. I develop significant side affects.
    d. I obtain pain medication from other sources or repeatedly request increased dosages or early refills.

13. If I do not follow the above contract I understand that my doctor will gradually reduce and discontinue my narcotics or refer me to an addiction specialist.

_____   _____

Patient Signature   Date

_____   _____

Witness Signature   Date

The Pain Clinic Manual, Second Edition,
edited by Stephen E. Abram and J. David Haddox.
Lippincott Williams & Wilkins,
Philadelphia, © 2000

17

Chronic Intrathecal Drug Delivery

Mark S. Wallace

*M. S. Wallace: Department of Anesthesiology, University of California, San Diego—
School of Medicine, La Jolla, California 92093.*

I. THEORETICAL CONSIDERATIONS

A. Small afferent input into the spinal cord is subject to modulation by a number of receptor systems. Repetitive stimulation of small, unmyelinated afferent fibers will result in a long, sustained partial depolarization of the dorsal horn cells, rendering the membrane increasingly susceptible to afferent input. This phenomenon is called "wind up." This wind up can be prevented by stimulating or inhibiting certain receptor systems within the spinal dorsal horn, thus resulting in analgesia.

B. Spinal dorsal horn pharmacology is an area of intense research in the treatment of pain. Modulation of dorsal horn activity involves receptor systems, enzyme inhibitors, and membrane channel blockers. Examples of each of these systems that may alter activity evoked by small afferent fiber input are as follows:

   1. Receptor systems
      a. Agonists
         (1) Opioid (mu, delta, kappa)
         (2) Alpha adrenergic (α2-agonists)
         (3) Serotonin
         (4) Adenosine
         (5) GABA B
         (6) Cholinergic (muscarinic)
         (7) Neuropeptide Y
      b. Antagonists
         (1) Glutamate
            (a) NMDA
            (b) non-NMDA
         (2) Tachykinin
            (a) NK-1
            (b) NK-2

    2. Enzyme inhibitors
       a. Cyclooxygenase inhibitors
       b. Nitric oxide synthase inhibitors
    3. Membrane channel blockers
       a. Sodium channels
       b. Calcium channels

II. PATIENT SELECTION
  A. Inclusion Criteria
    1. Failure of conservative therapies
       a. Failure to achieve adequate analgesia with adequate doses
       b. Intolerable side effects
    2. Further surgical intervention is not indicated or refused by patient.
    3. Patient has had a successful trial of intraspinal drug therapy (preferably a 1- to 2-week trial of a continuous infusion through an externalized catheter).
    4. Life expectancy of >6 months (for implantable pumps)
  B. Exclusion Criteria
    1. Active psychosis
    2. Major uncontrolled depression, anxiety
    3. Active suicidal behavior
    4. Active homicidal behavior
    5. Active alcohol or drug addiction
    6. Serious cognitive deficits
    7. Presence of active disease that preclude implantation such as coagulopathies, sepsis, etc.

III. TECHNIQUES OF CHRONIC INTRASPINAL DRUG DELIVERY
  A. Three Systems Used for Intraspinal Drug Delivery
    1. Externalized system
    2. Partially externalized system
    3. Totally implanted systems
  B. Externalized System
    1. Injection port and delivery system outside the body
    2. May be injected intermittently or connected to an external pump for chronic delivery
    3. There are no externalized catheters that are FDA approved for long-term intrathecal drug delivery
       a. Currently one externalized catheter approved for short-term intrathecal drug delivery (up to 4 days)—Algoline (Medtronic, Inc., Minneapolis, MN)
    4. Currently one externalized catheter approved for long-term epidural drug delivery (DuPen epidural catheter, CR Bard Inc., Salt Lake City, UT)
    5. All other epidural catheters may be used for up to 30 days.

C. Partially Externalized System
   1. Injection port implanted internally and delivery system is external.
   2. May be injected intermittently or connected to an external pump for chronic delivery.
   3. Currently one system with FDA approval for long-term epidural drug delivery—Port-a-Cath epidural port system (Pharmacia-Deltec, Inc., St. Paul, MN)
D. Totally Implanted Systems
   1. Catheter and delivery system implanted internally
   2. Much more expensive than the externalized or partially externalized system
   3. Generally reserved for patients with a life expectancy of more than 6 months
   4. Three devices on the market and one in clinical trials:
      a. FDA approved:
         (1) Synchromed Infusion System (Medtronic, Inc., Minneapolis, MN)
         (2) Arrow Constant Flow Implantable System (Arrow Int., Reading, PA)
         (3) Infusaid System (Pfizer, Norwood, MA)
      b. Not FDA approved:
         (1) Algomed Model 84112 (Medtronic, Inc., Minneapolis, MN)
   5. Synchromed Infusion System
      a. FDA approved for intrathecal morphine and baclofen
      b. Programmable (through an external radio-telemetry link) which allows for immediate rate adjustments without requiring pump access
      c. Allows for a variety of infusion modes
         (1) Continuous infusion
         (2) Continuous-complex infusion (increases and decreases throughout the day)
         (3) Single bolus
         (4) Intermittent bolus
      d. Pump refills are required every 30 to 90 days (depending on the flow rate).
      e. Battery operated with a battery life of 3 to 5 years, after which the entire pump must be replaced.
      f. Has both a pump refill port and a separate direct cerebrospinal fluid (CSF) access port.
   6. Arrow Continuous Flow Infusion System
      a. FDA approved for intrathecal morphine only
      b. Not programmable
      c. A factory preset flow rate (low, medium, and high)

     d. Because of the nonprogrammability, to increase the amount of drug delivered, the pump must be refilled with a higher or lower drug concentration.

     e. The infusion is driven by Freon; therefore it does not require replacement.

     f. Reservoir and direct CSF port are accessed through the same septum (there is a safety mechanism that prevents direct injection into the CSF when filling the pump).

7. Infusaid System
   a. FDA approved for intrathecal morphine only
   b. Similar to the Arrow system in all respects except that the pump refill port and direct CSF access port are separate (as with the Synchromed system).

8. Algomed Model 84112
   a. Currently in clinical trials
   b. Patient-controlled system activated by finger pressure on a control pad underneath the skin
   c. System includes three components:
      (1) Control pad
         (a) Reservoir fill port
         (b) Pumping chamber
         (c) Activation valve
      (2) Drug reservoir
      (3) Catheter
   d. The pumping chamber has a maximum volume of 1 ml and following a bolus, slowly fills over 60 to 90 minutes, thus limiting the amount of drug that can be administered.

IV. MORBIDITY OF INTRASPINAL DRUG DELIVERY
  A. Overall Incidence
    1. Postsurgical
      a. Minor: 5.4% to 44%
      b. Major: 2.7%
    2. Long-term
      a. Minor: 5.4% to 26.4%
      b. Major: 2.7% to 15.4%
  B. Catheter-Associated Morbidity
    1. Neurologic complications
      a. Incidence
        (1) Transient—0.1%
        (2) Permanent—0.02%
      b. Most often secondary to an abscess or fibrosis
    2. Infection
      a. Most often occurs with externalized long-term catheters and in patients who are immunosuppressed. Very rare with totally implanted systems.

    b. Insertion site infection is much more common than actual nervous system infection.

    c. The catheter hub is the main point of entry of bacteria leading to catheter colonization; however, hematogenous spread and tracking of bacteria from the insertion site may also occur.

3. Catheter fibrosis/inflammation
   a. Incidence of fibrosis
      (1) Epidural—0.5% to 19%
      (2) Intrathecal—9.5%
   b. Fibrosis occurs most often at the catheter tip, which may lead to encapsulation.
   c. Most patients can achieve long-term catheterization without significant fibrosis and altered drug delivery.

4. Catheter malfunction
   a. Incidence—10% to 40%
   b. Causes of malfunction
      (1) Disconnection from the pump or port
      (2) Large to small catheter disconnect (if present)
      (3) Kinks or holes in the catheter
      (4) Catheter breaks
      (5) Catheter dislodgments

C. Pump or Port Pocket Associated Problems
   1. Hematoma
      a. Usually occur immediately postoperatively
      b. Prevention
         (1) Meticulous control of bleeding intraoperatively
         (2) Proper screening of patients for coagulopathies
      c. Treatment
         (1) May require surgical exploration and removal
   2. Seroma
      a. Prevention
         (1) Abdominal binder worn for 1 month post pump implant
      b. Treatment
         (1) Percutaneous drainage using strict aseptic technique
   3. Infection
      a. Prevention
         (1) Pretreatment with a single dose of antibiotics prior to pump implant
         (2) Meticulous aseptic technique
      b. Treatment
         (1) Not all wound infections require pump or catheter removal, and if superficial, can be treated with antibiotics.
         (2) Careful aspiration of the pump or port pocket is useful to provide a culture and sensitivity.

  (3) If the infection is deep and severe (associated with fever and leukocytosis), the system should be removed.

  (4) Consultation with infectious disease physician may be necessary.

 4. Capsule formation

  a. Implanted pumps or ports may develop a capsule resulting in pain.

  b. Rarely requires intervention but some patients may require the system to be removed if the pain becomes severe.

D. Pump System–Associated Problems

 1. Filling errors

  a. Inadvertent side port access

   (1) Results in a large dose of drug delivered directly into the CSF, leading to drug overdose

   (2) The Synchromed 8615S pump has a screened side port that will only allow entry of a 25-gauge needle, which will prevent access from the usual 22-gauge huber type needle used for pump refill.

   (3) The Arrow model 3000 pump has a special bolus needle for bolusing directly into the CSF.

  b. Overfilling the pump

   (1) Overpressurization of the reservoir may lead to pump damage, failure, or overdose.

   (2) Most pumps come with a manometer system to alert the physician or nurse of an overpressurized system.

  c. Inadvertent placement of drug in the pump pocket

   (1) Most of the drugs used for intrathecal delivery are highly concentrated and can lead to very high plasma levels and drug overdose.

 2. Pump failure

  a. Most often occurs with battery failure (with Synchromed)

  b. Failure of the telemetry system (with Synchromed) may also occur.

   (1) This will convert the pump to a constant-flow system; to change drug delivery requires a change in concentration.

 3. Programming errors

  a. May lead to inadequate pain relief, abstinence syndrome, or drug overdose.

 4. Torsion or flipping of pump

  a. If the pump or port is not secured with sutures inside the pocket, the pump or port can flip or torque, leading to inability to refill or reprogram.

  b. May lead to catheter dislodgment or kink.

  c. Requires surgical revision.

V. DRUGS USED INTRASPINALLY FOR CHRONIC PAIN MANAGEMENT
  A. Opioids
    1. Morphine is the only opioid with FDA approval for chronic intraspinal use; however, based on the literature, other opioids are used "off label" for chronic intraspinal therapy. These include hydromorphone, fentanyl, Sufentanil, and meperidine.
    2. Side effects
       a. Side effects should be treated symptomatically, and if they do not resolve or are intolerable, a different opioid should be tried.
       b. Side effects include nausea, urinary retention, pruritis, constipation, sedation, polyarthralgia, amenorrhea, peripheral edema.
    3. Tolerance
       a. Patients may become tolerant to both analgesia and side effects. If tolerance to analgesia occurs, simple rotation to another opioid or the addition of a nonopioid analgesic (see later) may be beneficial.
    4. Equianalgesic doses: see Table 17-1.
    5. Highest commercially available drug concentrations
       a. Morphine—50 mg/ml
       b. Hydromorphone—10 mg/ml
       c. Meperidine—100 mg/ml
       d. Fentanyl—50 µg/ml
       e. Sufentanil—50 µg/ml
    6. Maximum recommended daily dose is based on the use of the commercially available drugs. If higher doses are desired, drug compounding is necessary to achieve higher concentrations.
       a. Morphine—25 mg
       b. Hydromorphone—5 mg
       c. Meperidine—50 mg
       d. Fentanyl—25 µg
       e. Sufentanil—25 µg
  B. Local Anesthetics
    1. Most often used in combination with the opioids
    2. The addition of a local anesthetic often allows a decrease in the dose of the opioid.

TABLE 17-1. *Equianalgesic doses*

	Oral	Parenteral	Epidural	Intrathecal
Morphine	300	100	10	1
Hydromorphone	100	20	2	0.2
Meperidine	4000	1000	100	10
Fentanyl	-	1	0.1	0.01
Sufentanil	-	0.1	0.01	0.001

    3. Bupivacaine is most commonly used, although lidocaine and tetracaine may also be used.

    4. Limiting side effect is sensory loss and motor weakness.

C. Baclofen

    1. GABA-B receptor agonist

    2. FDA approved for the treatment of spinal cord spasticity

    3. Commercially available in concentrations of 500 and 2000 µg/ml

    4. Maximum recommended daily dose—1000 µg

D. Clonidine

    1. Alpha-2-adrenergic receptor agonist

    2. FDA approved for cancer pain treatment only

    3. FDA approved for epidural use only

    4. Uses:

       a. Patients who become tolerant to the opioids

       b. Neuropathic pain

       c. Sympathetically mediated pain

       d. Spinal cord spasticity

    5. Side effects

       a. Hypotension

       b. Bradycardia

       c. Dry mouth

       d. Sedation

       e. Constipation

    6. Commercially available in a concentration of 100 µg/ml

    7. Maximum recommended intrathecal daily dose—50 µg

E. SNX-111

    1. N-type calcium channel blocker

    2. N-type calcium channels are located in the dorsal horn cells and blockade of these channels results in a powerful analgesia

    3. Currently in phase III trials

RECOMMENDED READING

De Lissovoy G, Brown RE, Halpern M, Hassenbusch SJ, Ross E. Cost-effectiveness of long-term intrathecal morphine therapy for pain associated with failed back surgery syndrome. *Clin Therapeut* 1997;19:96–112.

Krames ES, Schuchard M. Implantable intraspinal infusional analgesia: Management guidelines. *Pain Rev* 1995;2:243–267.

Krames ES. Intraspinal opioid therapy for chronic nonmalignant pain: Current practice and clinical guidelines. *J Pain Symp Manag* 1996;11:333–352.

Nelson DV, et al. Psychological selection criteria for implantable spinal cord stimulators. *Pain Forum* 1996;5:93–103.

The Pain Clinic Manual, Second Edition,
edited by Stephen E. Abram and J. David Haddox.
Lippincott Williams & Wilkins,
Philadelphia, © 2000

18

Adjuvant Analgesics

Donald C. Manning

D. C. Manning: Department of Anesthesiology, University of Virginia, Charlottesville, Virginia 22906; Novartis Pharmaceuticals Corp., East Hanover, New Jersey 07936

TABLE 18-1. Adjuvant analgesics

Generic name	Trade name	Starting dose	Dose range	Mechanism	$T_{1/2}$	Precautions/ adverse effects	Metabolism
Antiepileptic drugs							
Carbamazepine	Tegretol	100 mg BID	200–400 mg BID	Na⁺ channel inhibitor Reduces neuronal excitability	15–27 hr	Indicated for trigeminal neuralgia Monitor for bone marrow suppression	CYP2D6 Autoinduction of metabolism
Phenytoin	Dilantin	300 mg QD	300–400 mg QD	Na⁺ channel inhibitor	conc. dep. 16 hr	Gingival hyperplasia	
Valproic acid	Depakene	125 mg TID	500–1000 mg TID	GABA potentiation		Hepatotoxicity, thrombocytopenia, sedation, nausea, alopecia,	
Gabapentin	Neurontin	100 mg QID	100–900 mg QID	Ca²⁺ channel inhibitor Inhibits glutamate synthesis	5–7 hr	somnolence, ataxia, fatigue, dizziness	No metabolism
Lamotrigine	Lamictal	25 mg QD	200–400 mg QD	Na⁺ channel blockade	25 hr	Increase dose by 25/week to avoid rash/TEN Dizziness, ataxia, headache Inhibits dihydrofolate reductase	
Topiramate	Topamax	25 mg BID	25–100 mg BID	AMPA receptor blocker Reduces neuronal excitability Na⁺ channel blockade	21 hr	Sedation, ataxia, concentration and memory difficulties, nephrolithiasis Inhibits carbonic anhydrase	
Clonazepam	Klonopin	0.5 mg QD	2–8 mg QD	Benzodiazepine receptor agonist	39 hr	Taper slowly to D/C Active in atypical facial pain Sedation, weakness	

Continued

Tricyclic Antidepressants (3° and 2° amines)

3°	Amitriptyline	Elavil	25 mg QD	150–300 mg QD	NE and 5HT uptake inhibition	15–57 hr	Lowered seizure threshold, dry mouth, confusion, weight gain, closed angle glaucoma, urinary retention, constipation, orthostatic hypotension	CYP2D6
	Imipramine	Tofranil	25 mg QD	150–300 mg QD		13 hr		CYP2D6
	Doxepin	Sinequan	25 mg QD	150–300 mg QD	Na⁺and K⁺ channel inhibition	17–51 hr		CYP2D6
2°	Desipramine	Norpramin	25 mg QD	150–300 mg QD		18 hr	2° amines—less anticholinergic AE	CYP2D6
	Nortriptyline	Pamelor	25 mg QD	150 mg QD		31 hr	Dysrhythmias with desipramine	CYP2D6

Miscellaneous Agents

Baclofen	Lioresal	5 mg TID	15–120 mg QD	GABA-B agonist K⁺ Channel inhibitor	3–4 hr	Taper slowly to avoid seizures. Sedation, weakness	
Mexiletine	Mexitil	150 mg QD	150–300 mg TID	Na⁺ channel inhibitor with local anesthetic actions	10–12 hr	Baseline EKG and blood level monitoring suggested. Monitor for prolonged QT intervals. Dizziness, paresthesias, sedation, nausea, and vomiting	CYP2D6
Paroxetine	Paxil	10 mg QD	10–80mg QD	Serotonin uptake inhibitor. Weak anticholinergic	21 hr	Sedation, asthenia, nausea, insomnia	CYP2D6
Clonidine	Catapress	0.1 mg QD	0.1–0.3 mg TID	Alpha-2 adrenergic agonist	8.5 hr	Hypotension, sedation, bradycardia	
Calcitonin	Miacalcin	25 IU BID	25–150 IU BID	Unknown in pain	43 min	Nasal spray	

For drugs metabolized by the CYP2D6 system, combinations of agents can amplify side effects. For example, tricyclic antidepressants can reach toxic plasma levels when combined with another CYP2D6 substrate or inhibitor such as paroxetine or mexilitine.

Combinations of antiepileptic agents can lead to accentuated ataxia and sedation.

Plasma elimination half-life ($T_{1/2}$) estimates can be used to determine dose escalation schedules. Approximately $3.3 \times T_{1/2}$'s are required for steady-state plasma levels to assess a drug's effect. These are minimal estimates, as a particular drug's pharmacodynamics may dictate slower escalation schedules (e.g., lamotrigine or baclofen).

PART IV

Management of Specific Pain Syndromes

The Pain Clinic Manual, Second Edition,
edited by Stephen E. Abram and J. David Haddox.
Lippincott Williams & Wilkins,
Philadelphia, © 2000

19

Back Pain and Radiculopathy

Quinn H. Hogan

*Q. H. Hogan: Department of Anesthesiology, Pain Management Center,
Medical College of Wisconsin, Milwaukee, Wisconsin 53226.*

At any one time about 10% of adults will be suffering from some degree of back pain. Low back pain is the cause of between 10% and 40% of all sick days, and nearly all people will encounter this problem in their lifetimes. This results in an enormous cost and accounts for 3% of all doctor visits. More than 3% of American men will have a laminectomy.

Sensations from the axial skeleton are nonspecific, so diagnosis of the mechanism or source of low back pain is very challenging. Since back pain is so common, it requires special vigilance to identify the unusual and possibly fatal diseases among the customary presentations. The diagnosis and treatment of low back pain is the center of escalating controversies. This is due not only to the great cost of the problem, but also to the range of treatments, various backgrounds of practitioners treating back pain, and disagreement regarding the best approach. Governmental guidelines have been generated, and there is ever-growing attention by payers regarding documentation of outcomes.

I. RARE BUT IMPORTANT CONDITIONS NOT TO MISS
   A. Epidural Abscess
      1. May follow a few days to weeks after needle or surgical procedures of the vertebral column or after systemic infection; may also occur without previous events.
      2. Variable complaints may include back pain and tenderness, stiff neck, and progressive neurologic deficit.
      3. Systemic signs of infection may be absent.
      4. Diagnosis requires imaging by magnetic resonance imaging (MRI).
      5. Therapy requires surgery and intravenous antibiotics. Imaging and urgent surgical consultation are crucial to achieving adequate recovery.
   B. Vertebral Osteomyelitis
      1. Systemic signs of acute or chronic infection may be absent.
      2. Should be suspected if there is back pain, muscle spasm, limitation of motion, and a source of infection or trauma.

3. Pain may be the only symptom. Erythrocyte sedimentation rate (ESR) is usually elevated. MRI is diagnostic.

C. Epidural Hemorrhage
   1. Usually associated with procedures or anticoagulation
   2. Prompt progression of back pain and incomplete neurologic deficit
   3. Diagnosis by MRI
   4. Surgical decompression is typically necessary within 12 hours

D. Vertebral Neoplasm or Metastasis
   1. Usual primaries are prostate, breast, lung, kidney, or thyroid.
   2. Cord or nerve compression may result from tumor mass or pathologic fracture.
   3. Diagnosis is by imaging.
   4. Radiation may control symptoms but surgical decompression may be necessary. Rarely, epidural steroids may be indicated to relieve pain.

E. Abdominal Aortic Aneurysm
   1. Pain may be intense in middle or upper back but may also present as mild pain in early case.
   2. Pulsatile abdominal mass may be evident.
   3. Initial presentation of back pain in elderly, especially with peripheral vascular disease, should arouse suspicion.

II. LOW BACK PAIN

The innervation of the deep somatic structures is comparatively sparse. Unlike the skin, stimulation of the various sensitive components of the axial skeleton produces broadly comparable sensations. Also, sensory information originating from various segmental levels results in minimally different patterns of pain. Spinal cord cells that receive input from the vertebral column also have receptive fields in the skin or other distant structures. This accounts for radiation of pain and confusing patterns of pain distribution. Subsequent to injury at one site within the vertebral column and associated ligaments and muscles, sensory pathways in the spinal cord become more sensitive to painful input from other noninjured sites. In the chronic setting, back pain often cannot clearly be attributed to a single mechanism.

A. Nonspecific Therapy for Low Back Pain
   1. Physical therapy. Strain of joints, ligaments, and muscle by excessive mechanical loading is a contributing factor to most cases of low back pain. Abnormal posture or incorrect lifting, as shown earlier; excess body weight; and poorly conditioned muscles can all lead to increased pain and slowed recovery. The goal of physical therapy (back stabilization) is to increase muscle endurance and strength so that a greater amount of load is shared by surrounding muscle groups instead of damaged joints.
   2. Education and reassurance that most cases of back pain, especially when not chronic, are self-limited.

3. Mild analgesics such as acetaminophen, NSAIDs. Muscle relaxants and opioids are of uncertain efficacy.
4. Decreased activity (e.g., avoid heavy lifting), to allow recovery from acute phase without further injury. Bed rest is rarely indicated for more than a few days.
5. If pain persists beyond about a month without evidence of improvement:
   a. Confirm no dangerous condition exists (see earlier).
   b. Avoid injection therapy or surgery in the absence of specific indications.
   c. Consider TENS (see Chapter 12).
   d. Consider psychotherapy and rehabilitation program.
   e. Evaluate for a specific condition (see later).
6. Pain that persists after laminectomy can be very challenging. There may be progression of the disease or mistaken original diagnosis. Further imaging may be necessary, and an intensive rehabilitation program should be considered.

B. Sacroiliac Joint Pain

The sacroiliac (SI) joint is subjected to formidable forces and is stabilized by heavy ligaments. Stimulation of the joint causes pain that is felt locally and radiates into the adjacent paramedian pelvic area and into the buttock. This large joint is subject to systemic arthropathy such as osteoarthritis, rheumatoid arthritis, gout, ankylosing spondylitis, and Crohn's disease. Injury through stress is probably most common.

1. Diagnosis is by typical area of pain, tenderness over the joint, and provocation of pain by maneuvers:
   a. Compression of the iliac bones toward each other.
   b. Gaenslen's, in which the patient holds his or her knee on the healthy side, bent and pulled up against the chest while the examiner extends the hip on the painful side
   c. Fabere test, in which the ankle of the involved side is placed on the opposite knee and pressure is placed simultaneously on the flexed knee and the opposite iliac crest
2. Diagnosis may be aided by injection of anesthetic into the joint.
3. Treatment is by general measures (above) or by injection of steroids
   a. Injection into the ligaments posteriorly may be adequate.
   b. If ligamentous injection fails to produce relief, intraarticular injection using radiologic imaging may be helpful.

C. Facet Pain

There is no doubt that the facets are well innervated and can produce pain. When hypertonic saline is injected into the facet joints, pain is produced that spreads into the adjacent buttock and thigh. The area of perceived pain from stimulation of different facets broadly overlaps, so diagnosis of the particular site of pathology cannot be based purely upon the patient's report.

1. Diagnosis is supported by
   a. Localized pain in the back that may radiate into the paravertebral area, buttock, and proximal thigh.
   b. Pain that is worse with movement, especially back extension or rotation
   c. Tenderness in the area of the facet
   d. No evidence of nerve dysfunction
   e. Arthritic changes in the joint that are often evident by imaging. Tc99 scanning may show increased uptake.
   f. Findings may not produce a clear diagnosis. Diagnostic block may be helpful in confirming a facet pain site.
2. Treatment includes general measures (above) and the following:
   a. Consideration of steroid injections
   b. Surgical fusion in rare cases
   c. Neural ablation of facet nerves by radiofrequency lesion. Efficacy of this therapy is incompletely proved.

D. Myofascial Pain

Local pain in the back is often at least in part due to involvement of the muscles.

1. May be secondary to disease of other components of the axial skeleton via reflex increase in muscle activity or may be the primary cause of pain.
2. May be initiated by trauma or overuse, or without any obvious provocation.
3. Treatment is same as that for myofascial pain elsewhere (see Chapter 20).

E. Bony Damage

Loss of integrity of the complicated mechanical structure of the vertebrae and joints may lead to local pain.

1. Spondylolisthesis is due to a defect (spondylolysis) in the portion of the posterior elements between the superior and inferior articular processes where sheer stress is maximal. This may allow forward slippage of the upper vertebra relative to the lower.
   a. Most common level is L_5/S_1, usually between ages 7 and 20 years.
   b. Pain and restricted motion of the back are most common complaints. Radiculopathy may accompany local pain.
   c. Diagnosis is by imaging.
   d. Treatment is avoiding stress to the site through restriction of activity, physical therapy for strengthening, and rarely steroid injection into the epidural space or the injury site.
2. Osteoporosis that results in collapse of a vertebra causes sudden onset of local pain, usually in postmenopausal women.

       a. Diagnosis is by x-ray.

       b. Treatment is conservative. Hormonal therapy and calcium supplements may be of benefit.

   3. Ankylosing spondylitis

       a. Most common between ages 17 and 35 years.

       b. Morning stiffness accompanies local back pain that gradually progresses.

       c. May be primary or present with psoriasis or colitis.

       d. X-ray findings (sclerosis, erosion and fusion of joints, osteopenia) follow onset of symptoms.

       e. Blood tests include elevated ESR and alkaline phosphatase level, and positive HLA-B27 serology.

       f. Treatment is conservative. In advanced cases, immunosuppressive therapy may be used.

III. NECK PAIN

A similar array of conditions can produce pain originating in the cervical vertebral column, including facet arthropathy, myofascial processes, and bony trauma.

  A. Initial treatment is by conservative measures as outlined earlier.

  B. Physical therapy plays a key role in improving range of motion and decreasing muscle tightness.

  C. Facet disease is a diagnostic possibility for local neck pain.

    1. Pain may radiate into low neck and shoulder area.

    2. Decreased range of motion is a prominent feature.

    3. Tenderness at the level of the facet may be found.

    4. Spurling's test may be positive: with the head leaning slightly to the involved side; downward pressure on the head increases pain.

    5. Conservative measures are usually adequate.

    6. Facet injection for diagnosis and treatment (with steroid) may be useful.

    7. Rarely, surgery or facet neurolysis are indicated.

  D. The theory that neck pathology is a frequent cause of headache (cervicogenic headache) is unproved.

IV. RADIATING PAIN

Although most pain that is focused in the back also radiates to adjacent areas, conditions that involve irritation or injury to roots and proximal nerve trunks are characterized by pain that is primarily shooting and localized to the extremities. Other findings indicating neural dysfunction are usually also evident, such as loss of strength or reflexes, loss of sensation, or paresthesias. Pathophysiology involves inflammatory changes and altered function of the spinal cord, such that spontaneous signals are generated and nociceptive pathways are sensitized.

  A. Acute Lumbar Radiculopathy

    1. Etiologies of radiculopathy:

   a. Herniated nucleus pulposus, the most common. Peak incidence in ages 30 to 45 years. L_5/S_1 and L_4/L_5 discs are the most common levels.
   b. Foraminal stenosis and hypertrophy of facet or ligamentum flavum may contribute mechanical irritation to cause pain in an inflamed root.
   c. Tumor and epidural abscess are rare causes that should be kept in mind.
2. Signs and symptoms in a pattern consistent for a particular nerve (see Table 19-1).
   a. Pain with shooting or electrical quality in characteristic location for that nerve. Often provoked by movement or increased epidural pressure during cough, sneeze, or defecation.
   b. Diminished sensation (test touch, cold, scratch)
   c. Decreased strength and atrophy of muscles
   d. Loss of reflexes
   e. Tension signs producing pull on irritated nerve
      (1) Straight leg lift (identify level at which pain begins, drop the leg to relieve pain, and confirm pain can be produced by ankle dorsiflexion)

TABLE 19-1. *Signs and symptoms of radiculopathy secondary to disc herniation*

Clinical Signs of Cervical and Lumbar Disc Herniation

Level of herniation	Pain distribution and sensory Loss	Weakness	Reflex changes
C4–C5 Disc C5 Root	Lateral upper arm	Deltoid; biceps	Biceps
C5–C6 Disc C6 Root	Lateral forearm, thumb; forefinger	Biceps; wrist extensors	Brachioradialis
C6–C7 Disc C7 Root	Middle finger	Triceps; wrist flexors; finger extensors	Triceps
C7–T1 Disc C8 Root	Medial forearm, fourth, fifth fingers	Interossei; finger flexors	
T1–T2 Disc T1 Root	Medial portion, mid-arm	Interossei	
L3–L4 Disc L4 Root	Lateral thigh, medial calf and ankle	Quadriceps (mild)	Patellar
L4–L5 Disc L5 Root	Lateral thigh and calf, big toe	Foot dorsiflexors	Tibialis posterior
L5–S1 Disc S1 Root	Posterior thigh and calf, lateral foot	Foot plantar flexor	Achilles

      (2) Sitting straight leg lift (extend knee of sitting patient)

      (3) Lesegue's test (flex hip of recumbent patient and extend knee to produce pain)

      (4) Deep palpation of sciatic notch or popliteal fossa

3. Testing to support diagnosis of radiculopathy

   a. Electromyelogram and nerve conduction study confirming neuropathy of suspected root

   b. Imaging to identify lesion producing injury

      (1) MRI most useful

      (2) Myelography for surgical planning in complex cases

4. Treatment objectives

   a. Reduced neural sensitivity

   b. Reduced mechanical irritation

   c. Muscle strengthening and improved flexibility

   d. Improved activity level

5. Initial treatment: conservative (as outlined earlier)

   a. Bowel or bladder dysfunction may result from compression of the cauda equina by a large midline disc herniation and requires intense evaluation and possibly prompt surgery.

   b. Physical therapy should be pursued if it does not worsen pain. Flexion or extension program can be chosen on basis of pain response.

   c. Recovery in 3 months is typical of 75% of patients with acute radiculopathy.

6. Epidural steroids

   a. Response is most favorable in patients without previous surgery, nonsmokers, patients who are employed and not on disability financial support, and patients with pain that is of less than 6 months duration.

   b. Extremity pain is more likely to be relieved than the back pain that may also exist.

   c. Should be used as a component of a program including general measures (see earlier).

   d. Technique: See Chapter 37.

      (1) Document pain level and functional status (back range of motion, straight leg lift) prior to injection to allow comparison with initial response to local anesthetic.

      (2) Consider caudal approach with catheter and fluoroscopic imaging in patients who have had previous laminectomy.

   e. Risks

      (1) Postdural puncture headache

      (2) Spinal anesthesia after unrecognized subarachnoid injection of local anesthetic; dose should be limited to low end of typical spinal dose (e.g., 60 mg of lidocaine, 10 mg bupivacaine).

(3) Arachnoiditis following unrecognized subarachnoid injection of steroid

(4) Bleeding in patients with abnormal coagulation

(5) Hypertension, fluid retention, or elevated blood glucose in susceptible patients

(6) Infection, rarely reported in diabetics

f. Epidural steroid treatment plan

(1) If no relief 30 minutes after injection (local anesthetic plus steroid), either there was a technical problem with the injection or the diagnosis is incorrect.

(2) On return visit (7 to 10 days):

(a) If pain is relieved, no further injection is necessary.

(b) If relief is present but inadequate or not persistent, repeat injection (up to three).

(c) If the patient notes no response to steroids, repeat the injection only if epidural placement was uncertain or if alternative therapy is unavailable. Consider foraminal steroid injection.

B. Chronic Lumbar Radiculopathy

1. Continue general measures.

2. Address concomitant problems.

a. Physical deconditioning

b. Psychological distress

c. Myofascial pain

3. Epidural steroids

a. Unlikely to be beneficial, especially after previous laminectomy

b. May be helpful to treat a flare-up of pain.

c. May be indicated if all other therapy has been exhausted and patient recognizes low probability of success.

4. Pharmacologic management

a. Tricyclic antidepressants, especially for sleep regulation; may also help neuropathic pain component.

b. Anticonvulsant or systemic local anesthetic may rarely be useful.

c. Opioids are problematic but may occasionally be helpful in increasing activity level.

5. Dorsal column stimulation

a. High cost and frequent failure even after initial improvements

6. Coordinated behavioral and rehabilitative program

C. Cervical Radiculopathy

The pathophysiology, presentation, and treatment of radiculopathy at cervical levels is similar to lumbar radiculopathy.

1. Signs and symptoms (see Table 19-1)

a. Pain with shooting or electrical quality radiating in a dermatomal pattern

      b. Decreased sensation

      c. Loss of strength or atrophy of muscles

      d. Diminished reflexes

      e. Pain may be provoked by a particular head position.

   2. Testing and treatment objectives are the same as for lumbar levels.

   3. Initial conservative treatment may include soft collar or traction.

   4. Epidural or foraminal steroids may be indicated (technique: see Chapter 37).

      a. Greater risk: cord injury by needle or cardiovascular changes with needle placement and injection

      b. Starting an IV probably indicated

D. Other Causes of Radiating Pain

Not all radiating pain is due to injury or irritation of a nerve root. These are much more rare but should be considered in the differential diagnosis.

   1. Spinal cord tumor or syringomyelia. Diagnosis is made by the setting and imaging.

   2. Arachnoiditis

      a. Inflammatory changes in the arachnoid may follow trauma, myelography, hemorrhage, surgery, infection, or disc disease.

      b. Imaging shows thickened membranes and clumped nerve roots.

      c. Treatment is difficult, with some degree of relief from TCAs, opioid analgesics, and occasionally surgical neurolysis.

   3. Zoster and postherpetic neuralgia

   4. Piriformis syndrome

      a. Findings include tenderness over the muscle and pain elicited by resisted abduction/external rotation or passive adduction/internal rotation

      b. Treatment includes general measures and the following:

         (1) Stretching exercises with internal rotation and adduction of the hip (above).

         (2) Local anesthetic injection may be helpful in persistent cases, but it is hard to be certain of needle entry into the muscle.

         (3) Surgical release is rarely required.

   5. Spinal stenosis. The vertebral canal is narrowed in a concentric fashion by osteoarthritis and degenerative disc disease, producing impingement upon the entire cauda equina and the spinal cord at higher levels.

      a. Compression of the nerve roots results in the condition of neurogenic claudication, in which bilateral lower extremity pain develops after walking.

      b. Pulses are normal.

      c. Back pain may be present.

      d. Pain may be relieved by forward flexion of the vertebral column.

      e. Diagnosis is confirmed by imaging.

      f. Epidural steroids are occasionally effective, but surgery is the definitive therapy.

6. Pain may be referred from retroperitoneal structures (e.g., ureteral stone). Hip pain may be mistaken for radiating pain. Central pain may produce similar presentation.

RECOMMENDED READING

Abram SE, O'Connor TC. Complications associated with epidural steroid injections; a review. *Anesthesiol Reg Anesth* 1996;21:149–162.

Benzon HT. Epidural steroid injections for low back pain and lumbosacral radiculopathy. *Pain* 1986; 24:277–295.

Destouet JM, Gilula LA, Murphey WA, Monsees B. Lumbar facet joint injection: Indication, technique, clinical correlation, and preliminary results. *Radiology* 1982;145:321–325.

Haddox JD. Lumbar and cervical epidural steroid therapy. *Anesth Clin North Am* 1992;10:179–203.

Hoppenfeld S. *Physical Examination of the Spine and Extremities.* Norwalk, CT: Appleton-Century-Crofts; 1976.

Mooney V, Robertson J. The facet syndrome. *Clin Orthop* 1976;115: 149–156.

The Pain Clinic Manual, Second Edition,
edited by Stephen E. Abram and J. David Haddox.
Lippincott Williams & Wilkins,
Philadelphia, © 2000

20

Myofascial Pain Syndrome

Martin Grabois

*M. Grabois: Department of Physical Medicine and Rehabilitation,
Baylor College of Medicine, Houston, Texas 77030.*

I. INTRODUCTION
  A. General Remarks
     One finds acceptance of a disease entity and consensus in regard to etiology, evaluation, and treatment is usually inversely proportional to the amount of literature on the subject. A review of this subject indicates an extraordinary amount of literature and controversy. In spite of these controversies, this chapter will attempt to present a review of the subject along classic myofascial pain syndrome concepts.
  B. Goals of the Chapter
     1. To understand myofascial syndrome and how it differs from similar entities.
     2. To understand the etiology and pathophysiology of myofascial pain syndrome in order to have a better grasp of modalities utilized in treatment.
     3. To discuss clinical evaluation of the syndrome with emphasis on objective, quantity evaluation, if possible, in order to better diagnose myofascial pain syndrome and measure the success of treatment modalities utilized in treatment.
     4. To describe and evaluate treatment approaches with emphasis on rationale and success of each treatment in regard to etiology and clinical evaluation
  C. Definition
     1. The definition of myofascial pain syndrome is pain and/or autonomic phenomena referred from active myofascial trigger points. The presence of taut bands in muscles, trigger points, local twitch responses, and decreased active and passive range of motion is often seen.
     2. To better define myofascial pain syndrome, it is helpful to compare and contrast it with association of syndrome of fibromyalgia (Table 20-1)

TABLE 20-1. *Similarities and differences between primary fibromyalgia syndrome and myofascial pain syndrome due to trigger points*

Primary fibromyalgia syndrome	Myofascial pain syndrome
Similarities	
Muscle pain present	Muscle pain present
Muscle tenderness on palpation	Muscle tenderness on palpation
Very Common	Very Common
Differences	
Diffuse pain involving many muscles, ligaments, bones	Referred pain pattern specific to each muscle; pain is usually local or regional
Pain is chronic	Pain may be acute or chronic
Trauma may perpetuate local symptoms but is not a cause	Physical stress to muscle, including obvious trauma, is a cause
Nonmusculoskeletal symptoms (e.g., fatigue, poor sleep, chronic headaches) are common	Nonmusculoskeletal symptoms are unusual
Signs	
Tender points are present in muscles and other tissues, including tendon insertions and bones; radiation of pain, twitch response, and surrounding taut band in a tender point are unusual but have not been well studied. Tender points are usually more than 4 among 4 specific sites.	Myofascial trigger points are limited to muscle(s) with radiation of pain to a referred zone, twitch response, and accompanying taut band. Number of trigger points may be 1 or more.
Skin roll tenderness and cutaneous hyperemia are frequent.	
Laboratory tests	
Usual laboratory tests are normal; nonspecific pathologic changes are seen by muscle biopsy.	Laboratory tests are normal but not contributory to diagnosis; differences in muscle pathology are unclear at this time.
Theory and concept	
Pathogenesis is not well understood; disturbed sleep is a factor in most cases; psychological factors in about 25% of patients.	Pathogenesis is presumed to be acute or chronic. Muscle stress; poor sleep patterns may result; pain; psychological status usually not a factor.

D. Incidence. Simon reports that myofascial pain syndrome is a far more common cause of both chronic and acute musculoskeletal pain than generally recognized. Apparently, it is the most common cause of pain that brings patients to chronic pain treatment centers. One study reported 30% of the patients presenting at a university primary general internal medicine practice with pain had a diagnosis of myofascial pain syndrome.

E. Etiology and Pathophysiology

1. There is no generally accepted etiology for myofascial pain syndrome, but many proposed theories on the pathophysiology of the syndrome. There are probably multiple primary and secondary factors that can contribute to the etiology.

2. Fricton proposed that macrotrauma or microtrauma events may disturb the normal or weakened muscle through muscle injury or sustained muscle contraction leading to trigger points and myofascial pain syndrome (Fig. 20-1).

3. Escobar and Ballesteros noted in 200 asymptomatic patients that 54% of women and 45% of men had latent trigger points in the shoulder girdle muscles but only 13 female and 12 male subjects had active trigger points. Thus they proposed the concept of latent trigger points being activated by a primary or secondary event.

II. CLINICAL AND DIAGNOSTIC EVALUATION

A. General Concept

1. Because signs and symptoms of myofascial pain syndrome resemble many other musculoskeletal and arthritic entities, a large differential diagnosis is usually involved, as noted in Table 20-2.

2. Because of the lack of specific diagnostic tests, careful review of the complaints with a thorough physical examination is needed to make the diagnosis of myofascial pain syndrome.

B. History (Table 20-3)

1. If one believes that myofascial pain syndrome is caused by trigger points, then signs and symptoms are strongly muscle oriented. To make the diagnosis one needs to identify a myofascial trigger point and an appropriate referral pain pattern.

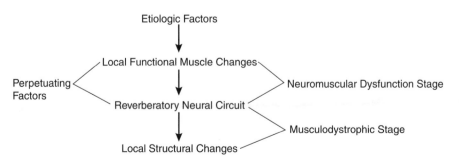

FIG. 20-1. Pathophysiology of myofascial pain syndrome.

TABLE 20-2. *Differential diagnosis in myofascial pain syndrome*

Myopathies	Polymositis, dermatomyositis, myositis due to infection
Arthritides	Osteoarthritis, rheumatoid arthritis, gouty arthritis, psoriatic arthritis, ankylosing spondylitis, polymyalgia rheumatica
Musculoskeletal	Tendinitis, bursitis
Neurological	Neuralgias (trigeminal), radiculopathies, nerve entrapments
Visceral	Ischemic heart disease, peptic ulcer, gall bladder
Infections and infestations	Viral (pleurodynia), bacterial (leptospirosis) infestations (trichinosis)
Neoplasm	Referred pain
Pyogenic Pain and behavior	

    2. Identify perpetuating factors if present.

    3. Pain and tenderness constitute a trigger point with radiation in a characteristic distribution. Trigger points have the following characteristics:

        a. Achy (dull or intense)

        b. Variable in intensity

        c. Pain that is often increased with muscle activity or abnormal posture

        d. Frequent association with perpetuating factors

    4. Associated signs and symptoms may be present and may be autonomic in character.

    5. Concomitant social, behavioral, and physiologic disturbance may precede or follow the initiation of myofascial pain syndrome.

C. Physical Exam

    1. The examination needs to concentrate on identification of trigger point and related analgesic movements, postures, and restricted range of motion of muscle.

TABLE 20-3. *Clinical Characteristics of myofascial pain syndrome*

A. Trigger points: ropeline band of muscle, tenderness on palpation, palpation alters pain, consistent palpable points of tenderness

B. Zone of reference: constant dull ache, fluctuating intensity, consistent patterns of referral, local or distant trigger points, alleviation with extinction of trigger point

C. Associated symptoms: otological symptoms, paresthesias, GI distress, visual disturbances, dermal flushing

D. Perpetuating factors: physical disorders, parafunctional habits, postural strains, disuse syndrome, nutritional disorder, sleep disturbance, stress

2. The strength is usually ratchety or breakaway.
3. Pressure on trigger point should cause a jump sign with grimacing and/or vocalization of the patient, as well as reproducing the patient's pain referral pattern.
4. A number of investigators now believe that quantification of the sensitivity of a trigger point is possible using algometers.

D. Diagnostic Tests
1. There is no laboratory or imaging test diagnostic for myofascial pain syndrome or trigger points.
2. Thermography alone cannot diagnose myofascial pain syndrome but can document what is identified by clinical examination (a 5- to 10-cm diameter hot spot over trigger point) and/or referral zone.
3. Magnetic resonance imaging may have promise for imaging change in the vicinity of an active myofascial trigger point.
4. Routine electromyography studies are normal and nondiagnostic.

III. TREATMENT
A. Concept of Treatment
1. Fricton notes that there is a critical need to match the level of complexity of treatment programs with the complexity of the patient (Table 20-4).
2. A major characteristic of the myofascial pain syndrome patient is continued pain and failure of traditional approaches for long periods of time. One study suggests approximately 5 to 7 years of pain, seeing 4.5 clinicians before adequate treatment and results.
3. Another problem with such chronic pain syndromes as myofascial pain syndrome is that patients vary in their response to different treatment techniques. Therefore a trial of therapy is often in order.

B. Patient Education
One needs to stress patient education, especially because of the perpetuating factors involved with myofascial pain syndrome. This is particularly true in preventing an acute situation from becoming recurrent and chronic. If a patient understands what activates the syndrome, he or she can better address prevention.

C. Trigger Point Inactivation
1. Simon notes the key to treatment of myofascial pain syndrome is identification of the specific muscles harboring active trigger points and treating appropriately. Lasting success depends on inactivation of the responsible trigger point by restoring full range of motion, pain-free function, and changing contributing factors.
2. Inactivation of the trigger point is usually accomplished by counterstimulation coupled with active and passive muscle stretching and postural rehabilitation. Counterstimulation usually includes spray and stretch and trigger point injections.

TABLE 20-4. *Conservative treatment*

Acute onset with rapid resolution

Clinical characteristics	Treatment (3 months)	Control of contributing factors
Onset is less than 2 months ago	Fluorimethane spray and stretch (office)	Reduce muscle tension habits
No previous treatment	Home stretching and postural exercises	Improve postural habits
Defined behavioral factors		Evaluate for other perpetuating factors
Few trigger points		
Prognosis is excellent		

Subacute

Clinical characteristics	Treatment (6 months)	Control of contributing factors
Onset is 1–6 months age	Fluorimethane spray and stretch (office and home)	Reduce tension-producing habits
Minimal previous treatment	Home exercises: jaw, head, neck, and body stretching and posture	Reduce postural habits
Some psychosocial or behavior factors	Stabilization splint	Behavioral therapy for habit change, relaxation and pacing skills training if indicated
Various trigger points bilaterally	Nonsteroidal anti-inflammatory drug for 2 weeks (optional)	If no continuing success, use physical therapy, trigger point injections, or acupuncture and reevaluation for perpetuating factors
No other symptoms		
Prognosis is good		

Chronic

Clinical characteristics	Treatment (1 year)	Control of contributing factors
Onset of more than 6 months ago	Physical therapy: mobilization with heat, ultrasound, or other modality	Reduce bruxism and clenching
Many previous unsuccessful therapies and medication	Home stretching and postural exercises: jaw, head, neck, and body	Improve postural habits Behavioral therapy for dietary and habit change, relaxation, and pacing skills training
Many psychological, behavioral, and social factors	Stabilization splint	Biofeedback, stress management training, or hypnosis if indicated and desired
Other symptoms may include diminished sensation, dizziness,	Eliminated medications, except short-term antidepressant if	

continued

TABLE 20-4. *Continued*

Clinical characteristics	Chronic Treatment (1 year)	Control of contributing factors
tinnitis, flushing, joint pathology, migraine Prognosis is guarded for long-term reduction of pain and improvement in function and depends on patient compliance	there is reactive depression with sleep difficulties; L-tryptophan for sleep disturbance only	Education and change of social contributing factors If depression or chemical dependency is present, manage first If no long-term success, consider trigger point injections, reevaluate contributing factors, reevaluate home program, enroll in inpatient chronic pain program

From Fricton JR, Awad EA. *Advances in Pain Research,* Vol 17. *Myofascial Pain and Fibromyalgia.* New York: Raven Press; 1990.

3. Spray and stretch technique is achieved by application of a vapocoolant like fluromethane with simultaneous passive stretching of the muscle. Travell and Simon originally described the technique, and Jaeger and Reeves found that both the trigger point sensitivity and referred pain intensity were reduced by utilization of the technique. The technique is demonstrated in Fig. 20-2.

4. Trigger point injection. Fricton reports that a number of authors have shown reduced pain, increased range of motion, increased exercise, and increased circulation of muscles with trigger point injections. The important factor is believed to be the mechanical disruption of the trigger point by the needle rather than injection of an anesthetic agent. Therefore accurate placement of the needle is vital (Fig. 20-3). However, it is recognized that dry needling is more painful than injections associated with local anesthetic. Simon recommends this treatment when a noninvasive (spray and stretch) approach is ineffective.

D. Muscle Rehabilitation

Muscle rehabilitation involves muscle stretching, modifying posture, and strengthening. It includes the following:

1. Stretching the muscle to reduce activity of remaining trigger points.
2. Postural exercise to reduce continuous mechanical strain.
3. Strengthening to increase muscle conditioning and reduce muscle susceptibility to reactivation of trigger point.

E. Behavioral, Biologic, and Mechanical Treatment

1. Control of contributing factors is vital, especially when perpetuating factors are present. These can be behavioral, biologic, and mechanical.

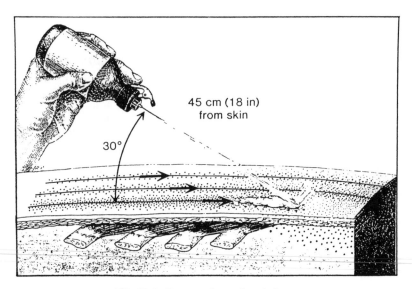

FIG. 20-2. Spray and stretch technique.

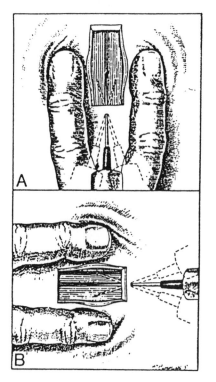

FIG. 20-3. Trigger point injection technique. (Reprinted with permission from Travell JG, Simons D. *Myofascial Pain and Dysfunction: The Trigger Point Manual.* Baltimore: Williams & Wilkins; 1983.

2. Failure to recognize or treat these factors may perpetuate muscle restriction and tension, leading to recurring activity of trigger points.

3. Travell and Simon emphasize the need to treat systemic biologic contributing factors, especially vitamin deficiency, to prevent recurrence of trigger points.

4. Stress management techniques such as biofeedback, hypnosis, and meditation have been reported to be of some help. For selected patients, antiolytic medication may be useful. Sedating antidepressants, reduction of caffeine, and good sleep hygiene are frequently employed to facilitate restorative sleep.

F. Other Treatment Modalities

1. Pleno et al. discussed in detail the rationale and technique for the use of transcutaneous electrical nerve stimulation (TENS) in myofascial pain syndrome. It should be noted that this treatment is not a cure but an adjunctive treatment. Graff-Radford suggests that high-frequency, high-intensity TENS is effective in reducing myofascial pain syndrome. Pain reduction does not reflect changes in local trigger point sensitivity by a central inhibition mechanism.

2. Waylonis et al. found no significant difference between low-output helium neon laser therapy and placebo in patients with myofascial pain syndrome when applied to acupuncture or trigger point. However, Snyder-Machler et al. did show that helium neon laser significantly increased skin resistance in musculoskeletal trigger points and noted that this may accompany the resolution of pathologic conditions.

3. If medication is to be used, NSAIDs are preferred in association with muscle relaxants, but only for short periods of time.

IV. PROGNOSIS

Two patterns of resolution are seen: (a) full recovery with possible intermittent relapses and (b) a waxing-and-waning pattern without full recovery. Results seem to correlate with a number of perpetuating factors and their resolution and the competence with which active trigger points are located and inactivated. Early intervention also seems to be important because one decreases some of the subsequent contributing factors.

V. SUMMARY

If one appreciates the etiologic factors and pathophysiology of myofascial pain syndrome and performs a comprehensive evaluation that identifies trigger points and perpetuating factors, a treatment program can be set up with adequate results. That treatment program usually consists of inactivation of trigger points by spray and stretch techniques and/or trigger point injections combined with muscle rehabilitation and control of contributing factors. Traditional physical therapy techniques as well as modalities such as newer types of transcutaneous electrical stimulation may be appropriate adjunctive treatment.

RECOMMENDED READING

Escobar PL, Ballesteros J. Myofascial pain syndrome. *Orthop Rev* 1987;16(10):16–21.

Fischer AA. Myofascial pain: Update in diagnosis and treatment. *Phys Med Rehab Clin North Am.* February 1997.

Fricton JR, Awad EA. *Advances in Pain Research,* vol 17. *Myofascial Pain and Fibromyalgia.* New York: Raven Press; 1990.

Gerwin RD. Myofascial pain syndrome. In: Grabois M, Garrison SJ, Hart KA, Lehmkuhl LD, eds. *Physical Medicine and Rehabilitation.* Cambridge, MA: Blackwell Science, in press.

Graff-Radford SB, Reeves JL, Baker RL, Chiu D. Effects of transcutaneous electrical nerve stimulation on myofascial pain and trigger point sensitivity. *Pain* 1989;37(1):1–5.

Irving A. Myofascial pain. In: Gordon A, et al., eds. *Pain Management for the Practicing Physician.* New York: Churchill Livingston; 1997: Chapter 18.

McCain GA. Fibromyalgia and myofascial pain syndromes. In: Wall PD, Melzack R, eds. *Textbook on Pain,* 3rd ed. Edinburgh: Churchill Livingston; 1994:475–493.

Newman LDI. Myofascial pain syndrome: A comprehensive review. *Clin J Pain* 1998;14(1):74–85.

Pleno JC, Raj PP, McDonald JS. Transcutaneous electrical nerve stimulation and myoneural injection therapy for management of chronic myofascial pain. *Dent Clin North Am* 1987; 31(4):703–723.

Rachlin ED. *Myofascial Pain and Fibromyalgia.* St. Louis: Mosby; 1994.

Simons DG. Myofascial pain syndrome due to trigger points. International Rehabilitation Medical Association Monograph Number 1, November 1987.

Simons DG. Single-muscle myofascial pain syndromes. In: *Pain Management in Selected Disorders.* Chapter 41.

Simons DG, Simons LS. Chronic myofascial pain syndrome. In: Tollison CD, ed. *Handbook of Chronic Pain Management.* Baltimore: Williams & Wilkins; 1989:509–529.

Snyder-Mackler L, et al. Effect of helium-neon laser on musculoskeletal trigger points. *Phys Ther* 1986; 66:1087–1090.

Thompson JM. The diagnosis and treatment of muscle pain syndrome. In: Braddom RL, ed. *Physical Medicine and Rehabilitation.* Philadelphia: WB Saunders; 1966:893–914.

Waylonis GW, et al. Chronic myofascial pain management by low output helium-neon laser therapy. *Arch Phys Med Rehabil* 1988; 69(12):1017–1020.

Yunus MB, Kalyan-Raman UP, Kalyan-Raman K. Primary fibromyalgia syndrome and myofascial pain syndrome: Clinical features and muscle pathology. *Arch Phys Med Rehab* 1988;69:451–454.

The Pain Clinic Manual, Second Edition,
edited by Stephen E. Abram and J. David Haddox.
Lippincott Williams & Wilkins,
Philadelphia, © 2000

21

Complex Regional Pain Syndromes and Sympathetically Maintained Pain

M. Alexander Gupta, J. David Haddox, and Srinivasa N. Raja

*M. A. Gupta: Critical Care Health Systems, Carolina Pain Consultants,
Raleigh, North Carolina 27619.
J. D. Haddox: Atlanta, Georgia; Pain and Policy Studies Group,
University of Wisconsin, Madison, Wisconsin
S. N. Raja: Department of Anesthesiology and Critical Care Medicine,
The Johns Hopkins University School of Medicine; Department of Anesthesiology and
Critical Care Medicine, Division of Pain Medicine,
Johns Hopkins Hospital, Baltimore, Maryland 21287.*

The sympathetic nervous system plays an important adaptive role in humans in preparing them for physically and emotionally stressful events. However, it is now well recognized that the sympathetic nervous system may play an important role in the pathogenesis of certain debilitating acute and chronic pain conditions, particularly those following traumatic injuries. The first vivid description of this clinical syndrome was by Weir Mitchell. He coined the term *causalgia* to describe the characteristic burning pain observed in Union soldiers with gunshot injuries to nerves during the Civil War. Since that time, a number of terms have been applied to these pain syndromes. Most recently, the International Association for the Study of Pain has grouped all of these related conditions under the term *Complex Regional Pain Syndrome* (CRPS). Subclassifications of CRPS include CRPS-I, previously called *reflex sympathetic dystrophy,* and CRPS-II, previously called *causalgia.* The term *sympathetically maintained pain* (SMP) is defined as that aspect of pain that is maintained by sympathetic nervous system activity, including circulating catecholamines. Clinically, it is often determined by pain relief following blockage of the efferent sympathetic nervous system. In contrast, sympathetically independent pain (SIP) is not relieved by blockage of the efferent sympathetic nervous system. It is now postulated that in patients with CRPS, there may be a varying component of SMP or SIP. Defining the SMP and SIP components of the overall pain in a given patient is important from a clinical perspective because it may affect treatment plans.

A common point of confusion in clinical practice and the literature is the mistaken belief that CRPS-I (RSD) and SMP are the same. In fact, several discrete pain states have been demonstrated occasionally to have sympathetically maintained components, such as diabetic neuropathy, myofascial pain, and herpes zoster. Therefore SMP is best conceptualized as a feature of some painful conditions that may influence treatment rather than a diagnosis or disease unto itself.

This chapter details some of the precipitating causes of CRPS and SMP, describes some of the presenting features, and outlines some of the pharmacologic, interventional, and psychological approaches to treatment.

I. PRECIPITATING FACTORS

In most patients there is a history of trauma with or without involvement of nerves, but in many patients a precipitating event may not be identified. There also seems to be no definitive relationship between occurrence of injury and onset of the pain syndrome. The following are more common causes:

A. Trauma

The severity of the trauma may range from a mere sprain to a gunshot wound. There is no correlation between the severity of the initial insult and the severity of the ensuing pain syndrome.

B. Postprocedural Factors

May commonly follow venipuncture, carpal tunnel surgery, or immobilization of extremities in splints or casts.

C. Neurologic Injury

Such as the following peripheral nerve injuries, cerebrovascular compromise, Parkinson's disease, head injuries.

D. Psychological Factors

This remains controversial. The exact contribution of psychological factors to the development of a particular patient's pain syndrome is unclear. Future studies may help to define further the contribution of predisposing psychological factors.

E. Neoplasm

The most commonly associated neoplasms include lung, breast, CNS, and ovarian.

F. Myocardial Infarction

II. PATHOGENESIS

The pathogenesis of SMP is not fully understood. There has been a recent resurgence of interest into the basic cellular mechanisms of SMP using animal models. Most of the current theories revolve around interactions between the sympathetic nervous system and the sensory system. Current theories involve both peripheral and central sites of involvement in the pathophysiology of pain. The traditional notion of the consistent involvement of the sympathetic nervous system in CRPS is now being challenged.

A. Peripheral Sympathetic/Sensory Interaction

May involve direct coupling of the two systems. Sensitization of the nociceptive afferent fibers may occur through an alpha-adrenergic mechanism. There also may be indirect coupling in which the nociceptive afferents are sensitized through mediators such as prostaglandins released from the sympathetic terminals. The theory of actual "crosstalk" between the two sets of neurons has also been proposed (ephaptic transmission).

B. Sympathetic/Sensory Interaction in the Dorsal Root Ganglia (DRG)
   Following peripheral nerve injuries in rats, sprouting of sympathetic post-ganglionic fibers around sensory neurons has been demonstrated immuno-histochemically. Thus the DRG could be another potential site of direct coupling between sensory neurons and sympathetic efferent fibers.

C. Dorsal Horn Interaction
   An injury stimulus activates unmyelinated afferent C fibers and impulses are transmitted to the dorsal horn of the spinal cord. In the dorsal horn, second-order neurons such as the wide dynamic range (WDR) neurons are activated and sensitized by activity in these C fibers. It is postulated that the sensitized WDR cells may subsequently be activated by light touch, thus explaining the allodynia seen in many CRPS patients. It was further proposed in SMP that activity in nociceptors may be maintained via an alpha-adrenergic mechanism, resulting in central pain signaling neurons being maintained in an activated state.

D. Autonomic Denervation Theory
   Proposes that the initial insult leads to autonomic denervation, which in turn leads to increased sensitivity to circulating catecholamines.

III. CLINICAL PRESENTATION AND WORK-UP OF CRPS
   The clinical presentation of CRPS can be quite variable. The traditional classi-fication of CRPS into the acute hyperemic, dystrophic, and late atrophic has recently fallen into disfavor. However, there are certain clinical characteristics that are more commonly seen.

A. History
   There may or may not be a history of antecedent trauma. The patient may not even recall a precipitating event. Pain is the presenting symptom in more than 90% of cases. CRPS-I and CRPS-II are characterized by spontaneous pain with or without associated hyperalgesia to mechanical or thermal stimuli. The pain is often burning and not relieved by rest and may be exacerbated by min-imal emotional or physical stimuli. The pain may also continue long after the initial stimulus has been stopped (part of the condition known as hyper-pathia). The pain may also spread to involve the entire extremity and in severe cases the entire ipsilateral side of the body. It has been reported as "spread-ing" to involve other body parts as well, such as the contralateral extremity.

B. Physical Findings
   1. Inspection. The clinician may notice that the patient often protects the involved extremity, holding it close to the body. There also may be sudomotor and vasomotor changes that are evident upon inspection, such as cyanosis; mottling; edema; localized sweating; smooth, shiny skin; and changes in hair growth and nails. Contractures may be seen in severe cases.

2. Palpation. May reveal coolness or warmness of the involved extremity. The patient may not initially allow the physician to touch the involved extremity because of allodynia (pain to normally innocuous stimuli). A cooling stimulus such as a drop of alcohol in the affected region is often perceived as painful. There is sometimes markedly impaired range of motion of the joints and marked tenderness to palpation. Decreased perfusion of the affected region is sometimes seen when compared with the unaffected extremity.

C. Special Tests

There is no single test that the clinician may order to establish the diagnosis, but certain tests may help confirm clinical impressions.

1. Blood tests. There are no pathognomic blood tests, but hypercholesterolemia and hypertriglyceridemia are often seen. Other blood tests may be ordered to exclude other diagnoses.

2. Radiographic studies. These also aid diagnosis and are more helpful in chronic disease where severe periarticular demineralization may be evident (Sudeck's atrophy of bone).

3. Nuclear medicine. Scans such as triple phase bone scan have been used to diagnose CRPS-I. Early stages of CRPS may show an increase in total blood flow, whereas later stages may demonstrate decreased total blood flow. Periarticular pooling during the late phase of the scan is considered to be diagnostic. The specificity of this test, particularly with regard to SMP, has been questioned.

4. Thermography. This may demonstrate increased or decreased temperatures between the affected and unaffected limbs. A temperature difference of at least 1°C is considered significant. Temperature asymmetries should raise an index of suspicion and may be useful in facilitating early diagnosis.

5. Skin conductivity tests. These may be increased with an exaggerated sympathogalvanic reflex as compared with the unaffected extremity.

6. Tests of sweat gland function, such as with ninhydrin and starch iodide. Sweat secretion may be increased or decreased. Abnormalities in sweat secretion can be quantified using quantitative sudomotor axon reflex test (QSART).

7. Local anesthetic sympathetic blocks. These help determine the degree of involvement of the sympathetic nervous system in CRPS. The classical block for CRPS involving the upper extremity is a stellate ganglion block. In the lower extremity the lumbar sympathetic block is most commonly used. Before the results of the blocks are interpreted, it is imperative to consider several factors that may alter interpretation:

   a. Degree of sympathetic blockade. It is important to know whether the sympathetic blockade is complete via objective measures such as skin temperature measurement. An optimal block should result in the skin temperature approaching core temperature. With "stellate ganglion block" or cervicothoracic sympathetic block, the development of Horner's syndrome (meiosis, ptosis, anhydrosis, and enophthalmos) is evidence of some degree of blockade of sympathetic fibers to the head. No inference about sympathetic blockade of the upper extremity can be based on the presence of Horner's syndrome following an injection.

b. Presence of motor or sensory blockade. The local anesthetic injected during stellate ganglion or lumbar sympathetic block may spread to the nearby cervical or brachial plexuses or lumbar plexus, respectively. If the patient develops any concomitant motor or sensory deficit, it is difficult to ascertain whether the patient's pain relief is a result of blockade of the sympathetic nervous system or secondary to blockage of the somatic nerves. Thus a meticulous sensory and motor exam must be carried out after a "sympathetic" block.

c. Systemic uptake of local anesthetic. This may also cause analgesia. Thus the total dose of local anesthetic used is important.

d. Placebo effect. This may also play a role in false-positive results from diagnostic sympathetic blocks.

e. Phentolamine test. This also helps determine the contribution of the sympathetic nervous system to CRPS. Phentolamine is a mixed α-1 and α-2 adrenergic antagonist. It is infused systemically via a peripheral vein in an unaffected extremity. If the patient experiences significant analgesia during infusion of the drug but not during the placebo infusion, then the sympathetic nervous system is likely to be involved in the maintenance of pain. Major advantages of the phentolamine test include minimal risk or discomfort to the patient, lack of invasive injections, no chance of analgesia due to unintentional somatic blockage or systemic uptake of local anesthetic, ease of obtaining repetitive pain assessments, and placebo control.

IV. DIAGNOSIS OF CRPS AND THE PRESENCE OF SMP

The diagnosis of CRPS is primarily based on a constellation of findings on history, physical exam, and special tests. There is no single test that is pathognomic for CRPS. The previously mentioned findings, studies, and blocks together with carefully elicited history will establish the diagnosis.

V. TREATMENT

It is important to determine in the CRPS patient how much of the pain is sympathetically maintained. This is important because SMP has occasionally been shown to be effectively treated with series of sympathetic blocks, which may lead to long-term attenuation of pain. SIP has an entirely different treatment regimen and is not responsive to sympathetic blockade by local anesthetic, phentolamine, or surgical sympathectomy.

A. Techniques for Sympathetic Blockade

1. Local anesthetic sympathetic blocks. These include stellate ganglion block for head, neck, and upper-extremity pain and lumbar sympathetic

blockade for lower-extremity pain. A series of local anesthetic blocks is indicated if significant relief is obtained with each block. It is a favorable prognosticator when the duration of analgesia is longer with each successive block. A trial of continuous epidural infusion for continuous sympathetic blockade is indicated if no relief is obtained with periodic local anesthetic blocks.

2. Phentolamine infusion on a repeated basis. This may also be an alternative way to achieve sympathetic blockade if favorable response is obtained with each infusion. Some investigators have reported good long-term results.

3. Epidural infusions. The role of continuous epidural infusions on long-term treatment of SMP has not been well studied. More studies are needed comparing this technique with repeated local anesthetic sympathetic blockade. Beneficial effects of epidural infusion of clonidine in treatment of refractory CRPS have been reported.

4. Intravenous regional blocks with guanethidine, reserpine, and bretylium. This has also been used in treatment of SMP. However, these drugs are not always readily available to the clinician for this indication in the United States.

5. Oral sympatholytic agents, including phenoxybenzamine, prazosin, and terazosin. These have been used effectively in treatment of SMP; however, their efficacy is limited by postural hypotension, and this may limit titration to therapeutic dosages.

6. Topical clonidine. This has been successfully used to treat patients with localized areas of SMP. Some authors report that the analgesia produced by clonidine spreads beyond the confines of the patch. Further studies are needed to fully assess these observations.

7. Spinal cord stimulation and intrathecal infusion devices. These should be considered after the diagnosis of SMP is made and all other conservative therapies have failed. Recent data have been very favorable in the usage of spinal cord stimulation in the treatment of SMP when confined to one or even two limbs. Although SMP has been traditionally thought to respond poorly to intrathecal opioids, the advent of intrathecal clonidine may make intrathecal infusion techniques more beneficial. A formulation of this drug for epidural use is now available.

8. Surgical sympathectomy. This may also be considered when less conservative therapies have failed. Surgical sympathectomy has been reported to be successful in treatment of SMP; however, failure to achieve long-term benefit has been attributed to collateral reinnervation and failure to extend the sympathectomy to adequate levels. Percutaneous techniques for ablation of the stellate ganglion using radiofrequency or neurolysis have been described.

B. Pharmacotherapy for Treatment of SIP
   This includes several classes of medications (Table 21-1).

TABLE 21-1. *Pharmacologic agents for treatments of CRPS*

Antidepressants

Tricyclics	*SSRIs*	*Mixed reuptake inhibitors*
Amitriptyline	Paroxetine	Venlafaxine
Nortriptyline		Nefazodone
Desipramine		Maprotiline
Doxepin		

Anticonvulsants/antiarrhythmics

Sodium channel blockers	*Other mechanisms of action*
Carbamazepine	Valproic acid
Phenytoin	Clonazepam
Lamotrigine	Gabapentin
Lidocaine	
Mexiletine	

Opioids

Oral long-acting opioids	*Transdermal opioids*	*Intraspinal opioids*
Controlled-release opioids (oxycodone, morphine)	Fentanyl	Morphine
Methadone		Fentanyl
Levorphanol		

Sympatholytics

Adrenergic receptor blockers	*Alpha-2 agonists*
Phenoxybenzamine	Clonidine
Phentolamine	
Prazosin	
Terazosin	
Doxazosin	

Topical Agents
Capsaicin
Local anesthetics
NSAIDs

Other agents
Corticosteroids
Nifedipine
Calcitonin
Baclofen
NSAIDs

NSAIDs: nonsteroidal antiinflammatory drugs.
Adapted from Wesselmann U, Raja SN. Reflex sympathetic dystrophy and causalgia. *Anesthesiol Clin N Amer* 1997; 15:407–427.

Many patients have a component of both SIP and SMP, and a combination of sympathetic blockade and pharmacotherapy should be used. Each of the drug classes has different mechanisms of action and an adequate trial of each class of drug should be undertaken. Many of the side effects associated with these drugs often improve with time, and it is important to reinforce the importance of the limited nature of the untoward effects and the potential benefit these drugs may have. The initial dose should be low and titrated in a controlled fashion, noting all side effects and beneficial effects.

VI. CONCLUSIONS

The pathophysiology behind SMP is still not fully elucidated. It is important to understand that patients with CRPS may or may not have SMP. The best diagnostic tool to discern the role of the sympathetic nervous system in a patient with CRPS is by a selective sympathetic blockade either through careful local anesthetic blockade or phentolamine infusion. Repeated sympathetic blockade has been shown to be a useful tool in patients with SMP. Invasive procedures such as spinal cord stimulation or intrathecal infusion therapies should be reserved for those patients who have failed more conservative therapies.

RECOMMENDED READING

Campbell JN, Meyer RA, Raja SN. Is nociceptor activation by alpha-1 adrenoreceptors the culprit in sympathetically maintained pain? *APS J* 1992;1:3–11.

Devor M, Jänig W, Michaelis M. Modulation of activity in dorsal root ganglion neurons by sympathetic activation in nerve-injured rats. *J Neurophysiol* 1994;71:38–47.

Drummond PD, Finch PM, Smythe GA. Reflex sympathetic dystrophy: The significance of differing plasma catecholamine concentrations in affected and unaffected limbs. *Brain* 1991;14:2025–2036.

Galer BS. Neuropathic pain of peripheral origin: Advances in pharmacologic treatment. *Neurology* 1995;45:S17–S25.

Hughes JH. Reflex sympathetic dystrophy—causalgia. In: Dolin J, Padfield NL, Pateman JA, eds. *Pain Clinic Manual*. Oxford: Butterworth-Heineman; 1996:461–497.

Jänig W. The sympathetic nervous system in pain: Physiology and pathophysiology. In: Stanton-Hicks M, ed. *Pain and the Sympathetic Nervous System*. Boston: Kluwer; 1990.

Jänig W. The puzzle of "reflex sympathetic dystrophy": Mechanisms, hypotheses, open questions. In: Jänig W, Stanton-Hicks M, eds. *Reflex Sympathetic Dystrophy: A Reappraisal, Progress in Pain Research and Management*. Seattle: IASP Press, 1996.

Jänig W, Levine JD, Michaelis M. Interactions of sympathetic and primary afferent neurons following nerve injury and tissue trauma. *Prog Brain Res* 1996;113:161–184.

Löfström JB, Cousins MJ. Sympathetic neural blockade of upper and lower extremity. In: Cousins MJ, Bridenbaugh PO, eds. *Neural Blockade in Clinical Anesthesia and Management of Pain*. Philadelphia: JB Lippincott; 1988:461–497.

Stanton-Hicks M, Jänig W, Hassenbusch S, et al. Reflex sympathetic dystrophy: changing concepts and taxonomy. *Pain* 1995;63:127–133.

Wesselmann U, Raja SN. Reflex sympathetic dystrophy and causalgia. *Anesthesiol Clin N Amer* 1997; 15:407–426.

The Pain Clinic Manual, Second Edition,
edited by Stephen E. Abram and J. David Haddox.
Lippincott Williams & Wilkins,
Philadelphia, © 2000

22

Acute Herpes Zoster and Postherpetic Neuralgia

Nabil M. K. Ali

N. M. K. Ali: The New Mexico Center for Pain Management; Anesthesia Specialists of Albuquerque; St. Joseph Healthcare, Albuquerque, New Mexico 87102.

I. INTRODUCTION

Herpes zoster (HZ) manifests itself as an acute neuropathic painful condition caused by the reactivation of the dormant varicella zoster virus (VZV) in the dorsal root or trigeminal ganglia. For this to happen, the patient must have had a prior varicella (chicken pox) infection. VZV was identified as a single etiologic agent that is responsible for both conditions. Postherpetic neuralgia (PHN) is characterized by the persistence of dermatomal neuralgic pain associated with acute HZ following the healing of vesicular lesions. Severe pain may continue for extended periods of time, especially in the elderly. It is known to be one of the most intractable and difficult chronic pain conditions to treat in this patient population.

II. CLINICAL FEATURES

A. Distribution

Herpes zoster is most commonly seen in a thoracic dermatomal distribution affecting one or several segments, usually unilateral. The ophthalmic division of the trigeminal nerve is the second most common site of HZ infection. Other dermatomes—such as the maxillary and mandibular divisions of the trigeminal nerve, cervical, brachial, and lumber plexuses—are affected less commonly.

B. Symptoms and Signs

Following viral reactivation, patients first notice hyperaesthesia and dysaesthesia in the affected dermatomes associated with itching, burning, and aching pain. Skin rash might begin with the onset of pain or shortly after. As the disease progresses, symptoms becomes more intense and are accompanied by severe lancinating and shooting pain that is precipitated by touching the skin in the affected area. Patients have difficulty tolerating touch by their clothing because the skin becomes exquisitely sensitive. If pain is not controlled during the acute phase of the disease, patients will suffer from severe behavioral and mood disturbances, such as anxiety, insomnia, restlessness, depression, and other complex psychologic changes. Vesicular eruption progresses into ulceration and possibly secondary infection. Healing is manifested by dark scab formation and scarring. When scabs fall, the skin underneath is pinkish in color, soft, and raw. As healing continues, the area appears slightly hypopigmented. Pain gradually subsides with treatment and healing.

C. Postherpetic Neuralgia (PHN)

If pain continues after complete healing of the HZ skin lesions, the condition is labeled PHN. The older the patient, the greater the likelihood that he or she will develop PHN. There are no reported cases of PHN under the age of 20 years. While the overall incidence of PHN in patients who had suffered from acute HZ is 10% to 20%, it is 50% or higher in patients over the age of 60. It has been suggested that PHN is the foremost cause of intractable, debilitating pain in the elderly and that it is a principal factor leading to suicide in patients over the age of 70 suffering from chronic pain.

D. Ophthalmic Division HZ and Eye Complications

In addition to severe pain caused by corneal HZ involvement, serious eye complications might result from herpes zoster ophthalmicus. The viral infection might lead to keratitis, corneal ulceration, iritis, and iridocyclitis—a devastating complication that might result in a permanently blind and severely painful eye.

III. PATHOPHYSIOLOGY

The latent varicella zoster virus is thought to be reactivated in response to various stressors and systemic conditions, such as stress, surgical procedures, trauma, radiotherapy, malignancy, toxic chemicals, ultraviolet light, ingestion of arsenic or lead, systemic corticosteroid therapy, tuberculosis, syphilis, human immunodeficiency virus (HIV) infection, and other immune system suppressors. The reactivated virus spreads from the ganglion, by retrograde axonal transport along the affected nerve, to the skin, resulting in vesicular eruption and inflammation. At this stage, the virus is detected in the skin lesions. The virus might disseminate systemically if the immune system is greatly compromised. Intense sympathetic activation in the affected dermatomes is produced by this acute inflammatory process, leading to vasoconstriction, intravascular thrombosis, and ischemia of the involved nerves.

IV. MECHANISMS OF NEUROPATHIC PAIN ASSOCIATED WITH HZ

A. Acute Phase

Severe neuropathic pain in acute herpes zoster is caused by the pathologic changes resulting from direct viral attack of the involved structures. Secondary inflammatory changes in the dorsal root ganglia, nerves, and skin, nerve roots, leptomeninges, and spinal cord activate the nociceptive primary afferents, manifesting as intense neuropathic pain in the affected dermatomes. Associated sympathetic hyperactivity contributes significantly to the perceived pain.

B. Chronic Phase

Postherpetic neuralgia, on the other hand, is caused by permanent damage to the central and peripheral nervous systems:

1. Pathologic sections of postherpetic nerves show preferential loss of large-diameter nerve fibers, which are replaced by fibrous tissue, and the relative preservation and proliferation of small-diameter nerve fibers. This finding had been termed *Fiber Dissociation.* Partial nerve damage could explain the occurrence of hyperaesthesia for the following reasons: Large-diameter fast-conducting nerve fibers are necessary to produce an inhibitory effect in the substantia gelatinosa on noxious pain impulses transmitted by the small, slow-conducting nerve fibers.

2. Additionally, postherpetic neuralgia is caused by spinal cord damage manifested in dorsal horn atrophy, as was shown in post-mortem pathologic sections of the spinal cord of patients suffering from postherpetic neuralgia.

3. Central pain mechanisms and psychologic changes interact with the peripheral factors, making postherpetic neuralgia a complex phenomenon to treat.

V. MANAGEMENT OF ACUTE HERPES ZOSTER

It is now clear that aggressive and prompt early treatment of acute HZ will not only control pain and enhance the healing process, but also help prevent its dreaded complications, namely, postherpetic neuralgia and serious eye complications, as in herpes zoster ophthalmicus. Typically, the combination of a newer antiviral agent and sympathetic blocks provides the best results in controlling pain and preventing complications.

A. Antiviral Agents

1. Acyclovir: effective in treating pain and enhancing healing but does not prevent the occurrence of postherpetic neuralgia.

2. Famciclovir: a "prodrug" that provides higher serum levels, is more effective than acyclovir, and has been shown to prevent PHN.

3. Valacyclovir: next generation "prodrug" more effective than famciclovir in treating the acute manifestations of the disease and preventing PHN.

B. Sympathetic Blocks

By increasing blood flow to the involved nerves and by interrupting sympathetically mediated pain, blocks are thought to enhance healing, pain is controlled promptly, and permanent nerve damage caused by ischemia is likely to be prevented, as described in the "pathophysiology" section of this chapter. Additionally, in herpes zoster ophthalmicus, sympathetic blocks will assist in prevention and treatment of associated uveitis by increasing blood flow to the eye. Usually the frequency of blocks will depend on the patient's response. In a number of patients two or three blocks over a period of 3 to 5 days will suffice; however, more may be necessary if pain is not completely controlled and/or rash eruption and ulceration continue. Usually, a long-acting local anesthetic, such as bupivacaine 0.25%, is used.

1. Stellate ganglion blocks: used for HZ affecting the head, neck, cervical plexus, brachial plexus, and upper thoracic dermatomes.
2. Intercostal blocks or thoracic/high lumbar epidural blocks: for HZ affecting the thoracic dermatomes.
3. Lumbar sympathetic or lumbar epidural blocks: for lumbar, groin, and lower-extremity involvement.

C. Subcutaneous Infiltration

This is another option to treat limited dermatomal distribution in patients who might be at more risk from sympathetic blocks or in those who will not consent to invasive block procedures. The subcutaneous tissue under the affected dermatomes is infiltrated with a mixture of dilute bupivacaine and dexamethasone.

D. Analgesics

Mild narcotic and nonnarcotic antiinflammatory analgesics can be used during the acute phase of the disease if necessary and as tolerated by the patients.

VI. MANAGEMENT OF POSTHERPETIC NEURALGIA

Treatment strategy should always be directed at prevention of PHN because all available evidence suggests that once PHN is established, it is extremely difficult to treat. It is hoped that with the increased use of vaccination against varicella (chicken pox) infection during childhood, herpes zoster will become extinct in future generations. In a busy pain medicine practice, physicians will encounter a number of elderly patients who continue to suffer from unremitting neuropathic pain that is refractory to most forms of therapy. The following therapeutic modalities should be considered with great caution and wisdom because patients will have variable responses to treatment. Because of the patients' advanced age, side effects and complications of some of the drugs used in treating neuropathic pain are often seen. Such drugs should be used in the lowest possible effective dose and patients should be carefully monitored during treatment. A combination of different drugs may be necessary if the pain is complex in character and intensity.

A. Sympathetic and Somatic Nerve Blocks

These blocks are not as effective as during the acute phase of the disease. In a great number of cases they will provide pain relief only for the duration of the block. In a small number of patients pain relief may be accomplished for days or even weeks. This would be best judged by assessing the individual patient's response to blocks and deciding whether or not they should be continued.

B. Antidepressants

Tricyclic antidepressant drugs such as amitriptyline and doxepin in small doses may be effective in some patients. Their action is mainly through their analgesic norepinephrine and serotonin reuptake inhibiting effect rather than their antidepressant properties. Sufficient time should be allowed for patients to be on such drugs before a decision is made regarding their ineffectiveness. Patients who develop significant side effects with these drugs might benefit from selective serotonin reuptake–inhibiting drugs such as sertraline.

C. Sodium Channel Blockers

Mexiletine may be effective in some patients. Prior to starting this, an intravenous lidocaine test will show whether or not such patients would benefit from oral mexiletine. It should only be used if the patient gets sufficient pain relief after small doses of intravenous lidocaine. A baseline electrocardiogram (ECG) to rule out conduction problems is also necessary prior to initiation of this therapy. It is also prudent to obtain ECG tracings during follow-up visits while the patient is on mexiletine.

D. Anticonvulsants

Newer anticonvulsants such as Gabapentin are preferable to older ones (carbamazepine and phenytoin) because of their safer profile and lack of some serious side effects seen in older drugs. Gabapentin also appears to be more effective in controlling neuropathic pain, particularly when it is paroxysmal, shooting, and lancinating.

E. Phenothiazines

May be effective, but their major side effects, such as extrapyramidal manifestations and confusion, especially in elderly patients, preclude routine use.

F. Behavioral Therapy

Biofeedback, behavior modification, relaxation therapy, and hypnotherapy may be effective in conjunction with other forms of treatment. This should always be considered in view of the complex nature of PHN and the psychologic factors that result from the severity and chronicity of the disease.

G. Analgesics

Narcotic analgesics in small or moderate doses may be effective in certain patients who do not respond or who have serious side effects to other forms of therapy. They should not be used in patients with history of drug or alcohol addiction. Nonnarcotic analgesics are rarely effective in PHN.

H. Electric Stimulation

Transcutaneous electric nerve stimulation (TENS) is occasionally effective in combination with drug therapy in mild cases. After prolonged use, pain may become refractory to TENS. Pain relief may be reestablished after a period of treatment interruption. Implanted spinal cord dorsal column stimulators have also been used in some severe cases.

I. Implanted Spinal Catheters and Pumps

Implanted intrathecal catheters for continuous opioid and/or small-dose local anesthetics infusions via implanted pumps may provide pain control in rare patients who do not get pain relief by any other form of therapy and in whom pain is of great severity that leaves them incapacitated. Proper trial period and documentation of pain relief are essential prior to permanent implantation.

J. Dorsal Root Entry Zone Lesion (DREZ)

Neuroablative surgical procedures may prove useful in hopeless cases that show no response to any other form of therapy. Following DREZ lesions, some patients may have recurrence of pain in addition to having developed loss of sensation in the involved area.

VII. CONCLUSIONS

It is becoming quite evident that the most crucial factor in the management of herpes zoster is very early and aggressive treatment of acute HZ, especially in the elderly patient. If this is not accomplished, a significant number of patients may be left with an intractable neuropathic pain condition that is extremely difficult and frustrating to manage. It is unfortunate that the majority of patients referred to anesthesiologists for treatment are beyond their acute illness and a number of them will not benefit from the usual available interventions. Vaccination against varicella zoster virus infection should be enforced during childhood.

RECOMMENDED READING

Ali NMK. Does sympathetic ganglionic block prevent postherpetic neuralgia? *Reg Anesth* 1995;20: 227–233.

Burgoon CF, Burgoon JS, Baldridge GD. The natural history of herpes zoster. *JAMA* 1957;164:265–269.

Colding A. The effect of regional sympathetic blocks in the treatment of herpes zoster. *Acta Anaesth Scand* 1969;13:133–141.

Colebunders R, Mann JM, Francis H, et al. Herpes zoster in African patients: A clinical predictor of human immunodeficiency virus infection. *J Infect Dis* 1988;157:314–318.

Loeser JD. Herpes zoster and postherpetic neuralgia. In: Bonica JJ, ed. *The Management of Pain*. Philadelphia: Lea & Febiger; 1990:257–263.

Mahalingam R, Wellish M, Wolf W, et al. Latent varicella-zoster viral DNA in human trigeminal and thoracic ganglia. *N Engl J Med* 1990;323:627–631.

Tenicela R, Lovasik D, Eaglstein W. Treatment of herpes zoster with sympathetic blocks. *Ciln J Pain* 1985;1:63–67.

Tyring S, Barbarash RA, Nahlik JE, et al. Famciclovir for the treatment of acute herpes zoster: Effects on acute disease and postherpetic neuralgia. A randomized, double-blind, placebo-controlled trial. Collaborative Famciclovir Herpes Zoster Study Group. *Ann Int Med* 1995;123:89–96.

Weller TH. Varicella and herpes zoster: A perspective and overview. *J Infect Dis* 1992;166:S1–S6.

Winnie AP, Hartwell PW. Relationship between time of treatment of acute herpes zoster with sympathetic blockade and prevention of post-herpetic neuralgia: clinical support for a new theory of the mechanism by which sympathetic blockade provides therapeutic benefit. *Reg Anesth* 18:277–282,1993.

The Pain Clinic Manual, Second Edition,
edited by Stephen E. Abram and J. David Haddox.
Lippincott Williams & Wilkins,
Philadelphia, © 2000

23

Painful Peripheral Neuropathies

David J. Hewitt

*D.J. Hewitt: Department of Neurology, Emory University;
Section of Neurology, The Emory Clinic, Inc., Atlanta, Georgia 30322.*

Peripheral neuropathies represent a large subset of the neuropathic type pains encountered in a pain clinic. Not all polyneuropathies are painful, but the pain of peripheral neuropathy can be disabling and is often difficult to treat. Adjuvant analgesics are considered the first-line medications for the treatment of neuropathic pain, but other analgesics (e.g., opioids) as well as nonpharmacologic techniques should be considered.

I. BACKGROUND
  A. Signs
     1. Decreases in sensation to primary sensory modalities in a stocking/glove distribution
     2. The absence of deep tendon reflexes
     3. Distal weakness
     4. NB: These neurologic findings can be absent even in the presence of severe pain.
  B. Symptoms
     1. Determining the character of the pain can help.
        a. Define the etiology.
        b. Guide treatment.
     2. Lancinating pain refers to a sharp, shooting, electrical type pain that can be paroxysmal in nature.
     3. Dysesthetic pain refers to abnormal and disagreeable sensations.
     4. Paresthesias refers to abnormal sensations described as a burning, pins and needles, tingling, prickly or tickling sensation.
     5. Hyperalgesia refers to an extreme sensitivity to noxious stimuli.
     6. Allodynia refers to pain or discomfort brought on by a non-painful stimulus.
     7. Neuropathic pain can be provoked or spontaneous.

C. Etiology of Neuropathic Pain
   1. Results from injury to neural structures, including the peripheral nerve trunk, plexus, dorsal root ganglion, nerve root, dorsal horn, spinal cord, brain stem, thalamus, and parietal lobe.
   2. The two major pathologic processes in peripheral neuropathy are axonal degeneration and segmental demyelination.
   3. Neuropathies can therefore be classified as axonal, demyelinating, or mixed.
   4. Peripheral neuropathies can affect either large or small fibers.
   5. Pain is not related to fiber size distribution alone.
   6. Rapidly progressive neuropathies are more likely to be painful.
   7. Small fiber involvement is often associated with pain.
   8. Pain may be sympathetic dependent.
   9. Nerve ischemia may exacerbate paresthesias and contribute to pain following peripheral damage.
   10. Severe ischemia can cause painful neuropathies.
D. Pain Assessment
   1. Believe the patient's pain complaint.
   2. Perform a good history of the pain complaint and concurrent illnesses.
   3. Perform a directed medical and neurologic examination.
   4. Define the temporal character of the pain.
      a. Constant versus intermittent
      b. Aggravated by activity
      c. Worse at night (very typical of neuropathic pain)
      d. Exacerbating and alleviating factors
   5. Review pertinent laboratory work and previous medical records.
   6. Review all diagnostic studies.
   7. Order the appropriate diagnostic work-up.
   8. Determine a pain diagnosis.
   9. Determine if definite therapy is available and warranted.
   10. Treat the pain complaint concurrently as the diagnostic work-up or definitive therapy proceeds.
E. Special Studies
   1. Electromyography and nerve conduction studies
      a. Help isolate the location of an entrapped nerve.
      b. Distinguish between axonal and demyelinating neuropathy.
      c. Focus further investigations to determine the etiology of the neuropathic process.
II. POLYNEUROPATHIES
   A. Toxic Neuropathies
      1. Alcohol-induced polyneuropathy
         a. Burning and tenderness in feet and legs: nonselective fiber loss
         b. Abstinence from alcohol

  c. Consumption of a normal diet
  d. Thiamine (vitamin B_1) 100 mg po qd
2. Mercury—two forms: elemental and organic
  a. Organic—toxic to central nervous system, with distal paresthesias
  b. Elemental mercury does not cause peripheral neuropathy.
3. Arsenic neuropathy
  a. Sometimes painful
  b. Pure sensory or mixed sensorimotor neuropathy
  c. Axonal degeneration
4. Isoniazid
  a. Painful deep ache and burning in calf muscles
  b. Worse with walking followed by spontaneous pain and paresthesias
  c. Often worse at night with spontaneous pain and paresthesias
  d. Cutaneous hyperesthesia
  e. Selective large-fiber loss
  f. Possible response to pyridoxine administration
5. Other medications known to cause or aggravate peripheral neuropathy
  a. Adriamycin—for cancer
  b. Vincristine—for cancer
    (1) Symmetric, progressive sensorimotor distal neuropathy beginning in legs with areflexia
  c. Cis-platinum—for cancer
    (1) Pure sensory distal neuropathy, paresthesia, impaired vibration sense, and loss of Achilles tendon reflexes
  d. Amiodarone—for irregular heartbeat
  e. Chloramphenicol antibiotic
  f. Dapsone—for chronic and certain rare skin diseases
  g. Diphenylhydantoin (Dilantin)—for seizures and neuropathic pain
  h. Disulfiram (Antabuse)—for alcoholics
  i. Ethionamide—for tuberculosis
  j. Flagyl (Metronidazol)—for trichomonas infection
  k. Gold—for rheumatoid arthritis
  l. Hydralazine (Apresoline)—for high blood pressure
  m. Nitrofurantoin (Furadantin, Macrodantin)—for urinary tract infection
  n. Nitrous oxide (chronic repeated inhalation)—for an anesthetic
  o. Perhexiline (Pexid)—for angina
  p. Pyridoxine (vitamin B_6)—both a treatment for neuropathy produced by INH and a cause of neurotoxicity at higher doses
B. Nutritional Neuropathies
  1. Vitamin deficiencies
    a. Beriberi: "dry beriberi"
      (1) Common, painful, sensorimotor polyneuropathy

(2) Severe spontaneous burning pain in feet and sometimes hands
(3) Allodynia
(4) Possible cause: thiamine deficiency
(5) Degeneration in distal nerves and posterior columns, dorsal root ganglion, and anterior horn cells
(6) Distal muscle wasting with trophic change
b. Strachan's syndrome—Jamaican neuropathy
(1) Pain, paresthesias, sensory loss in feet and hands
(2) Pain proximally around shoulders and hip girdles
(3) Visual impairment, deafness, orogenital dermatitis
c. Burning feet syndrome—seen during World War II
(1) Prisoners of war: severe aching or causalgic-like burning pains, unpleasant paresthesias involving soles of feet and legs worse at night relieved by cold.
(2) Amblyopia, orogenital dermatitis, hyperhidrosis of feet
(3) No single nutritional deficit determined
d. Pellagra
(1) Niacin deficiency
(2) Sensorimotor neuropathy
(3) Tenderness in the calf muscles
(4) Spontaneous pain and cutaneous hyperesthesia of the feet
(5) Selective large-fiber loss
(6) Hyperkeratotic skin lesions
(7) Treat by adding thiamine and pyridoxine to diet
e. Vitamin B_{12} deficiency
(1) Subacute combined degeneration of the spinal cord
(2) Pain likely due to spinal cord involvement
C. Neuropathies Associated with Chronic Diseases
1. Diabetic neuropathy
a. Several types
b. Numbness and distal sensory loss
c. Burning and hyperesthesia
d. Spontaneous deep, aching pain and lightning pain
e. Pain possibly troubling even when sensory and motor loss is mild
f. Symptoms of autonomic neuropathy
g. Selective small-fiber loss
h. Demyelination is usually primary pathology and axonal degeneration is less common.
i. Laboratory tests include a serum glucose level, hemoglobin A-1C, glucose tolerance test.
j. Treatment includes obtaining better glycemic control.
2. Renal failure
a. Can be painful.

    b. May complain of restless leg syndrome, distal numbness, and paresthesia.

    c. Axonal degeneration

    d. Neuropathy resolves after renal transplant.

3. Hypothyroidism

    a. Sensorimotor neuropathy

    b. Pain in feet

    c. Progressive difficulty walking

    d. Possible development of entrapment neuropathies

    e. Painful paresthesias in the hands and feet

    f. Tendon reflexes possibly reduced or absent and possibly characteristic delayed or "hung-up" response

    g. Possible myoedema

4. Paraproteinemia—polyclonal or monoclonal IgM autoantibodies that react with glycoconjugates in peripheral nerve

    a. IgM antibodies react with myelin associated glycoprotein (MAG).

      (1) Treat with plasmapheresis, chemotherapy, or IV Ig to reduce autoantibody concentrations.

    b. Monoclonal gammopathies: IgA, IgG

      (1) Primary amyloidosis

        (a) Fragments of monoclonal light chains deposited as amyloid in peripheral nerve

      (2) Cryoglobulinemia types 1 and 2

        (a) Monoclonal immunoglobulins are components of cryoprecipitates.

        (b) Treat with plasmapheresis, prednisone, and chemotherapy.

      (3) Chronic B-cell lymphocytic leukemia or lymphoma monoclonal B-cells infiltrate nerves.

5. Amyloid neuropathy

    a. Painful

    b. Possible deep, aching pain with superimposed shooting pain

    c. Small-fiber neuropathy

    d. Inherited and sporadic varieties

    e. Sensory loss of pain and thermal sensations

    f. Often with autonomic involvement

    g. Progression to involve all modalities

    h. Loss of reflexes and motor involvement

    i. Selective small-fiber loss

6. Myeloma

    a. Osteosclerotic type with IgG or IgA monoclonal gammopathies

    b. Multiple and solitary types

    c. Variable in severity and rate of progression

    d. Chemotherapy may provide definitive treatment and pain control.

    e. Nonselective fiber loss

7. Infectious
   a. HIV disease
      (1) Symmetric painful peripheral neuropathy of AIDS
      (2) CMV radiculomyelitis
      (3) Cause—antiretroviral medication
   b. Lyme neuropathy
      (1) Tick-borne spirochete infection: *Borrelia burgdorferi*
      (2) Painful sensory radiculitis
      (3) Three weeks after erythema migrans
      (4) Variable pain from day to day
      (5) Movement from one area to another
      (6) Unpleasant areas of dysesthesiae
      (7) Inflammatory changes in the cerebrospinal fluid with specific intrathecal *Borrelia burgdorferi* antibodies or antigen detection
      (8) High-dose penicillin treatment
   c. Herpes zoster will be discussed elsewhere.
D. Hereditary Neuropathies
   1. Dominantly inherited sensory neuropathy
      a. Involvement mainly in the feet
      b. Pain and temperature loss
      c. Severe lancinating pain
      d. Selective small-fiber loss
E. Acute Inflammatory Polyneuropathy (AIP)
   1. Guillain-Barré
      a. Pain—an early symptom preceding sensory impairment or weakness
      b. Distal, generalized muscular, or root pain
      c. Pain—usually transient
F. Mononeuropathies and Multiple Mononeuropathies (Mononeuropathy Multiplex)
   1. Postherpetic neuralgia—see specific section.
   2. Diabetic mononeuropathy—pain is common but transient.
      a. Extraocular muscles
         (1) Pain may precede weakness.
         (2) Third nerve—pupil-sparing, most common
         (3) Pain around and behind eye, often severe
      b. Median
      c. Ulnar
      d. Peroneal
      e. Femoral
      f. Lateral cutaneous nerve of the thigh
   3. Diabetic amyotrophy
      a. Asymmetric motor neuropathy
      b. Associated with poor diabetic control

      c. Often acute

      d. Pain possibly associated with nervi nervorum

G. Entrapment Neuropathies Pain and Paresthesias in Early Stages

Damage to myelin. Nerve trunk pain mediated by nervi nervorum produces local pain and tenderness.

    1. Radiculopathies—pain follows the distribution of the sensory nerve and can be the result of compression on a nerve root.

    2. Meralgia paresthetica—result of compression of the lateral femoral cutaneous nerve

    3. Carpal tunnel syndrome—compression of the median nerve within the carpal tunnel

    4. Ulnar neuropathy—at the elbow. Conservative treatment requires not putting pressure on elbows.

    5. Peroneal nerve affected at the knee

    6. Tarsal tunnel syndrome—pain from entrapment of the tibial nerve in the tarsal tunnel

    7. Morton's neuralgia—plantar digital nerve compressed in the region of the metatarsal heads in the foot

    8. Acromegalic neuropathy—develop entrapment neuropathies

    9. Cachexia is also associated with focal neuropathies due to compression.

H. Ischemic Neuropathy

Microangiopathic; central fascicular degeneration

    1. Polyarteritis nodosa

    2. Rheumatoid arthritis

    3. Systemic lupus erythematosis

I. Neuralgic Amyotrophy

Cryptogenic brachial plexus neuropathy

    1. Acute onset of severe pain around the shoulder girdle or in the arm in a root distribution

    2. Weakness follows within 2 weeks

    3. Occasionally preceding viral illness

    4. Recovery within 2 years

    5. Most often occurs as a mononeuropathy multiplex

    6. Etiology unknown

    7. Predominantly axonal

J. Neuropathies Associated with Cancer

    1. Nonmetastatic complication of cancer

      a. Progressive sensory neuropathy

      b. Occasionally painful

      c. Subacute onset

      d. Associated with small cell carcinoma of the lung

      e. Autoantibodies against the Hu antigen

    2. Direct invasion of peripheral nerves by carcinoma causing compression or from direct infiltration

     3. Radiation neuropathy
       a. Brachial plexus after radiation—for lung or breast cancer
       b. Caudal roots and lumbosacral plexus after radiation—for testicular cancer or Hodgkin disease
       c. Severe pain and paresthesias and sensory loss
       d. Possible latent period of 12 to 20 months
       e. Possible myokymia

III. TREATMENT

  A. Goal of Therapy
     1. Improve overall function and activity level.
     2. Achieve acceptable level of pain control.
     3. Set appropriate expectations regarding level of pain control and treatment methodology.
  B. Treat the underlying cause if possible (e.g., surgery for entrapment neuropathies, chemotherapy for cancer).
     1. Pharmacologic approaches
       a. Tricyclic antidepressants
         (1) First-line treatment when pain is of burning dysesthetic type
         (2) Amitriptilyne most studied
         (3) Antimuscarinic side effects: dry mouth, orthostatic hypotension, constipation, worsening of narrow angle glaucoma
         (4) Arrhythmogenic effects
         (5) Start low, titrate slowly until analgesic efficacy is achieved or intolerable side effects occur.
       b. Anticonvulsants
         (1) First-line medication for neuropathic pain dominated by lancinating character
         (2) Phenytoin and carbamazepine
           (a) Follow serum drug levels.
           (b) Complete blood counts.
           (c) Do liver function test.
           (d) Electrolytes
         (3) Gabapentin
           (a) Fewer side effects
           (b) No need to check serum levels
           (c) Treatment of diabetic neuropathy and postherpetic neuralgia
         (4) Opioid analgesia
           (a) For the treatment of neuropathic pain—has been controversial.
           (b) A number of studies and anecdotal experience support the use of opioid analgesia for the treatment of peripheral neuropathy.

(c) Long-acting agents should be given by around-the-clock dosing.

(d) Shorter-acting opioid analgesics should be used for break-through pain.

(5) Sodium channel blockers

(a) Mexiletine—450 mg a day in three divided doses

(b) Tocainide—400 mg tid

(c) Intravenous infusions of lidocaine have been helpful in the treatment of diabetic neuropathy

(i) Requires the use of continuous EKG monitoring.

(ii) A loading dose of 2 mg/kg lidocaine is infused over 5 minutes, followed by an infusion of 50 mcg/kg/min for 30 minutes.

(6) Topical local anesthetics

(a) EMLA—the eutectic mixture of lidocaine and prilocaine

(i) Apply thickly over the area of allodynia.

(ii) Cover with a thick, occlusive dressing.

(iii) Sometimes pain relief can be obtained without the occlusive dressing.

(7) Anesthetic approaches

(a) Infiltrate involved nerve with local anesthetic (e.g., 2 to 3 ml of lidocaine—1% or bupivacaine 0.25% to 0.50%). Can repeat at weekly intervals.

(b) Add small amount of corticosteroid to local anesthetic for infiltration (e.g., triamcinolone 12.5 mg or dexamethasone 2 mg). Steroid may stabilize the neuronal membrane.

(c) Sympathetic blocks if burning pain and hyperpathia are the predominant physical findings. If successful, repeat series of blocks.

(d) Prolonged local anesthetic blockade while inpatients.

(i) Lower extremities: continuous lumbar epidural analgesia

(ii) Upper extremities: continuous brachial plexus blockade by an indwelling catheter

(iii) Maintain blockade for 3 to 6 days with concurrent vigorous physical therapy.

(8) Transcutaneous electrical nerve stimulation (TENS)

(9) Physical therapy

(a) Restore and maintain function.

(b) Prevent disuse atrophy and soft tissue dystrophy. Restore central neural input.

The Pain Clinic Manual, Second Edition,
edited by Stephen E. Abram and J. David Haddox.
Lippincott Williams & Wilkins,
Philadelphia, © 2000

24

Facial Pain

J. David Haddox and David M. Biondi

*J. D. Haddox: Atlanta, Georgia; Pain and Policy Studies Group,
University of Wisconsin, Madison, Wisconsin.
D. M. Biondi: Michigan Head, Pain, and Neurological Institute,
Ann Arbor, Michigan 48104; Department of Neurology, Michigan State University
College of Osteopathic Medicine, East Lansing, Michigan 48824.*

Facial pain may be due to a variety of causes. Many diseases and syndromes discussed elsewhere in this manual are also represented in the facial area. This chapter focuses on the description and management of several syndromes that may present to a pain clinic. The treatment of herpes zoster of the trigeminal distribution is not substantially different from that occurring in the thoracic dermatomes and therefore will not be addressed here. The treatment of most facial pain should be a multidisciplinary effort coordinating the efforts of the anesthesiologist with those of the psychologist, the dental consultant, and other medical specialists.

I. EXAMINATION OF THE PATIENT WITH FACIAL PAIN
   A. Anatomic Focus
      Examination of patients with facial pain should address all systems of the head and neck. Special attention should be paid to the muscular system, including the muscles of mastication, looking for myofascial trigger points that may be sites of complaints or the origin of pain referred elsewhere. The technique for examination of the pterygoid muscles may need to be learned from a competent dental practitioner, as this may be foreign to the average physician.
   B. Sensory Distribution
      The sensory distribution of the face should be examined with reference to which division of the trigeminal nerve is involved and which peripheral branches are implicated. The trigeminal dermatomes are contiguous with cervical innervations near the ears, the top of the forehead, and the inferior aspect of the mandible. The auriculotemporal nerve (a branch of the third division) innervates the temporomandibular joint.
   C. Cranial Nerve Function
      All cranial nerve function should be assessed. To be adequately tested, the ophthalmic division of the trigeminal nerve must demonstrate intactness of

the corneal reflex. All muscles of mastication are supplied by the mandibular division, while the muscles of facial expression are innervated by the branches of the facial nerve. The ability to elevate the eyelid is partially mediated by sympathetics traveling with the third nerve.

D. Occlusal Analysis

Although a thorough discussion of occlusal analysis is beyond the scope of this manual, several aspects can be helpful. A good rule for mandibular range of motion is that the average adult will be able to achieve an interincisal distance of between 35 and 50 mm (approximately three finger-breadths). Closure of the mandible should be a relatively smooth event with no side-to-side deviation of the mandibular midline. As teeth come into contact, there should be no midline shift when the teeth are moved to maximum closure. The teeth should be inspected for wear facets, and the masseters should be observed for hypertrophy, indicating bruxism.

E. Joint Motion

Joint motion should be nonpainful and should occur without pops or clicks, although some sounds may have no clinical significance. Palpation anterior to the ear will allow one to feel the condyle first rotate in place, then translate forward out of the glenoid fossa as the patient opens wider. Palpation of the joint capsule can be accomplished indirectly by placing the examiner's small finger in the patient's external auditory canal while his mouth is closed and pulling anteriorly.

F. Soft-Tissue Examination

Examination of the soft tissues of the mouth is also important in the assessment of facial pain, primarily because of the possibility of an undiagnosed malignancy. A thorough visual inspection, especially at the posterolateral borders of the tongue, is followed by manual palpation of the cheeks, tongue, and floor of the mouth.

G. Psychologic Factors

Because almost all facial pain syndromes have been associated with stress or other psychologic findings, care must be directed to this aspect. A high incidence of depression has been noted in facial pain patients.

II. TEMPOROMANDIBULAR DISORDERS (TMD)

A. General Considerations

This is a poorly defined group of problems that are related to or referred to the temporomandibular joint (TMJ). The aid of a competent dental practitioner should be enlisted in the evaluation of these patients. A dentist can rule out the more discrete causes of TMJ pain, such as a perforated meniscus or arthritis, and provide or coordinate appropriate therapy. If a patient describes "locking" of the jaw, either in the open or closed position, there is almost always associated joint pathology. Elimination of these diagnoses will still leave a large group of patients with an entity known as myofascial pain dysfunction syndrome (MPDS), also known as Costen's syndrome, myofascial pain syndrome, facial arthromyalgia, and, loosely, TMJ syndrome.

B. Symptoms
  1. Pain in or near the TMJ (usually a dull, deep ache that is exacerbated by chewing)
  2. Clicks or pops on mandibular movement
  3. Limitation of mandibular range, either opening and closing or lateral excursions
  4. Tenderness to palpation of the muscles of mastication, especially the pterygoids; frequently with discrete trigger points
  5. Most frequent occurrence in females (up to 80% of cases)

C. Pathophysiology

  TMJ syndromes are essentially a variant of myofascial pain syndromes. The TMJ is unique in that it is the link between a complex array of muscles and ligaments; it is the only sliding-hinge joint in the body; it has a meniscus that has muscle-guided movement; and its action must allow the dentition to achieve intercuspation. This intricate functional unit is subject to many anatomic and functional variations that may impair its operation.

  1. A multifactorial theory of myofascial pain dysfunction syndrome is illustrated in Fig. 24-1.
  2. Critical components
     a. Joints themselves
     b. Occlusion of the teeth
     c. Muscles of mastication
     d. Stress factors
  3. The muscles have predetermined length when they are at rest. Myofascial trigger points will shorten the muscles and make them more likely to be symptomatic (see Fig. 24-1).

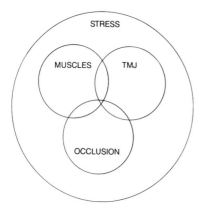

FIG. 24-1. Multifactorial model of myofascial pain dysfunction syndrome.

    4. The contribution of occlusion abnormalities to TMD is a hotly debated issue in the dental community. Proponents of this theory grind (equilibrate) teeth interferences and use repositioning splints. They believe that if the occlusion is abnormal, muscle strain will evolve in response to avoidance of interference to closure or incomplete closures (such as a high amalgam restoration), keeping some muscles from reaching resting length, thereby causing symptoms. Opponents, who are presently in the majority, say that there are scant data to support this idea and disagree with permanent alteration of the teeth to cure the problem.

    5. The TMJs may have internal restriction to movement, caused by degenerative changes.

    6. Stress will alter the threshold for any of the preceding abnormalities to become symptomatic. This may strongly contribute to an intermittent nature of symptoms.

D. Treatment Objectives

    1. Eliminate obvious occlusion interferences.

    2. Rule out TMJ itself as a precipitant for symptoms.

    3. Minimize stress.

    4. Treat muscles of mastication.

        a. Decrease muscle tenderness.

        b. Restore muscles to normal working length.

        c. Allow unstressed resting length to be obtained.

        d. Eliminate trigger points.

    5. Restore sleep.

E. Management

Presumably, a patient referred to a pain clinic will have had a thorough dental evaluation and treatment of occlusal and joint factors. The management of myofascial pain dysfunction syndrome can be facilitated by conceptualizing the disorder as a psychosomatic problem in the purest sense—an anatomic or physiologic substrate that can be made more symptomatic by various psychologic factors. Of primary importance is education of the patient. Surgery for muscle pain symptoms in the absence of clear joint pathology is not indicated.

    1. Muscle symptoms (most of the techniques that are applicable for other myofascial pain apply to MPDS)

        a. Trigger point injections

        b. Spray and stretch

        c. Ischemic compression of trigger points can be taught to patient to help control symptoms

        d. TENS (do not place over carotid sinus or transcranially)

        e. Physical therapy (aimed at stretching muscles to normal length—can be helpful if done on a regular basis at home)

        f. Restoration of restful sleep

2. Stress
   a. Psychologic/psychiatric evaluation to identify sources of stress that may make patient more likely to be symptomatic
   b. Progressive muscle relaxation protocols may teach the patient to relax muscles of mastication as well as enable a state of generalized relaxation.
   c. Biofeedback, especially EMG biofeedback of masseters and temporalis muscles, can be useful.
   d. Hypnosis may benefit selected patients by relaxation or by suggestion of analgesia.
3. Pharmacologic Management
   a. Tricyclic antidepressants, in doses of 10 to 50 mg hs amitriptyline or equivalent, can be useful for sleep and analgesia.
   b. Nonsteroid antiinflammatory drugs (NSAIDs) may benefit some patients. Nonacetylated salicylic acid derivatives (salsalate, choline magnesium trisalicylate) may have better gastrointestinal tolerance and are less likely to contribute to platelet dysfunction.
   c. Muscle relaxants such as metaxolone chlorzoxazone, orphenadrine, cyclobenzaprine, and methocarbamol have generally not proven useful, especially in protracted cases, but anecdotally may help some patients.
   d. Benzodiazepines should be avoided because of their unproven efficacy in muscle relaxation long term, their dependence liability, and their possible "algesic" (pain-enhancing) effects.
   e. The role of opioids in managing severe pain that is refractory to other therapy is undergoing redefinition. In complaint patients with no history of addictive disorders, opioids, especially long-acting forms, may play a role.
   f. In a patient who reports a burning quality, such as the individual who has failed TMJ surgery, trial of a gabapentin either alone or in conjunction with a tricyclic antidepressant, may prove beneficial.

III. NEUROMAS
   A. Symptoms
      1. Neuromas may be seen after facial trauma, especially "blowout" orbital fractures or Le Fort III injuries.
      2. Pain is generally discretely localized and of a sharp, electric, or burning nature in the distribution of a branch of the trigeminal nerve. It may be constant or episodic.
      3. An area of exquisite tenderness (the neuroma) can usually be demonstrated at or near the site of bony exit of the involved nerve. The supraorbital and infraorbital nerves are particularly susceptible to injury because they exit from bony canals or notches and abruptly turn 90° to supply their skin innervation.

    4. Hypoesthesia, hyperesthesia, hyperalgesia, paresthesia, dysesthesia, or allodynia may be present.

    5. Neuromas typically do not respond well to opioid analgesics, although some studies have shown opioid responsivity in certain similar neuropathic pain syndromes.

    6. If sympathetically maintained pain is proven, treatment can follow the principles outlined in Chapter 21.

B. Pathophysiology

    1. Neuromas are areas of damaged nerve and myelin sheath. They are thought to be neural regenerative efforts gone awry.

    2. Microscopically, neuromas are characterized by disrupted sheathing and sprouting of nerve ends.

    3. Electrophysiologically, areas of damaged nerve tend to discharge spontaneously and have exuberant and prolonged discharge in response to mechanical stimuli.

    4. Receptor analysis shows a proliferation of adrenergic receptors at the site of a neuroma, making these areas more responsive to circulating catecholamines.

C. Treatment Objectives

    1. Avoid further neural damage.

    2. Minimize spontaneous discharge from neuroma.

    3. Optimize functional outcomes.

D. Management

    1. After initial examination and mapping of the sensory abnormality to delineate which nerve is involved, a diagnostic local anesthetic block can confirm the diagnosis.

        a. In performing blocks of nerves of the face, it is helpful to remember that the supraorbital, infraorbital, and mental nerve exits lie along a vertical line that intersects the pupil.

        b. The supraorbital nerve typically does not lie in a foramen, but rather exits through a groove or notch at the superior medical aspect of the orbital rim, whereas the infraorbital and mental nerves exit from canals that end in discrete foramina.

        c. Block can usually be established with a 25-gauge or smaller needle and 1 to 3 ml of 1% to 2% lidocaine.

    2. If diagnostic block relieves the pain, it can be followed at another appointment by a block of local anesthetic and a corticosteroid (25 mg of triamcinolone acetate or 1 mg of dexamethasone).

        a. In this instance, the local anesthetic serves as a diluent and a marker; immediate relief indicates correct deposition of the steroid.

        b. Steroids have been known to suppress spontaneous discharges of neuromas in laboratory experiments.

      c. Repeated injections of steroids carry the risk of Cushing syndrome and adrenal suppression.

   3. As with other pains of primarily neural origin, certain pharmacologic aspects may be tried.

      a. Antidepressants

      b. Anticonvulsants (gabapentin is the first choice)

IV. TRIGEMINAL NEURALGIA (TIC DOULOUREUX)

  A. Symptoms

    1. Lightninglike, lancinating pain that occurs paroxysmally, with pain-free intervals

    2. Onset in middle age

    3. Pain that is usually limited to one trigeminal division, although multiple divisions can be involved

    4. A trigger zone (not to be confused with myofascial trigger point) exists, stimulation of which will precipitate an attack

      a. These zones may be small or somewhat diffuse.

      b. They may be intraoral as well as facial.

      c. A classic feature of the trigger zone is that stimuli that are normally innocuous (light touch, breeze) but are sufficient to activate a painful episode.

    5. The pain is typically not responsive to opioid analgesics.

    6. Behavioral alterations in this population are quite common and include

      a. Avoidance of toothbrushing or even eating, for fear of setting off an attack

      b. Wearing of hoods, hats, and so on, to prevent breeze from blowing against skin

      c. Staying indoors to prevent exposure to stimuli

      d. Self-imposed social isolation because of embarrassment

      e. Depression

      f. Suicidal thoughts, which are not infrequently considered by patients as a realistic method of coping with the pain

  B. Pathophysiology

  This is disrupted, but most investigators agree that the trigeminal ganglion is implicated.

    1. May be a sensory processing error in which peripheral stimuli are summed or otherwise altered to be perceived as nociceptive when they normally would not be.

    2. One theory espouses the notion that a pulsatile loop of artery irritates the ganglion or a division and creates a local neuritic process that causes the nerve to respond aberrantly to peripheral stimuli.

  C. Treatment Objectives

    1. Treatment directed peripherally is generally not successful.

2. Central approaches may be pharmacologic or surgical.
3. Behavioral treatment is not successful primarily. The behavioral abnormalities will resolve when the painful attacks are terminated.

D. Management
1. Carbamazepine is still the standard medical therapy.
   a. The drug was initially tried because some thought the paroxysmal nature of tic douloureux had an epileptiform pattern.
   b. Dose range is 400 to 1200 mg/day. It should be started slowly (100 mg bid) and increased until effect occurs.
   c. Toxicity is significant. Hematologic abnormalities such as thrombocytopenia and aplastic anemia can occur and may be profound or, occasionally, irreversible.
   d. Baseline complete blood count with differential and liver function tests should be obtained prior to instituting therapy. These should initially be checked frequently and at least every 3 months during treatment.
   e. Serum levels should be monitored periodically. Specimens should be obtained prior to a scheduled dose to avoid spurious elevations caused by recent dosing.
   f. Coadministration of carbamazepine and propoxyphene can result in excessive serum levels of carbamazepine.
2. Gabapentin is rapidly becoming the anticonvulsant of choice for neuropathic pain because it does not have significant toxicity.
3. Glycerol injections into the trigeminal ganglion have been useful for some patients because of its mild neurolytic properties.
4. Radiofrequency lesioning of the ganglion may result in symptom relief.
5. Surgical decompression of the ganglion by placing a nonresorbable shock-absorbing sponge between the arterial loop and the neural structures has been reported to be efficacious.
6. On occasion, local anesthetic block of the nerves supplying the trigger zone can be useful in confirming diagnosis and temporizing a situation.

V. ATYPICAL FACIAL PAINS
A. Symptoms
1. This is a vague clinical entity that may actually represent several syndromes.
2. Chronic pain, which is unaffected by movement and is usually characterized by a deep ache, is the patient's presenting complaint.
3. The pain is frequently poorly localized, may migrate or spread, and is often described in quite vivid terms by the patient.
4. Multiple dental and facial surgeries, all to no avail, are common features in the patient's history.
5. Another characteristic historic finding is the preponderance of normal examination and unrevealing diagnostic procedures.

6. Atypical facial pain occurs predominantly in females.
7. Symptoms of depression are frequent in this group, and some have considered the syndrome to be a depressive variant or a psychogenic problem.
   a. Frequent sleep disturbance
   b. Fatigue
   c. Irritability
   d. Tension or anxiety
   e. Crying spells and mood swings
8. Obsessive personality traits have been linked to the syndrome.

B. Pathophysiology
1. The mechanism of these pains is unclear.
2. It is likely to be a centrally mediated phenomenon because it is quite common for the pain to cross the midline or involve other areas inconsistent with known neuroanatomic distribution.
3. A somewhat controversial etiology for some pains has been proposed. The theory is that microabscesses occur in bone of the maxilla or mandible and cause sensitization of trigeminal afferents. It is called neuralgia-inducing cavitating osteonecrosis, or NICO.

C. Treatment Objectives
1. A primary goal of treatment should be education of the patients with regard to the poor record of continued surgical interventions in this syndrome.
2. A supportive environment should be maintained in the clinic—one that focuses on the patient, not the pain.
3. Review of diagnostic studies must be thorough to rule out the possibility of undiagnosed organic disease such a oropharyngeal malignancy, recurrent sialolithiasis, cracked tooth syndrome, and so on.

D. Management
1. Antidepressant therapy (tricyclic antidepressants and monoamine oxidase inhibitors) has been helpful in up to 75% of these cases.
2. Formal psychotherapy may be needed.
3. A psychologic/psychiatric evaluation may be useful.
4. Depression psychometrics may be helpful (e.g., Hamilton, Beck, Zung).
5. Behavioral pain management techniques can be useful for decreasing pain behavior and improving function.
6. Detoxification from habituating substances is often required.
7. Providing a comfortable environment in which the patients can find compassionate, supportive physicians may serve to keep them from "doctor shopping" and participating in therapies that are useless or harmful.
8. If NICO is suspected, some oral surgeons advocate opening and correcting the involved area.

VI. GLOSSOPHARYNGEAL NEURALGIA
  A. Clinical Features
   1. Onset typically during the fourth decade
   2. Women and men equally affected
   3. Pain distribution: posterior tongue, tonsillar fossa, larynx, ear, and face
   4. Unilateral (2% bilateral)
   5. Pain description: stabbing, sharp, shocklike, burning
   6. Pain triggers: swallowing, coughing, yawning, talking
   7. Associated signs and symptoms: syncope, cardiac dysrhythmia, seizure mediated through the vagus nerve
   8. Possible spontaneous remissions and exacerbation
  B. Treatment
   1. Medical
      a. Same as for trigeminal neuralgia
   2. Surgical interventions
      a. Extracranial avulsion of the glossopharyngeal nerve
      b. Intracranial sectioning of the glossopharyngeal nerve and the upper rootlets of the vagus nerve
      c. Microvascular decompression

VII. SPHENOPALATINE NEURALGIA (SLUDER'S NEURALGIA)
  A. Clinical Features
   1. Onset at any age
   2. Women affected more commonly than men (2:1)
   3. Pain distribution: middle one-third of the face, retroorbital, upper jaw, teeth, nose, soft palate, temple, neck
   4. Unilateral
   5. Pain description:stabbing, sharp, shocklike, burning
   6. Pain triggers: none recognized
   7. Associated signs and symptoms: lacrimation, rhinorrhea, salivation, sneezing
  B. Treatment
   1. Medical
      a. Same as for trigeminal neuralgia
   2. Anesthesiologic and surgical interventions
      a. Sphenopalatine ganglion blockade with local anesthetic (spray, drop, swab)
      b. Sphenopalatine chemical or thermal (radiofrequency) gangliolysis
      c. Surgical resection of the sphenopalatine ganglion

VIII. POSTHERPETIC NEURALGIA
Postherpetic neuralgia is defined as neuropathic pain that persists longer than 3 months after lesions heal in an area infected by herpes zoster. Herpes zoster

affects the trigeminal nerve in 10% to 15% of all cases, and of these 80% involve the ophthalmic division. Slightly more than 20% of all herpes zoster cases will have pain persisting more than 1 year.

A. Clinical Features

    1. Increased incidence with age (majority are more than 60 years old) and immune system compromise

    2. Pain distribution: most commonly trigeminal ophthalmic division

    3. Pain description: constant, burning, tearing, stabbing, shocklike

    4. Triggers: shaving, light touch, or cool breeze over affected area

    5. Other pain characteristics

        a. Allodynia: the perception of pain from nonpainful stimuli

        b. Hyperpathia: the exaggerated perception of intense pain from mildly painful stimuli

    6. Spontaneous remissions can occur.

B. Treatment

    1. Medical

        a. Tricyclic antidepressants

        b. Antiepileptic drugs

            (1) Gabapentin

            (2) Carbamazepine

            (3) Phenytoin

            (4) Clonazepam

        c. Clonidine

        d. Analgesics

            (1) NSAIDs

            (2) Opioids

        e. Other systemic medications

            (1) Intravenous lidocaine

            (2) Mexiletine

            (3) Amantadine (NMDA antagonist)

            (4) Phenothiazines

        f. Topical treatment

            (1) Local anesthetics

            (2) Capsaicin

    2. Anesthesiologic treatments

        a. Local nerve blockade

        b. Superior stellate ganglion blockade

        c. Neurolytic blockade

    3. Surgical intervention

        a. There is little evidence to support the use of surgical procedures for the treatment of facial postherpetic neuralgia.

RECOMMENDED READING

Anderson G, Haddox JD, eds. Orofacial pain: Guidelines for diagnosis and management. American Academy of Orofacial Pain and American Academy of Pain Medicine, Quintessence (in preparation).

Bell WE. *Orofacial Pains: Differential Diagnosis,* 2nd ed. Chicago: Year Book Medical Publishers; 1979.

Fricton JR, Kroening R, Haley D, et al. Myofascial pain syndrome of the head and neck: A review of clinical characteristics of 164 patients. *Oral Surg Oral Med Oral Pathol* 1985;60:615–623.

Lascelles RG. Atypical facial pain and depression. *Br J Psychiatry* 1966;112:651–659.

Rees RT, Harris M. Atypical odontalgia. *Br J Oral Maxillofac Surg* 1978;16:212–218.

Sharau Y, Singer E, Schmidt E, et al. The analgesia effect of amitriptyline on chronic facial pain. *Pain* 1987;31:199–209.

Terezhalmy GT, ed. Treatment for temporomandibular joint dysfunction. *Ear Nose Throat J* 1982;61(12): entire issue.

The Pain Clinic Manual, Second Edition,
edited by Stephen E. Abram and J. David Haddox.
Lippincott Williams & Wilkins,
Philadelphia, © 2000

25

Headache

David M. Biondi

*D. M. Biondi: Michigan Head, Pain, and Neurological Institute, Ann Arbor,
Michigan 48104; Department of Neurology, Michigan State University
College of Osteopathic Medicine, East Lansing, Michigan 48824.*

Headache is one of the most frequent complaints presented to a physician regardless of specialty. It is estimated that only 5% of the general population will never experience headache. About 45 million Americans suffer with chronic recurrent headaches that are severe enough to cause impairment or require medical attention. Of these, an estimated 18 million women and 5.6 million men in the United States are affected with headaches that meet the diagnostic criteria for migraine.

Headache brings with it a high economic and social burden. In the United States, headache accounts for more than 18 million outpatient visits per year and 3 million patient-days bedridden each month. Migraine headaches alone cause an annual loss of $6.5 to $17 billion in labor costs and productivity. A California-based managed health care system reported that patients with migraine generated 1.7 times more medical claims, 3 times more pharmacy claims, 3.8 times more emergency department visits, and 5 times more diagnostic procedures performed when compared with an age-and sex-matched nonmigraine control group.

Despite these dramatic statistics, the prevalence of migraine and severe recurrent headache is thought to be significantly underestimated. People often do not report recurrent headaches unless specifically asked by the medical practitioner.

I. HEADACHE CLASSIFICATION

There are literally hundreds of causes for head and face pain. Pain-sensitive structures of the head include the scalp, muscles, periosteum, dura, and blood vessels (extracranial and intracranial). The brain parenchyma itself is pain insensate. Secondary headaches are those that are associated with underlying disease processes such as tumor, infection, trauma, hemorrhage, systemic disease, or other medical conditions. Primary headaches are those that have no identifiable structural or disease-related etiology and include the diagnostic categories of migraine, cluster, and tension-type headaches. Primary headache disorders are the etiology of head pain in 90% of cases. In 1988, the International Headache Society (IHS) established criteria for the classification and diagnosis of headache. The IHS Classification of Headache has 13 categories of head pain that are further subdivided into 129 different subtypes.

A. International Headache Society Categories of Head Pain
  1. Migraine
      a. Migraine with aura (previously called classic migraine)
          (1) Accounts for approximately 20% of all migraines
      b. Migraine without aura (previously called common migraine)
          (1) Accounts for seventy-five percent to 80% of all migraines
      c. Migraine aura without headache (migraine equivalent)
      d. Migraine with prolonged aura (previously called complicated migraine)
      e. Basilar migraine (Bickerstaff migraine)
      f. Hemiplegic migraine
  2. Tension-type headache
  3. Cluster headache and chronic paroxysmal hemicrania
  4. Miscellaneous headache unassociated with structural lesion
  5. Headache associated with head trauma
  6. Headache associated with vascular disorders
  7. Headache associated with nonvascular intracranial disorder (includes abnormal CSF pressure syndromes and CNS infection)
  8. Headache associated with substances or their withdrawal
  9. Headache associated with noncephalic infection
  10. Headache associated with metabolic disorder
  11. Headache or facial pain associated with disorder of the cranium, neck, eyes, ears, nose, sinuses, teeth, mouth, or other facial or cranial structures
  12. Cranial neuralgias, nerve trunk pain, and deafferentation pain
  13. Headache not classifiable

II. HEADACHE HISTORY

A comprehensive medical and headache history is required to establish an accurate headache diagnosis. The final diagnosis will require confirmation by the performance of a complete general physical and neurologic examination. Diagnostic testing is necessary if the clinical history and examination suggest an underlying disease process or structural abnormality. Although not intended to be comprehensive, some important elements of history for the accurate classification of headaches are outlined.

A. Initial Headache Presentation and Progression
  1. Acute, fulminant, or cataclysmic
  2. Subacute or gradual
  3. Chronic or protracted

       4. Paroxysmal
       5. Cyclic
  B. Pain Location
       1. Generalized
       2. Unilateral
       3. Focal or discretely localized
       4. Bitemporal or band-like
  C. Pain Expression
       1. Intermittent
          a. Frequency
          b. Duration
       2. Constant
       3. Intensity (mild, moderate, severe)
  D. Pain Characteristic
       1. Throbbing, pounding
       2. Squeezing, viselike, tightening, pressure
       3. Boring, drilling, knifelike
       4. Jabbing, jolting, shocklike, shooting
       5. Burning, searing
  E. Associated Signs and Symptoms
       1. Nausea, vomiting, diarrhea
       2. Photophobia, phonophobia, osmophobia
       3. Paresthesia, numbness
       4. Dizziness, vertigo, disequilibrium
       5. Blurred vision, visual scotoma, visual field cuts
       6. Autonomic symptoms and signs
          a. Eye tearing, rhinorrhea, nasal congestion, miosis, ptosis, flushing, diaphoresis, blood pressure alterations, syncope
       7. Cognitive inefficiency, fatigue, irritability, confusion, altered consciousness
  F. Triggers and Ameliorating Factors
  G. Complete Medical and Surgical History
  H. Medication History
       1. Current medications, including over-the-counter analgesics
       2. Dose and frequency of medication use
       3. Medications found to be effective in the past
  I. Psychosocial History
  J. Family History
  K. Historic Information Warranting Urgent Medical Attention
       1. More than two severe headaches per week
       2. Daily or near-daily use of pain relievers or the need to take more than the recommended dosage of pain relievers to control headache symptoms
       3. Fever or stiff neck (meningismus) associated with the headache

4. Dizziness, unsteadiness, dysarthria, weakness, or changes in sensation (numbness or tingling)
5. Presence of confusion or drowsiness
6. Headache triggered by exertion, coughing, bending, or sexual activity
7. Headache that is progressive and resistant to treatment
8. Change in the headache's typical characteristics or accompaniments
9. Persistent or severe vomiting that accompanies the headache
10. Patient has the worst headache of his or her life.
11. Headaches beginning after the age of 50 are associated with a higher risk of arteritis and intracranial tumors. Therefore head scanning and laboratory tests should be done early in the course of an evaluation. Specifically, ask about the typical accompaniments of giant cell (temporal) arteritis including unexplained weight loss, sweats, fevers, myalgia, arthralgia, and jaw claudication.
12. Frequent emergency department or acute-care utilization

III. MIGRAINE HEADACHE

Migraine is one of several specific primary headache disorders. It is a paroxysmal disorder of the central nervous system that may or may not be associated with headache and has typical identifying characteristics. Written history describing symptoms of migraine date back more than 3000 years. Clear descriptions of migraine are found in medical writings from the second century. Despite the historic longevity of migraine and the medical community's awareness of the condition, much is still unknown about its pathophysiologic mechanisms, and the search continues for more reliable, effective, and safe treatments.

A. Diagnostic Criteria (adapted from the IHS Classification)
   1. Migraine without aura (common migraine)
      a. One-sided headache or pain predominant on one side
      b. Pulsating or throbbing quality
      c. Nausea
      d. Sensitivity to light and sound
      e. Moderate to severe intensity
      f. Untreated headache typically lasts 4 to 72 hours
      g. Similar headaches in the past
      h. No evidence of an underlying disease process or structural pathology
   2. Migraine with visual aura (classic migraine)
      a. Same as above but headache is preceded by a visual warning of scintillating scotoma or fortification spectra (aura).
      b. The aura should last less than 60 minutes.
      c. The aura can occur 1 to 2 hours before the onset of a headache but may occur without a following headache.

B. Clinical Features
  1. An estimated 18 million women and 5.6 million men in the United States have migraine headaches.
  2. The peak incidence of migraine occurs within the 25- to 34-year age group, and 90% will experience their first migraine before the age of 40 years.
  3. Migraine affects girls and boys equally, but during adolescence and early adult life, women experience migraine at a prevalence 3 to 4 times greater than men.
  4. Contrary to popular belief, migraine prevalence is considerably higher in groups with low household income complicated by factors such as inadequate medical care, poor diet, and emotional and physical stress.
C. Pathophysiology
  Migraine is a "neurovascular" headache. Its pathophysiologic mechanism is associated with cranial perivascular inflammation mediated through the trigeminal nerve (trigeminovascular system) as well as alterations in cerebral blood perfusion, neurochemical transmitter activities, and cerebral electrophysiology. For the most part its precise cause is unknown. The hypothesized pathophysiology of migraine is a complex cascade of neurovascular and neurochemical activities that has several components.
  1. Vascular component
    a. Blood vessel caliber
      (1) Phases of vascular constriction or dilation do not strictly correlate with the phases of a migraine attack.
    b. Cerebral perfusion
      (1) Cerebral hypoperfusion or hyperperfusion occurring during a migraine attack do not strictly follow cerebrovascular territories; therefore the alterations in cerebral perfusion are likely to be neurologically mediated.
  2. Neurogenic component
    a. Cerebral cortex
      (1) Suppressed cerebrocortical electrophysiologic activity
    b. Reticular formation of the upper brain stem
      (1) Activation of brain stem neurons that may act as a generator of the migraine cascade or represent modulation of pain signals from higher cerebral centers
    c. Trigeminal nerve
      (1) Activation of the trigeminal nerve and subsequent release of vasoactive and inflammatory neuropeptides
  3. The integrated theory of migraine pathophysiology (trigeminovascular theory)
    a. Intrinsic or extrinsic factors trigger the migraine cascade.

b. Neurons in the reticular formation of the upper brain stem are activated.
c. Electrophysiologic changes occur in the brain stem and cerebral cortex.
d. The trigeminal nerve is activated and releases vasoactive neuropeptides from its terminals that surround cranial blood vessels.
e. The vasoactive neuropeptides cause vasodilatation directly and through the actions of nitric oxide.
f. Trigeminal sensory nerve terminals are activated by the vasodilatation, inflammatory neuropeptides, and nitric oxide.
g. Nociceptive signals are transmitted back through the trigeminal nerve to the brain stem and cerebral cortex, giving rise to the perception of pain within the trigeminal sensory fields of the face and head.

4. Neurochemical and neuromodulator component. Many different neurochemicals, transmitters, modulators and hormones are involved in the trigeminovascular model of migraine.
   a. Monoamine peptides
      (1) Serotonin, norepinephrine, dopamine
   b. Vasoactive or inflammatory chemicals and peptides
      (1) Calcitonin gene-related peptide (CGRP), neurokinin A, vasoactive intestinal peptide (VIP), nitric oxide (NO)
   c. Nociceptive or inflammatory transmitters and modulators
      (1) Substance P, prostaglandins, endorphin, cholecystokinin, histamine
   d. Hormones
      (1) Estrogen
   e. Excitatory neuroamino acids
      (1) Glutamate, aspartate
   f. Voltage gated channels
      (1) Calcium, sodium, potassium

5. Serotonin (5-HT) Receptors
   a. 5-HT_{1B} receptors
      (1) Found on the dural, cerebral, and coronary blood vessels
      (2) 5-HT_{1B} receptor agonists cause vasoconstriction
   b. 5-HT_{1D} receptors
      (1) Found on the trigeminal nerve terminals and within the brain stem
      (2) Agonists of 5-HT_{1D} receptors on the trigeminal nerve act to inhibit the release of vasoactive peptides from the trigeminal nerve terminals and thereby reduce neurovascular inflammation.

       (3) Agonists of 5-HT$_{1D}$ receptors in the central nervous system (brain stem) decrease neurotransmission of signals through the pain pathways of the brain stem sensory nuclei or inhibit activity of the migraine generator within the upper brain stem. (The raphe nuclei have a high density of serotonergic neurons.)

   c. The triptan class of migraine medications are selective agonists at the 5-HT$_{1D}$ and 5-HT$_{1B}$ receptors in the brain, trigeminal nerve, and cranial and extracranial blood vessels.

   d. The ergotamine class of migraine medications are agonists at 5-HT receptors (including 5-HT$_{1D}$ and 5-HT$_{1B}$ receptors) as well as dopamine and adrenergic receptors.

   e. 5-HT$_2$ receptors

       (1) Agonists at the 5-HT$_2$ receptor on the trigeminal nerve terminal facilitate pain transmission.

       (2) Antagonists at 5-HT$_2$ inhibit pain transmission, and it is through this mechanism that many preventive medications are believed to derive their benefit in reducing headache frequency, intensity, and duration.

   f. 5-HT$_{1F}$ receptors

       (1) They are found in the trigeminal nucleus caudalis.

       (2) Their action in migraine pathophysiology is still under study.

D. Genetics

   1. Migraine may be inherited in 80% to 90% of cases.

   2. A parent with migraine has a 50/50 chance of passing the trait onto his or her children.

   3. Genes for familial hemiplegic migraine have been localized to chromosomes 19 and 1.

E. Comorbid Medical Conditions

Several medical and psychiatric conditions coincidentally occur with migraine at a higher prevalence than would be expected by pure chance. The presence of comorbidity suggests a common pathophysiology among the coexisting conditions. It is important to recognize these associations so that overlapping pharmacologic interventions can be selected to reduce the total number of medications required and iatrogenic worsening of a comorbid condition can be avoided or minimized. Selected comorbid conditions are listed.

   1. Sleep disturbance

   2. Depression, bipolar disorder

   3. Anxiety, panic disorder

   4. Obsessive-compulsive behavior

   5. Personality disorders

   6. Epilepsy

    7. Fibromyalgia syndrome

    8. Mitral valve prolapse

F. Diagnostic Studies

Diagnostic imaging and laboratory tests are necessary if the medical history or physical examination suggests an underlying disease process or structural cause for the headache. Tests may also be done to evaluate certain risk factors, such as cardiovascular risks, which may significantly influence therapeutic interventions or necessitate a change in the pain treatment plan.

    1. Diagnostic imaging and other tests

        Imaging is necessary when neurologic deficits occur that had not been experienced previously (i.e., diplopia, dysequilibrium, vertigo, altered consciousness confusion or encephalopathy), significant changes occur in the quality or severity of the headache, significant changes occur in the response to previously effective treatments, and unusual headache presentations or characteristics are present. Other studies are ordered as clinically indicated.

        a. Computerized tomography (CT)

           (1) CT is particularly useful to evaluate for acute intraparenchymal or subarachnoid hemorrhage.

           (2) Unless contraindicated, always obtain a contrasted study after completing the noncontrasted study.

        b. Magnetic resonance imaging (MRI)

           (1) Provides very detailed views of the brain, especially in the posterior fossa, where the thicker bone of the skull often obscures CT images.

           (2) Always obtain a contrasted study unless contraindicated.

        c. Magnetic resonance angiography (MRA)

           (1) A noninvasive procedure for evaluation of vascular pathology such as arteriovenous malformations (AVMs), aneurysm, or thrombosis

        d. Electroencephalography (EEG)

           (1) Not generally required unless the headache is accompanied by unusual neurologic presentations, loss of consciousness, or altered mentation

           (2) Can be used to identify cerebrocortical effects of medication toxicity, brain injury, or brain tumor.

           (3) May be helpful in determining the potential risk of seizure induction from medications that lower seizure threshold (i.e., identifying a latent epileptogenic focus if the clinical history is favorable for its existence).

e. Lumbar puncture
    (1) Evaluation of cerebrospinal fluid (CSF) chemistry and cytology
    (2) Identification of high- or low-CSF pressure syndromes
    (3) Mandatory in all cases in which subarachnoid hemorrhage is suspected
f. Cerebral arteriography
    (1) More sensitive than MRA in the evaluation of vascular disease
g. Electrocardiography (EKG)
    (1) Cardiac abnormalities may limit treatment options because of cardiovascular risks, including cardiac ischemia, conduction block, or dysrhythmia
h. Ultrasonography and Doppler
    (1) Noninvasive extracranial and intracranial neurovascular diagnostic techniques
2. Laboratory testing (serum, blood, and urine).
    Blood and urine tests are obtained to evaluate for organic etiologies of head pain and assess for possible risks of headache treatments such as diseases of the liver, kidney, or blood.
    a. Initial laboratory evaluation
        (1) CBC, ESR, BUN, creatinine, AST, ALT, vitamin B_{12}, total protein, albumen, calcium, sodium, potassium, magnesium, glucose, cholesterol, triglycerides, thyroid function tests, serum estrogen for women, serum testosterone for men, urinalysis, and urine drug screen
        (2) Additional laboratory studies may be required to search for other headache etiologies, such as rheumatologic conditions (i.e., systemic lupus erythematosus), infections (i.e., Lyme disease, syphilis, or HIV), or inflammatory conditions of the blood vessels (i.e., temporal arteritis).
G. General Treatment Principles for Migraine
    1. Patients should keep a diary of the headache episodes and provide a detailed description of their headache characteristics.
    2. Patients should be encouraged to become actively involved in their treatment plan so that the medical practitioner can be more effective in providing care.
    3. Medical practitioners should insist on their patients complying with the prescribed pain treatment plan.
    4. An effective treatment plan is found by a trial-and-error process that may take weeks or months to develop.
    5. There is no cure, but preventive treatment will almost always bring a reduction in the frequency, duration, severity, and disability associated with future headache episodes.

6. Set realistic goals and expectations of treatment and openly discuss them with the patient to avoid future misunderstanding and frustration.
7. Identify, reduce, and withdraw triggering factors.
   a. Food triggers include chocolate, aged cheeses (cheddar, brie, gruyere), beer, wine (especially red and rose), sherry, champagne, buttermilk, processed meats (bacon, hot dogs, cold cuts, canned ham), sour cream, seeds, nuts and their products, including peanut butter.
   b. Excessive caffeine use can trigger or worsen headaches.
   c. Tobacco use can worsen headaches by reducing oxygen-carrying capacity of the blood, contributing the adverse pharmacologic actions of nicotine on the central nervous system, and inducing catabolic liver enzymes that lessen migraine medication efficacy.
8. Treat symptoms of anxiety and depression. Stress reduction, relaxation exercises, and biofeedback can be very helpful as an adjunct to pharmacologic therapy.
9. Treat sleep disorders; prescribe regular exercise and a healthy, well-balanced diet.
10. Overuse of prescribed or over-the-counter analgesic medications can trigger or worsen headache patterns. (Refer to the section in this chapter about transformed migraine and analgesic rebound headache.) This can also occur with overuse of ergotamine tartrate.
11. Certain prescribed medications may contribute to headaches; review the patient's use of prescribed and over-the-counter medication.
H. Abortive Medications (for the treatment of an active, acute headache)
   1. Simple over-the-counter analgesics containing aspirin, acetaminophen, or combinations of these with caffeine
      a. Overuse may lead to a chronic daily headache (analgesic rebound headache).
   2. Dihydroergotamine (DHE) injectable and nasal spray
      a. Several studies have shown parenteral DHE to be a more effective migraine pain reliever than narcotics.
      b. Often used in treating the drug rebound syndrome and persistent headache pattern (status migrainosis)
   3. Triptans (5-HT$_{1B/D}$ agonists)
      a. Sumatriptan injectable, nasal spray, and oral tablet
      b. Zolmitriptan oral tablet
      c. Naratriptan oral tablet
      d. Rizatriptan oral tablet and oral melt tablet
   4. Ergotamine tartrate
      a. Rectal suppository is the most effective delivery route.
      b. Nausea is often a side effect and may require medication.
      c. Overuse can lead to ergotamine rebound headaches.

   5. Butalbital-containing products
      a. Judicious and restricted use is necessary to avoid analgesic rebound syndrome and barbiturate dependence.
   6. Isometheptene mucate
      a. A vasoconstrictor typically found as a component in combination products
   7. Nonsteroidal, antiinflammatory drugs (ketorolac, naproxen, ibuprofen, indomethacin, and others)
      a. Particularly useful in menstrual migraine
      b. Less likely to cause drug rebound syndrome
      c. Ketorolac is available for parenteral delivery.
   8. Narcotic analgesics
      a. Butorphanol injectable and nasal spray
         (1) Butorphanol may be preferable to meperidine for treatment of infrequent acute headaches since it is longer-acting and has less potential for respiratory depression. Extreme caution and close monitoring of butorphanol use is required since it can cause strong physical dependence as well as severe rebound and narcotic abstinence syndromes.
      b. Nalbuphine injectable
      c. Injectable, transdermal, oral, and rectal opiates (morphine, hydrocodone, codeine, oxycodone, meperidine, fentanyl, and others)
   9. Oxygen (6 to 7 liters by face mask for 15 minutes)
      a. Most effective for cluster headaches
  10. Corticosteroids (dexamethasone, prednisone, or methylprednisolone)
      a. May be useful as an adjuvant medication in breaking a persistent headache pattern (status migrainosis) and is often very effective for short-term use in preventing cluster headaches.
      b. Caution and limited use is required to avoid the development of a Cushingoid syndrome and to reduce the risk of aseptic bone necrosis at major limb joints.
  11. Others
      a. Neuroleptics (Phenothiazines, butyrophenone)
      b. Hydroxyzine
      c. Muscle relaxants (baclofen, tizanidine, cyclobenzaprine)
      d. Magnesium sulfate (intravenous)
 I. General Guidelines for Preventive Pharmacotherapy
   1. Reasons to consider preventive treatment
      a. Headache-related disability occurs 3 or more days a month.
      b. Symptomatic medications are ineffective, contraindicated, or likely to be overused.
      c. Special circumstances exist such as profound migraine-associated disability, prolonged migraine auras, or history of migrainous cerebral infarction.

2. Reasons for failure of preventive treatment
   a. Inadequate dosage
   b. Insufficient duration of use
      (1) Each newly added medication or dosage change may require 4 or more weeks before a beneficial effect is recognized.
   c. Noncompliance with medication regimen
      (1) Patient education is very important to achieve a favorable outcome from a prescribed pain treatment plan.
      (2) To minimize medication side effects and improve patient compliance, start with a low dose and titrate the medication slowly upward until the desirable effect is attained or intolerable side effects occur.
   d. Analgesic or ergotamine overuse has caused a drug rebound syndrome.
   e. Incorrect initial diagnosis or development of a new, concurrent medical condition.
   f. Although monotherapy is preferred, many patients may require appropriate combinations of preventive medications ("co-pharmacy").
3. Address nonpharmacologic interventions and life-style modification such as diet, exercise, scheduling of daily routines, proper sleep, smoking cessation, and abstinence from alcohol.
J. Preventive Medications (medications taken daily to reduce the frequency, duration, and intensity of headaches)
   1. Beta-blockers
      a. Propranolol, nadolol, timolol, metoprolol
      b. First-line treatment alone or together with a TCA
      c. Contraindicated in cases of asthma, congestive heart failure, hypotension, diabetes mellitus, migraine with prolonged aura
   2. Tricyclic antidepressants (TCAs)
      a. Amitriptyline, nortriptyline, doxepin, protriptyline, desipramine, others
      b. Helpful in treating comorbid depression
      c. Sedation associated with many of these medications can be helpful in improving sleep patterns when used as a single nighttime dose.
      d. First-line treatment alone or together with a beta-blocker
      e. Contraindicated in cases of cardiac dysrhythmia, glaucoma, urinary retention, hypotension
   3. Antiepileptic drugs (AEDs)
      a. Divalproex sodium, gabapentin, carbamazepine, topiramate
      b. Effective in migraine and possibly cluster
      c. Helpful in treating comorbid epilepsy or bipolar disorder

4. Ergot derivatives
   a. Methysergide, methylergonovine
   b. Effective in migraine and cluster
   c. Retroperitoneal and organ fibrosis may rarely occur after prolonged use; therefore a 1-month drug holiday and diagnostic testing (abdominal CT, CXR, IVP) are recommended every 6 months.
5. Calcium channel blockers
   a. Verapamil, nimodipine, nicardipine, others
   b. Verapamil is a first-line treatment for cluster headache.
   c. Generally not as effective as beta-blockers for migraine but may be helpful if beta-blockers are contraindicated.
6. Nonsteroidal antiinflammatory drugs (NSAIDs)
   a. Useful as an adjunctive treatment for catamenial/menstrual migraine
   b. Indomethacin is the treatment of choice for benign paroxysmal hemicrania and hemicrania continua.
7. Selective serotonin reuptake inhibitors—SSRI antidepressants
   a. Fluoxetine, paroxetine, sertraline, others
   b. Generally not as effective as TCAs for migraine
   c. Possibly useful in the treatment of frequent or daily headaches, especially if depression or anxiety are comorbid conditions
8. Monoamine oxidase inhibitors (MAOI)
   a. Phenelzine, tranylcypromine
   b. Typically reserved for migraine that is refractory to other treatments
   c. Helpful in treating comorbid depression and anxiety
   d. Many dietary and medication contraindications
9. Other antidepressant medications
   a. Nefazodone, venlafaxine, mirtazapine, lithium, others
   b. Reserved for migraine that is refractory to other treatments or if comorbid psychiatric conditions warrant their use
10. Neuroleptics (major tranquilizers)
    a. Risperidone, olanzapine, others
    b. Reserved for migraine that is refractory to other treatments or if comorbid psychiatric conditions warrant their use

K. Interventional Treatments

Anesthesiologic and surgical interventions should not be performed routinely unless the headache history and findings of the physical and neurologic examinations strongly suggest their necessity. Interventional treatments may be considered if traditional headache treatments are ineffective, diagnostic studies do not reveal an underlying disease process, and the procedure appears indicated by the clinical evaluation.

1. Peripheral nerve or ganglion blockade
   a. Occipital nerves
   b. Upper cervical nerve roots

          c. Sphenopalatine ganglion
          d. Gasserian ganglion
          e. Trigeminal nerve
     2. Cervical facet joint blockade (refer to the following section in this chapter on cervicogenic headache)
          a. Consider especially in posttraumatic head pain syndromes and whiplash injuries
     3. Trigger point injections
          a. Regional myofascial pain syndrome with pain referred to the head
     4. Epidural blood patch (for low-CSF-pressure headaches)
     5. Repeated lumbar punctures or lumboperitoneal shunts (for idiopathic intracranial hypertension/pseudotumor cerebri)
 L. Transformed Migraine Headache and Analgesic Rebound Syndrome
     1. Periodic, acute migraine pattern that "transforms" or progresses to a more frequent and continuous headache pattern with superimposed acute migraine attacks
     2. Analgesic-rebound headache syndrome (drug-induced transformed migraine)
          a. Frequent use of over-the-counter or prescription analgesic medications, including acetaminophen, aspirin, caffeine, butalbital, and narcotics causes intractable headaches in which a vicious cycle of increasing analgesic use and worsening headache develops. This syndrome also occurs with ergotamine tartrate overuse.
          b. The risk for developing this syndrome occurs in headache-prone individuals who use analgesics or ergotamine more than 2 to 3 days of each week on a regular basis.
          c. The features of this syndrome include
               (1) Insidious increase of headache frequency and intensity
               (2) Ineffectiveness of alternative abortive or preventive medications to control headaches
               (3) Predictable early-morning awakenings because of headache
               (4) Predictable onset or worsening of headache intensity following the last dose of medication or prior to the next scheduled dose
               (5) Development of drug dependency or addictive behaviors
          d. An estimated 75% of patients with transformed migraine have the drug-induced variety.
          e. Studies have shown that 75% to 90% of those who experience chronic daily headache associated with drug overuse are able to gain total or significant pain control by simply withdrawing the overused drug.
 M. Hospitalization
     1. Suggested requirements for in-patient treatment
          a. Narcotic addiction/dependency
          b. Butalbital/barbiturate addiction/dependency

    c. Benzodiazepine addiction/dependency

    d. Ergotamine tartrate dependency

    e. Inability or unwillingness of the patient to discontinue analgesic medications due to rebound pain, dependency, addiction, or withdrawal symptoms

    f. Intractable headache not responding to appropriate, aggressive outpatient or emergency department interventions

    g. Poor psychosocial situation at home or lack of outpatient emotional support structure

    h. Comorbid medical condition(s) that would make outpatient medication withdrawal risky; unstable vitals

    i. Patient has dehydration, electrolyte imbalance, and prostration requiring IV fluids and monitoring.

    j. Severe comorbid psychiatric disease

IV. TENSION-TYPE HEADACHES

Tension-type headache is the most common form of headache. Many medical practitioners who specialize in the treatment of headache object to using the term *tension-type headache* because it implies that muscle or emotional tension is the pathogenesis of this headache type even though there is little evidence to support this implication. Muscle tension and myalgia are present in both migraine and tension-type headaches. Moreover, emotional distress is a common trigger for both headache types. Many headache specialists believe that migraine and tension-type headache fall at opposite poles of a headache continuum or headache spectrum, and these headache types, although distinct in their defining characteristics, share a common pathophysiologic basis. It is not uncommon for a headache-prone individual to experience both migraine and tension-type headaches independently or concurrently at some time during his or her life. Many common treatments are effective for both headache types. Chronic tension-type headaches can be just as disabling as migraine and result in a similar substantial socioeconomic burden.

  A. Diagnostic Criteria (adapted from the IHS Classification)

    1. Episodic tension-type headaches

      a. Generally occurring on both sides of the head

      b. Pressing, squeezing, or bandlike quality (throbbing during physical exertion)

      c. Sensitivity to light or sound but no nausea

      d. Mild-to-moderate intensity

      e. Headache lasting from 30 minutes to 7 days

      f. Less than 15 headache days per month

      g. No evidence of an underlying disease process or structural abnormality

    2. Chronic tension-type headaches

      a. Same as item 3 above but greater than 15 headache days per month and may have nausea when headache is more intense.

B. Pathophysiology
1. The precise mechanism of pathogenesis is unknown, but available evidence suggests that it is multifactorial and heterogeneous. There appears to be an activation of peripheral nociceptors within strained neck muscles or ligaments as well as alterations in central pain modulation. The pathophysiologic mechanisms in the central nervous system are likely the same as those described in the migraine section of this chapter.
C. Treatment Principles
1. Episodic tension-type headaches most often respond to simple analgesics and nonpharmacologic interventions.
2. Chronic tension-type headache requires a pain management plan employing nonpharmacologic and pharmacologic interventions. In clinical practice, the tricyclic and selective serotonin reuptake inhibitor antidepressants have been the most effective.
3. Since the treatment of migraine and tension-type headaches overlap, refer to the section on migraine treatment in this chapter.

V. CLUSTER HEADACHE

Cluster headache syndrome is an excruciatingly painful and devastating medical condition. The true prevalence of cluster headache is unknown, but it has been suggested that it affects between 0. 08% and 0.4% of the general population, or approximately 0.5 million people in the United States. The pain is often so severe that many people with cluster contemplate or commit suicide.

A. Diagnostic Criteria (adapted from IHS Classification)
1. Episodic cluster headache
a. Severe unilateral orbital, supraorbital, or temporal pain
b. Untreated headache lasts for 15 to 180 minutes
c. Associated with at least one autonomic sign on the side of pain
(1) Conjunctival injection, lacrimation, nasal congestion, rhinorrhea, sweating, miosis, ptosis, or eye edema
d. Attack frequency from 1 every other day to 8 per day
e. Cycles last from 7 days to 1 year
f. Cycles are separated by pain-free periods lasting at least 14 days
g. No evidence of an underlying disease process or structural pathology
2. Chronic cluster headache
a. Same as episodic cluster except that cycles last longer than 1 year or are separated by remissions lasting less than 14 days
B. Clinical Features
1. Cluster begins at any age, although the onset is typically between 20 and 40 years old
2. Cluster headaches are five to six times more prevalent in men than women.

3. Attacks frequently occur during sleep and at the same time each day.
4. The pain is constant and excruciating, with drilling or boring qualities.
5. Nausea and vomiting occur only in 2% to 5% of those with cluster as compared with 85% with migraine.
6. During an attack a cluster sufferer typically paces, cries, screams, pounds his fists, and strikes or rubs his face or head on furniture, walls, or floors.
7. Common phenotypic features are often observed, including leonine facies (thick, roughened skin with deep nasolabial folds and skin furrows) and blue or hazel eye color.
8. Alcohol is a consistent headache trigger while a cluster cycle is active.

C. Pathophysiology
   1. The pathophysiologic mechanism of cluster headache remains mostly unknown.
   2. There appears to be a complex association of changes in hypothalamic, brain stem, endocrinologic, and central nervous system functioning that involves the trigeminal nerve, facial nerve, parasympathetic autonomic nervous system, changes in cerebral blood flow, and alterations in neurochemical transmitter activity. It has been hypothesized that there is involvement of the trigeminovascular system.

D. Genetics
   1. Cluster headaches appear to be inherited in less than 10% of cases.

E. Treatment of Cluster Headaches
   The main goal of treatment is to prevent the cluster attacks. Since cluster attacks are frequent and relatively brief, many medications that are used to treat acute pain are not effective or convenient.
   1. General guidelines for the treatment of cluster headaches
      a. Recommend the discontinuance of alcoholic beverages during and between cluster attacks.
      b. Recommend the discontinuance of cigarettes and tobacco products.
      c. Begin preventive and abortive treatment as soon as possible at the onset of a cluster cycle.
   2. Abortive medications for the acute treatment of a cluster headache
      a. Oxygen (O_2) by inhalation via mask
      b. Sumatriptan injection or nasal spray
      c. Dihydroergotamine injection or nasal spray
      d. Ergotamine tartrate rectal suppository
      e. Chlorpromazine rectal suppository
      f. Lidocaine nasal spray
   3. Preventive medications for recurrent cluster attacks
      a. Corticosteroids (prednisone, methylprednisolone, dexamethasone)

(1) Steroids are rapidly helpful and are particularly useful for controlling cluster attacks for short periods of time while waiting for other appropriate medicines to take effect.

   b. Verapamil

   c. Lithium

   d. Methysergide, methylergonovine

   e. Divalproex sodium

   f. Cyproheptadine

   g. Methylphenidate

4. Nonsurgical treatment for cluster headaches

   a. Sphenopalantine ganglion blockade

   b. Radiofrequency sphenopalantine thermal gangliolysis

   c. Chemical neurolysis of the trigeminal nerve or gasserian ganglion

   d. Radiofrequency thermal neurolysis of the trigeminal nerve or trigeminal ganglion

   e. Gamma radiation directed specifically at the trigeminal nerve or trigeminal ganglion (gamma knife radiosurgery)

VI. HEADACHE ASSOCIATED WITH CHANGES IN CEREBROSPINAL FLUID PRESSURE

Alterations in cerebrospinal fluid pressure as a cause of chronic headache can be easily overlooked. The typical range for cerebrospinal pressure is between 70 and 200 millimeters of water pressure (mm H_2O), sometimes as high as 250 mm H_2O in an obese patient.

  A. Low-CSF-Pressure Headache

Headache due to low cerebrospinal fluid pressure is estimated to occur after 15% to 30% of all lumbar punctures. Low-pressure headaches can result from a dural tear and subsequent CSF leak caused by strenuous activity, heavy lifting, straining, sexual intercourse, surgery or head injury. Decreased CSF production and orthostatic headache can occur as a result of dehydration, severe infection, and poorly controlled diabetes mellitus. Spontaneous or idiopathic low-CSF-pressure headaches also occur.

   1. Clinical features

     a. Cerebrospinal fluid pressure

      (1) Typically between 0 and 30 mm H_2O

     b. Pain distribution: frontal, temporal, holocephalic

     c. Pain characteristics: severe, throbbing, similar to migraine or tension-type headache

     d. Pain triggers: occur daily, usually within minutes of sitting or standing, continuous while upright, dramatically relieved within minutes of lying supine although the positional features may be minimal or lost in chronic cases.

     e. Associated signs and symptoms: nausea, vomiting, dizziness, tinnitus, neck stiffness

2. Treatment
    a. Medical
        (1) Bedrest
        (2) Intravenous or forced oral fluids
        (3) Increased oral caffeine intake or intravenous caffeine sodium benzoate
        (4) Abdominal binder
        (5) Medication
            (a) NSAIDs
            (b) Mineralocorticoids
    b. Interventional
        (1) Epidural blood patch
        (2) Continuous epidural saline infusion
B. Idiopathic Intracranial Hypertension (pseudotumor cerebri)
    Headache is the most consistent complaint in idiopathic intracranial hypertension, formerly pseudotumor cerebri. It occurs eight times more commonly in women, especially overweight women of childbearing age (20 to 50 years old). Other risk factors for the development of idiopathic intracranial hypertension include oral contraceptive pills, hypervitaminosis A, naldixic acid, tetracyclines, steroid withdrawal, hypoparathyroidism, Addison's disease, renal failure, and systemic lupus erythematosus. Permanent visual loss is a sequela of this condition; therefore early diagnosis and treatment are imperative.
    1. Clinical features
        a. Cerebrospinal fluid pressure
            (1) Typically more than 250 mm H_2O
        b. Pain distribution: holocephalic, frontal, temporal
        c. Pain characteristics: daily, constant, similar to chronic migraine or tension-type headache
        d. Pain triggers: physical exertion and Valsalva maneuvers (straining, coughing, or sneezing)
        e. Associated signs and symptoms: nausea, vomiting, dizziness, blurred vision, brief episodes of visual loss, diplopia, pulsatile tinnitus, neck stiffness
        f. Visual loss occurring in up to 80% of cases, with most being reversible with effective treatment
    2. Physical examination
        a. Papilledema in approximately 90% of cases
        b. Abducens nerve palsy (lateral rectus extraocular muscle weakness)
        c. Enlargement of the physiologic blind spot
    3. Treatment
        Blindness can occur in up to 10% of cases if the elevated CSF pressure is left untreated.

  a. Medical
   (1) Weight loss
   (2) Treatment of underlying medical conditions and withdrawal of medications that may contribute to an elevation of cerebrospinal fluid pressure
   (3) Medications
      (a) Acetazolamide or other carbonic anhydrase inhibitors
      (b) Furosemide
  b. Interventional and surgical
   (1) Repeated lumbar punctures
   (2) Optic nerve sheath fenestration
   (3) Lumboperitoneal shunt
   (4) Temporal craniotomy and decompression

VII. CRANIAL ARTERITIS

Temporal arteritis needs to be considered in any person who develops new-onset headache later in life. The vasculitis of this condition affects the temporal arteries, but it can also involve carotid, vertebral, ophthalmic, and coronary arteries. Ischemic optic neuropathy resulting in permanent visual loss and blindness is generally the most significant sequela.

  A. Temporal Arteritis (giant cell arteritis)
   1. Clinical features
     a. Typically affects people more than 60 years old
     b. Pain distribution: holocephalic, temporal or bitemporal, occasionally occipital
     c. Pain characteristics: constant, dull, aching, throbbing
     d. Associated signs and symptoms: loss of appetite, malaise, low-grade fever, weight loss, jaw claudication
     e. Associated medical conditions or sequelae
      (1) Polymyalgia rheumatica
         (a) Arthralgias
         (b) Myalgias
         (c) Muscle fatigue
         (d) Stiffness
      (2) Transient ischemic attacks (TIAs)
      (3) Cerebrocortical infarction
      (4) Myocardial infarction
   2. Diagnostic evaluation
     a. Physical examination
      (1) Temporal tenderness
      (2) Temporal edema
      (3) Induration and inflammation surrounding temporal arteries
     b. Laboratory
      (1) Elevated erythrocyte sedimentation rate (ESR)

        (2) Elevated c-reactive protein

        (3) Anemia

        (4) Elevated liver transaminases

     c. Temporal artery biopsy

        (1) Required to confirm diagnosis since long-term corticosteroid treatment can cause significant morbidity

        (2) For immediate reduction of the risk of blindness or infarction, corticosteroids may be started 1 to 3 days prior to obtaining a biopsy specimen without affecting biopsy results.

  3. Treatment

     a. Medical

        (1) Corticosteroids

           (a) Rapid resolution of most signs and symptoms

           (b) One to 2 years of daily treatment typically required

           (c) ESR and clinical symptoms are followed to gauge effectiveness and further need of treatment

        (2) Symptomatic treatment of headache

           (a) Simple analgesics

VIII. OTHER HEADACHE DISORDERS

Special headache types are identified by their unique pain patterns, unusual characteristics, and distinct response to treatment. It is important to recognize these conditions because effective treatment can be very specific, such as with the indomethacin responsive syndromes of chronic paroxysmal hemicrania and hemicrania continua.

  A. Chronic Paroxysmal Hemicrania (CPH)

    1. Clinical features

     a. Affects women more commonly than men

     b. Pain distribution: strictly unilateral around the eye, temple, forehead, ear, occiput

     c. Pain characteristics: severe, sharp, jolting

     d. Pain features: 10 to 30 headache episodes per day, each lasting 5 to 30 minutes

     e. Associated signs and symptoms

        (1) Autonomic symptoms ipsilateral to the pain

           (a) Lacrimation, rhinorrhea, conjunctival injection

        (2) Restlessness

     f. Pain triggers: head and neck movement

    2. Treatment

     a. Indomethacin provides dramatic improvement.

  B. Hemicrania Continua

    1. Clinical features

     a. Affects women more commonly than men (5:1)

     b. Pain distribution: strictly unilateral around the eye, temple, forehead, ear, occiput

   c. Pain characteristics: continuous, severe, sharp jabbing, jolting, burning

   d. Associated signs and symptoms

    (1) Autonomic symptoms ipsilateral to the pain

     (a) Lacrimation, rhinorrhea, conjunctival injection, photophobia

   e. Pain triggers

    (1) Physical exertion

  2. Treatment

   a. Indomethacin provides dramatic improvement.

C. Carotidynia

  1. Clinical features

   a. Women primarily affected

   b. Often comorbid with migraine headache

   c. Pain distribution: unilateral or bilateral neck and carotid artery pain that can be referred to the ipsilateral jaw, face, ear, and head

   d. Pain characteristics: dull, throbbing, stabbing

   e. Pain features: daily and constant, lasting from days to months

   f. Associated signs and symptoms

    (1) Carotid artery tenderness

   g. Pain triggers: head and neck movement, swallowing, sneezing, yawning, coughing

  2. Treatment

   a. Medical

    (1) Medications

     (a) Indomethacin

     (b) Corticosteroid

     (c) Ergots derivatives

    (2) Typical treatments for migraine

D. SUNCT Syndrome

  1. Nomenclature: SUNCT = "Short duration, Unilateral, Neuralgic, Conjunctival injection and Tearing"

  2. Clinical features

   a. Pain distribution: strictly unilateral around the eye, temple, forehead

   b. Pain characteristics: severe, jolting, jabbing

   c. Pain features: 5 to 30 attacks per hour, each lasting between 15 and 60 seconds

   d. Associated signs and symptoms

    (1) Autonomic symptoms ipsilateral to the pain

     (a) Lacrimation, rhinorrhea, conjunctival injection, diaphoresis

   e. Pain triggers: head and neck movement, chewing

  3. Treatment

   a. Refractory to all typical medications, including indomethacin

E. Benign Exertional Headache or Effort Migraine
   1. Clinical features
      a. Pain distribution: usually bilateral or holocephalic
      b. Pain characteristics: abrupt onset, severe, throbbing
      c. Pain features: onset during physical exertion and lasting from 5 minutes to 24 hours
      d. Associated signs and symptoms: nausea, vomiting, dizziness, photophobia, phonophobia
      e. Pain triggers: physical exertion, heavy lifting, sexual intercourse, coughing, sneezing
   2. Diagnostic Evaluation
      a. Since intracranial tumors or vascular abnormalities may present identically to these benign headache types, diagnostic imaging studies are required in all cases of exertional headache.
   3. Treatment
      a. Medical
         (1) Medication
            (a) Indomethacin, other NSAIDs, or ergots 1 to 2 hours prior to exertion

IX. OCCIPITAL NEURALGIA

The greater occipital nerve receives sensory fibers from the C-2 nerve root and the lesser occipital nerve receives fibers from the C-2 and C-3 nerve roots. Neck trauma, cervical spine degenerative changes and cervical disc disease are common etiologies for this condition. Some cases of occipital neuralgia may actually be a C-2 or C-3 radiculopathy since these conditions have similar clinical characteristics.

A. Occipital Neuralgia
   1. Clinical features
      a. Pain distribution: occiput, posterior scalp, upper neck and occasionally pain referred to the temple, frontal regions, and periorbital region
      b. Pain characteristics: constant, burning, aching, shooting, shocklike
      c. Associated signs and symptoms: posterior scalp paresthesias, migraine or clusterlike headaches, photophobia, dizziness
      d. Pain triggers: neck movement especially extension and rotation, pressure applied directly to the nerve at the occiput
   2. Diagnostic evaluation
      a. Cervical spine and craniocervical imaging
      b. Brain (posterior fossa) imaging
      c. Diagnostic occipital nerve blockade
   3. Treatment
      a. Nonpharmacologic interventions
         (1) Physical and manual therapy
      b. Medications

      (1) NSAIDs
      (2) Muscle relaxers
      (3) Tricyclic antidepressants
      (4) Antiepileptic drugs
         (a) Carbamazepine
         (b) Gabapentin
         (c) Divalproex sodium
   c. Anesthesiological interventions
      (1) Greater and lesser occipital nerve blockade
   d. Surgical interventions
      (1) Surgical procedures should be reserved for cases of severe refractory pain
         (a) Occipital nerve decompression
         (b) Occipital cryoneurolysis
         (c) Avoid nerve sectioning and dorsal rhizotomy

X. CERVICOGENIC HEADACHE

Cervicogenic headache is defined as head pain referred from anatomic structures and soft tissues of the neck. The trigeminocervical nucleus is a region of the cervical spinal cord where sensory nerve fibers of the upper cervical roots converge with sensory nerve fibers of the descending tract of the trigeminal nerve, thereby creating a pathway by which pain emanating from the neck can be referred to the head. Despite the availability of diagnostic criteria, the presenting characteristics of cervicogenic headache may be difficult to distinguish from migraine, tension-type headache, cluster or paroxysmal hemicrania. Because neck pain is often an associated symptom of the primary headache disorders, its presence in association with head pain should not always actuate a diagnosis of cervicogenic headache. The etiology of cervicogenic headache is a heterogeneous group of disorders. Some common but often overlooked causes of chronic head pain include cervical facet joint pathology, upper cervical radiculopathy, occipital neuralgia, and regional myofascial pain.

  A. Diagnostic Criteria (adapted from the 1997 proposed diagnostic criteria of the Cervicogenic Headache International Study Group)
    1. Major criteria
      a. Head pain caused by neck movement, awkward head positioning, or pressure applied over the upper cervical or occipital region
      b. Restricted neck range of motion
      c. Ipsilateral neck, shoulder, or arm pain of nonradicular origin
      d. Confirmation by diagnostic anesthetic blockade
      e. Unilateral headache without sideshift, although the criteria allow for bilateral pain ("unilateral on both sides") in a clinical setting
    2. Pain characteristics
      a. Variable pain distribution, depending upon the source of the referred pain; neck, occiput, referred pain to the temple, frontal region, periorbital region

      b. Moderate to severe intensity, nonthrobbing, nonlancinating, originating in the neck, intermittent or constant
   3. Associated signs and symptoms
      a. Nausea
      b. Photophobia
      c. Phonophobia
      d. Dizziness
      e. Ipsilateral blurred vision

B. Clinical Features
   1. Structures from which head pain of cervicogenic origin may arise
      a. Atlantooccipital joint
      b. Atlantoaxial joint
      c. C-2–3 facet joint
      d. C-2–3 intervertebral disc
      e. Vertebral artery
      f. Suboccipital and upper cervical muscles
      g. Trapezius and sternocleidomastoid muscles
   2. Pain features
      a. May present with features identical or similar to those of migraine, tension-type headache, cluster, hemicrania, or occipital neuralgia.
   3. Pain triggers
      a. Neck movement, especially extension and rotation
      b. Valsalva, coughing, sneezing
      c. Pressure applied to the upper neck, trapezius, and sternocleidomastoid muscles

C. Pathophysiology
   1. Nociceptive signals emanating from anatomic structures and soft tissues of the neck are transmitted through the upper cervical nerve roots and converge with the descending tract of the trigeminal nerve in the trigeminocervical nucleus thereby allowing a referred sensation of pain from the neck to the corresponding trigeminal sensory receptive fields of the face and head.
   2. This convergence of nociceptive signals appears to have the ability to trigger the trigeminovascular cascade that hypothetically underlies the pathogenesis of migraine thereby causing migraine headaches.
   3. Also relevant is the convergence of sensorimotor fibers in the spinal accessory nerve (CN XI) with the upper cervical nerve roots that ultimately converge with the trigeminal nerve. These connections may be the basis for the well-recognized patterns of pain referred from the trapezius and sternocleidomastoid muscles to the face and head.

D. Diagnostic Evaluation
   1. Cervical spine imaging
   2. Diagnostic blockade
      a. Trigger point injections

        b. Peripheral nerve blockade
          (1) Greater occipital nerve
          (2) Selective nerve root
        c. Cervical spine facet joint blockade
        d. Cervical epidural steroid injection
    E. Treatment
       1. Nonpharmacologic
         a. Physical therapy
         b. Manual therapy
         c. Biofeedback
       2. Medication
         a. NSAIDs
         b. Muscle relaxers
         c. Tricyclic antidepressants
         d. Antiepileptic drugs
       3. Surgical interventions
         a. Radiofrequency facet joint rhizolysis
         b. Radiofrequency third occipital neurolysis

RECOMMENDED READING

Dalessio DJ, Silberstein SD, eds. *Wolff's Headache and Other Head Pain,* 6th ed. New York: Oxford University Press; 1993.

Davidoff RA. *Migraine: Manifestations, Pathogenesis, and Management* (Contemporary Neurology Series). Philadelphia: FA Davis; 1995.

Gershwin ME, Hamilton ME, eds. *The Pain Management Handbook: A Concise Guide to Diagnosis and Treatment.* Totowa, NJ: Humana Press; 1998.

Goadsby PJ, Silberstein SD, eds. *Headache* (Blue Books of Practical Neurology). Boston: Butterworth-Heinemann; 1997.

Saper JR, Silberstein SD, Gordon CD, et al. *Handbook of Headache Management: A Practical Guide to Diagnosis and Treatment of Head, Neck, and Facial Pain,* 2nd ed. Baltimore: Williams & Wilkins; 1999.

Wall PD, Melzack R, eds. *Textbook of Pain,* 3rd ed. London: Churchill Livingstone; 1994.

The Pain Clinic Manual, Second Edition,
edited by Stephen E. Abram and J. David Haddox.
Lippincott Williams & Wilkins,
Philadelphia, © 2000

26

Chronic Pelvic Pain

Daniel Brookoff

*D. Brookoff: Methodist Comprehensive Pain Institute,
Methodist Healthcare, Memphis, Tennessee 38104.*

I. OVERVIEW

Chronic pelvic pain is defined as any pelvic pain, continuous or episodic, that persists for more than 6 months. A recent Gallup poll of more than 5000 American women between the ages of 18 and 50 found that one in seven reported chronic pelvic pain and that the lifetime incidence of chronic pelvic pain in women was as high as 33%. Most of these women sought care from gynecologists and family practitioners. Fewer than 1% report using the resources of a pain management clinic.

II. ETIOLOGY OF CHRONIC PELVIC PAIN

The most common gynecologic causes of chronic pelvic pain in women under 30 are endometriosis and pelvic inflammatory disease. More than 20% of patients with pelvic inflammatory disease will have prolonged pelvic pain after the resolution of the acute episode. In women over 30, endometriosis and adhesions are still common causes, along with adenomyosis (growth of glandular tissue into the muscle wall of the endometrium). Many of these women can have pelvic pain from nongynecologic causes, emanating from the bowel, bladder, spine, or abdominal wall. In older women, lower abdominal pain accompanied by back pain may be a sign of pelvic relaxation associated with cystoceles, rectoceles, and enteroceles. Some causes of chronic pelvic pain are listed in Table 26-1.

A. Chronic Pelvic Pain Syndrome

Gynecologists still differentiate between pelvic pain with "anatomic" and "nonanatomic" (e.g., psychogenic) causes. Many hold to the tenet that chronic pelvic pain that does not have a cause that is identifiable on laparoscopy is psychogenic. This is a myth that has victimized many patients. Patients who have chronic pelvic pain without a remediable anatomic cause have been said to suffer either from chronic pelvic pain syndrome (CPP) or from chronic pelvic pain without obvious pathology (CPP-WOP). This syndrome, which is widely referred to in the gynecology literature, is characterized by

TABLE 26-1. *Causes of chronic pelvic pain*

Episodic pain
Dyspareunia
Mittleschmerz
Primary dysmenorrhea
Secondary dysmenorrhea
Adenomyosis
Endometriosis

Continuous pain
Endometriosis
Adhesions
Chronic pelvic inflammatory disease
Pelvic tumors
Uterine retroversion
Genital prolapse
Adenomyosis
Pelvic congestion syndrome
Vulvodynia
Ovarian remnant syndrome
Degenerating leiomyoma
Pelvic relaxation syndrome
Sympathetic pelvis syndrome
Obstructed menstrual flow (imperforate hymen or vaginal septum)

Nongynecologic causes of chronic pelvic pain
Irritable bowel syndrome
Colitis/proctitis
Interstitial cystitis
Urethral syndrome
Abdominal nerve disorders
Osteoporotic sacral fractures
Hematoma of the pyramidal muscle
Osteitis pubis
Pelvic joint instability (associated with precocious puberty and early use
   of oral contraceptives)

1. Duration of 6 months or longer
2. Incomplete relief with most treatments
3. Significantly impaired function at work or at home
4. Signs of depression, which can include anorexia, weight loss, and early-morning awakening
5. Pain out of proportion to pathology
6. Alteration in family roles
   CPP was originally meant to refer to those patients with no clear anatomic cause for their pain. It has also come to include patients who once had a clearly identifiable cause for the pain but who have failed to respond to accepted management and now present with continued pain for further care.

III. GOAL OF CARE

By the time a patient with pelvic pain presents to a pain clinic it may be more important to focus on the concept of treating chronic pain rather than an individual disease entity. At the same time, it is critical that pain clinicians be aware of specific pelvic pain syndromes so that treatable conditions do not go undiagnosed. For example, many women with interstitial cystitis—for which there are specific treatments—are subjected to gynecologic procedures and an average of 5 years of pelvic pain before the correct diagnosis is made. Patients should not be labeled "somatic" or "psychogenic." However, they do need to understand that it is normal for chronic pelvic pain to have a psychologic impact upon their lives and that these psychologic issues deserve attention and care.

IV. EVALUATION OF THE PATIENT WITH CHRONIC PELVIC PAIN

A. History

1. Location of pain

To ascertain the "Torso score" the patient is asked to rate pain from zero to 10 in any of the 30 locations on the diagram (Fig. 26-1). In patients who indicate pain in one or two areas and assign a high score, structurally remediable disease is likely to be found. Localization by the patient may be more revealing than the physical examination. For example, ovarian pain is often described as originating in the umbilical, periumbilical, or upper abdominal regions but is difficult to reproduce on physical examination. Patients who have a total score of more than 30 or indicate pain greater than 7 in more than four areas usually do not derive benefit from further laparoscopy.

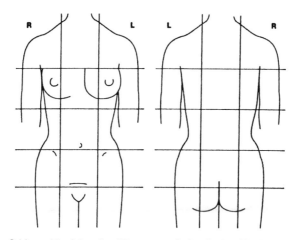

FIG. 26-1. Grid used to determine "Torso score" of patients with chronic pelvic pain. Patients put value from 1 (pain is just noticeable) to 10 (pain is so severe that working is impossible) in boxes where pain occurs. (Reprinted with permission from Nolan TE, Elkins TE. Chronic pelvic pain: Differentiating anatomic from functional causes. *Postgrad Med* 1993;94:125–128, 131–134, 138.)

2. Periodicity of pain

In addition to ascertaining whether pain is episodic or continuous, determine the relationship of the pain to the menstrual cycle. Many women who begin using oral contraceptives in their teens and stop after marriage in their mid-20s may never have experienced mittleschmerz pain or dysmenorrhea before the current episode of pain.

3. Exacerbating factors

The relationship of pain to changes in position or sexual activity may yield important clues to its origin. For example, the pain of pelvic congestion syndrome tends to worsen when the patient bends forward. A detailed description of dyspareunia may guide nerve block therapy. For example, "entry dyspareunia" suggests vaginismus and possible hymenal syndrome. Dyspareunia during deep thrusting is often a sign of endometriosis.

4. Review of previous therapies

Obtain a careful history of previous medications, hormonal manipulations, and surgical interventions. Patients who continue to have dysmenorrhea-type pain after a good trial of NSAIDs may have endometriosis or adenomyosis. Adhesions on previous laparoscopic examination may correlate poorly with severity or duration of pain but are often correlated with the location of pain and can guide nerve blocks.

5. Assessment of nongynecologic symptoms

Question the patient about bowel and bladder symptoms. For example, cramping pelvic pain with alternating bouts of constipation and diarrhea may be a sign of irritable bowel syndrome. Pelvic pain accompanied by urinary urgency may indicate interstitial cystitis.

B. Physical Examination

1. Abdominal examination

Differentiating between pelvic pain and abdominal pain can sometimes be difficult. Examine the abdominal wall with the patient's legs bent to assess for visceral sites of pain and then reexamine with rectus muscles stretched (legs hyperextended) to find abdominal trigger points typical of myofascial pain syndrome. Have the patient tense the rectus muscles by straight-leg raising or lifting her head and shoulders off the table. Tensing the rectus muscles usually reduces the pain of visceral disease.

2. Pelvic examination

Examine the external genitalia for signs of fistulae or herpes. Look for vulvar or perivulvar varices typical of pelvic congestion syndrome. If the patient complains of introital discomfort, examine the vulvar mucosa with a cotton-tipped swab, looking for tender areas and for areas of punctate, erythematous lesions characteristic of vulvar/vestibular syndrome. Many women who complain of vaginismus during intercourse will not have pronounced contractions on vaginal examination. On pelvic examination, begin palpating at the umbilicus and move downward. Palpable lesions with reproducible focal pain may indicate endometriosis. Palpate the uterus and adnexa for masses. Diffuse fullness may be a sign of pelvic congestion syndrome. A frozen pelvis is usually a sign of chronic pelvic inflammatory disease or endometriosis. Urethral tenderness may indicate urethral syndrome or interstitial cystitis.

3. Examination of other sites

Patients with chronic pelvic pain should be assessed for costovertebral angle tenderness, which can be a sign of indolent pyelonephritis. Rectal examination will allow for palpation of a thickened uterosacral ligament, which is a sign of endometriosis. Rectal tenderness can be a sign of proctitis or colitis. Look for evidence of spinal or muscle tenderness and check for signs of thyroid dysfunction.

C. Psychologic Evaluation

The psychologic interview forms the framework for recognition by the patient that this is a vital aspect of her health and well-being. Included in the psychologic evaluation is an assessment of sleep disorders, eating problems, excessive concern with body image, substance abuse, violence, and history of personal loss. Assess for dysfunctional marital, personal, or family relationships and for signs of depression.

The Minnesota Multiphasic Personality Inventory (MMPI) is often helpful in the psychologic evaluation as the Beck Depression Inventory. In addition to the usual pain-measurement surveys, women-oriented measurement tools such as the West Haven–Yale Multidimensional Pain Inventory (WHYMPI) have proved especially useful in assessing chronic pelvic pain.

1. Assessing for physical and sexual abuse

A history of sexual or physical abuse has been associated with a variety of pain syndromes, but the association is particularly strong in chronic pelvic pain. This relationship may be more than psychogenic, given the physical damage to the genital organs that often occurs during sexual abuse. Although patients with chronic pelvic pain with and without histories of sexual abuse do not generally differ in terms of description of pain or functional disability, patients with a history of abuse tend to have higher levels of somatization, greater psychologic distress, and poorer response to medications.

D. Diagnostic Testing

Women who are referred to pain clinics for pelvic pain have usually undergone extensive diagnostic testing, including laparoscopy. Additional laboratory testing rarely differentiates among different types of pelvic pain.

V. SPECIFIC PELVIC PAIN SYNDROMES

A. Endometriosis

Pelvic pain due to endometriosis is strongly associated with the presence of deep disease in which the lesions penetrate at least 5 mm beyond the peritoneal surface. The most common treatments are gonadotropin-releasing hormone agonists, androgens, and progestins. Oral contraceptives may be just as effective (especially when administered continuously instead of cyclically) and can be continued for longer durations. In successful medically treated cases, the pain resolves within 2 months but often returns when medical therapies are discontinued. Many patients who have had successful treatment of endometriosis with laser or thermal endocoagulator ablation may have increased pain for months after the procedure and may require analgesics. If pain persists, consider superior hypogastric plexus block, laparoscopic uterine nerve ablation, or presacral neurectomy.

B. Nerve Entrapment Syndromes

Many Pfannenstiel-type incisions cross-cut both the ilioinguinal and iliohypogastric nerves. Retraction of these nerves around the incision line may result in overstretching and avulsive-type nerve injuries and severe chronic pelvic pain. These patients can be treated by repeated local anesthetic nerve blocks. Abdominal wall catheters can be placed for continuous local irrigation of the nerves between the transversalis and oblique muscle groups if there is only a transient response to blocks. These nerves can also be ablated with cryotherapy. In instances where multiple nests of neuromas may be active and refractory to other treatments, surgical extirpation of the local nests can be considered. The risk of creating new neuromas must be considered.

Perineal pain may be due to pudendal nerve entrapment. Diagnostic pudendal nerve blocks with local anesthetic or electromyography and nerve conduction studies of the pelvic floor may be useful to confirm the diagnosis. Some patients will require surgical neurolysis.

C. Genitofemoral Nerve Disorders

The distribution of this nerve includes the lower abdomen and the perineum. The patient will often give a history of lower abdominal pain or back pain that has migrated into the perineum. There is often a good response to nerve blocks.

D. Hymenal Syndrome

Hymenal syndrome is characterized by pain at the introitus without visible lesions. The patient may appear distraught and histrionic during the gynecologic examination, and pain often prevents the examiner from getting past the introitus. There is no pain on examination of the vagina, cervix, uterus, or adnexae. These patients often have a history of infection with *Candida albicans*. Repeated yeast infections may cause irritation of superficial nerves around the hymenal ring. The pain leads to severe sexual dysfunction, but patients usually report that they were not dysfunctional before the onset of the pain syndrome. Hymenal blocks may prove effective, but definitive therapy may involve surgical extirpation of the hymenal ring.

E. Sympathetic Pelvic Syndrome

Patients with this syndrome, which is a sequela of endometriosis or chronic pelvic inflammatory disease, complain of deep pain originating in the pelvic organs not associated with physically detectable abdominal wall tenderness or myofascial disease of the abdominal musculature. There may be some cutaneous pain that is referred from visceral structures. Nerve blocks can prove both diagnostic and therapeutic, starting with a paracervical block, pudendal nerve block, and a block of one of the auxiliary nerves of the perineum. The last block in the series is a superior hypogastric ganglion block. Nerve ablation techniques may be considered for patients who get definite but temporary relief from these blocks.

F. Primary Dysmenorrhea

In this syndrome, pain is due to excessive production of prostaglandins and other inflammatory mediators at the end of the luteal phase of the menstrual cycle that promote myometrial contractility and vascular spasms leading to ischemia and pain. Treatment with NSAIDs or oral contraceptives is usually effective. In addition, calcium channel blockers (e.g., nifedipine 20 to 90 mg/day) magnesium or electrostimulation may be useful.

G. Pelvic Congestion Syndrome

This is an uncommon and frequently overlooked cause of debilitating pelvic pain. It is caused by dilated, incompetent ovarian veins in women with a history of two or more pregnancies. Symptoms include pelvic pain and heaviness that is most severe premenstrually and is exacerbated by prolonged standing or coitus. One of the most consistent symptoms is an increase in pain upon bending forward. Bladder irritability and urinary urgency are frequently present as well. A typical finding is vulvar or perivulvar varices that can extend into the posterior-medial thigh and buttock. The diagnosis is made by selective ovarian venography, which demonstrates dilated incompetent ovarian veins that often fill to the ovary. Transvaginal ultrasound with color duplex sonography shows promise as a less invasive way to make the diagnosis. The pain resolves with ovarian vein ligation.

H. Ovarian Remnant Syndrome

This is seen in patients who have had hysterectomy and bilateral salpingo-oophorectomy for severe endometriosis or pelvic inflammatory disease. It usually presents with episodic lateral pelvic pain, most often beginning 2 to 5 years after the initial oophorectomy. It responds to hormonal manipulation or surgical removal of the remnant.

I. Vulvodynia

Vulvodynia is characterized by chronic burning or stinging sensations in the vulvar area. It often has an acute onset. Half of these patients have long histories of entry dyspareunia and pain upon inserting tampons, pain on wearing pants, or pain on riding a bicycle. There are usually no abnormalities on physical exam. The pain can be elicited by touching the vestibule with a moist cotton swab. Corticosteroid-responsive dermatosis (usually characterized by redness, blisters, erosions) must be ruled out. Therapies for idiopathic vulvodynia include removal of the vulvar vestibule through perineoplasty or treatment with a flashlamp-excited dye laser. Success also has been reported using electromyographic biofeedback of the pelvic floor musculature.

J. Interstitial Cystitis/Urethral Syndrome

These syndromes are characterized by urinary urgency, frequency, dysuria (with sterile urine), and suprapubic pain. Urethral syndrome occurs in women during the reproductive years, and interstitial cystitis was classically thought to occur in perimenopausal women (though more than 25% of women are under 30 at presentation). The diagnosis of interstitial cystitis is often made by seeing pinpoint hemorrhages in the bladder submucosa after cystoscopic hydrodistension. Oral doses of pentosan polysulphate, bladder distension, and intravesicular instillation of antiinflammatory agents have sometimes proven useful for the treatment of interstitial cystitis.

VI. SPECIFIC MANAGEMENT TECHNIQUES FOR CHRONIC PELVIC PAIN

A. Medical Management

It is often useful to initiate some form of therapy on the first visit. Tricyclic antidepressants are often effective in reducing chronic pelvic pain. If tolerated, nonsteroidal analgesics should be part of the treatment regimen. Chronic pelvic pain sometimes responds to other medications used to treat neuropathic pain (e.g., gabapentin, mexiletine). The use of opioids for the treatment of chronic pelvic pain is controversial. There is growing evidence that long-term opioid treatment, using controlled-release formulations, is safe and appropriate in selected patients with intractable pain and no history of drug abuse.

B. Nerve Blocks and Nerve Ablation

1. Pudendal nerve block

Pudendal nerve block can relieve pain in the dermatomal distributions of S-2, S-3, and S-4. Blockade of the ganglion impar (ganglion of Walther) can be used to manage intractable perineal pain of sympathetic origin. Patients with presumed "intrapelvic ligamentous strain" can be treated with paracervical trigger point injections of 5 ml of 0.5% bupivacaine and 25 mg prednisolone. In resistant cases, 6% aqueous phenol has been used. Inject into the area where the needle point reproduces the patient's usual sharp pain. The pain is generally relieved within 5 to 10 minutes.

2. Uterosacral Nerve Block

To evaluate if pain is coming from uterosacral ligament, infiltrate 3 to 5 ml of 1% lidocaine into each ligament. If the pain is relieved on reassessment after 10 minutes, the patient may benefit from a uterosacral nerve ablation. Laparoscopic uterine nerve ablation is often offered to patients with centrally located pain who have failed medical therapy. This procedure has been effective for 3 months in a randomized double-blind trial in women with intractable primary dysmenorrhea and endometriosis, but the pain returned within a year in half of these women.

3. Superior hypogastric block

The superior hypogastric plexus block has been shown to be effective in chronic pelvic pain and in patients with pain due to endometriosis. This block generally helps centrally located pain but not adnexal discomfort. If blocks do not result in persistent analgesia, the sympathetic innervation to the uterus can be interrupted at the level of the superior hypogastric plexus by presacral neurectomy. This can be performed by laparotomy or laparoscopy. Presacral neurectomy has been effective in the treatment of dysmenorrhea and has yielded equivocal results for patients with chronic pelvic pain due to endometriosis. Presacral neurectomy works best in patients who have central pelvic pain. It can give relief when uterosacral nerve ablation has failed. The side effects can include constipation and urinary urgency.

C. Electrical Stimulation

Approximately one-third of women with chronic pelvic pain get some relief with electrical stimulators. Stimulation of A-delta myelinated fibers at the S-3 and S-4 roots may decrease spasm of the pelvic floor and may excite antinociceptive neurons. This modality has had excellent results in women with dysmenorrhea.

D. Intraspinal Medications

Intrathecal drug therapy may be an important option for selected patients with refractory pelvic pain. In our clinic we have seen good results using intrathecal opioids (e.g., morphine, hydromorphone, fentanyl) in combination with clonidine and local anesthetics delivered by implantable pumps.

RECOMMENDED READING

Duleba AJ, Keltz MD, Olive DL. Evaluation and management of chronic pelvic pain. *J Am Assoc Gynecol Laparascopists* 1996;3: 205–227.

Ling FW, Slocumb JC. Use of trigger point injections in chronic pelvic pain. *Obstet Gynecol Clin North Am* 1993;20:809–815.

Mathias SD, Kuppermann M, Liberman RF, Lipschutz RC, Steege JF. Chronic pelvic pain: prevalence, health-related quality of life and economic correlates. *Obstet Gynecol* 1996;87:321–327.

McDonald, JS. Management of chronic pelvic pain. *Obstet Gynecol Clin North Am* 1993;20:817–838.

Nolan TE, Elkins TE. Chronic pelvic pain: Differentiating anatomic from functional causes. *Postgrad Med* 1993;94:125–132.

Patt RB, Plancarte R. Superior hypogastric plexus block: A new therapeutic approach for pelvic pain. In: Waldman SD, Winnie AP, eds. *Interventional Pain Management.* Philadelphia: WB Saunders; 1996.

Robinson JC. Chronic pelvic pain. *Curr Opin Obstet Gynecol* 1993;5: 740–743.

Sant GR, ed. *Interstitial cystitis.* Philadelphia: Lippincott-Raven; 1997.

Wesslmann U, Burnett AL, Heinberg LJ. The urogenital and rectal pain syndromes. *Pain* 1997;73:269–294.

The Pain Clinic Manual, Second Edition,
edited by Stephen E. Abram and J. David Haddox.
Lippincott Williams & Wilkins,
Philadelphia, © 2000

27

Postdural Puncture Headache

Margaret Charsley

*M. Charsley: Department of Anesthesiology and Critical Care Medicine,
University of New Mexico, Health Sciences Center—School of Medicine,
Albuquerque, New Mexico 87131.*

Headache following dural puncture is related to the loss of cerebrospinal fluid (CSF) through the dural defect. The resultant decrease in CSF volume and pressure leads to sagging of the brain within the cranial vault and traction on pain-sensitive supporting structures such as the tentorium, falx cerebri, venous sinuses, and cerebral vessels. Furthermore, a compensatory mechanism to restore the intracranial volume results in dilatation of intracranial blood vessels. These features impart to the headache both postural and vascular characteristics.

Many factors affect the incidence of the headache. Smaller needles have a lower incidence overall, as do pencil-point or blunt-tip needles in some hands. The incidence is lower when the dura is punctured with longitudinal bevel orientation, a small or acute angle, or a lateral approach. Incidence is increased between the ages of 13 and 40 years, with a further increase in parturients.

I. CHARACTERISTICS
   A. Postural Headache
      1. Occurs only when the patient is upright, or minimally symptomatic when the patient is recumbent.
      2. Is reported as a dull ache, often throbbing in nature.
      3. May be occipital, frontal, occipitofrontal, or diffuse.
      4. Ranges from mild to severe.
      5. Is increased by jugular venous compression and head shaking.
      6. Is decreased by carotid artery compression, Valsalva maneuver.
   B. Associated Symptoms (more common with severe type)
      1. Stiff neck, pain radiating to neck and shoulders, low back pain.
      2. Eye symptoms such as diplopia, blurred vision, trouble focusing, spots before the eyes, photophobia.
      3. Diminished hearing, tinnitus, vertigo, hearing loss.
      4. Nausea and vomiting.

C. Duration
   1. Twenty-four percent subside within 48 hours.
   2. Greater than 50% subside spontaneously within 4 days.
   3. Approximately 72% subside within 1 week with minimal intervention.
   4. Rarely, may persist for weeks or months.
   5. Those patients whose headaches persist may go on to experience chronic headache and cervical pain.

   CAUTION: When headache is not postural or when it is accompanied by fever, look immediately for other causes (e.g., aseptic or bacterial meningitis, cortical vein thrombosis, subdural hematoma). A neurology work-up, including a computed tomography or magnetic resonance imaging, may be indicated.

II. MANAGEMENT SCHEMA
   A. Conservative Management (generally effective for mild type)
      1. Avoid dehydration
         a. Ensure patient is taking adequate p.o. fluids so that CSF production is not decreased.
         b. Probably not very important unless dehydration is severe, since CSF production is constant over a wide range of conditions, including dehydration (0.35 ml/min to 0.5 ml/min)
         c. Intravenous fluids if patient unable to take p.o. but no more than necessary
      2. Abdominal binder
         a. Increases epidural back pressure and may increase CSF pressure.
         b. Use has declined in recent years.
      3. Analgesics
         a. Aspirin, acetaminophen, ibuprofen
         b. May allow patient to ambulate.
      4. Bedrest
         a. If patient cannot tolerate erect position
         b. Lateral or prone position preferred
         c. Recumbency does not shorten duration of headache
         d. Some feel that the erect position hastens recovery by allowing the increased lumbar CSF pressure to approximate the dura to the rigid structures of the spinal canal and thereby help to seal the tear.
   B. Caffeine Sodium Benzoate
      1. Reported to provide effective, lasting relief in 75% of patients
      2. Reported by others to be merely palliative, while permanent relief depended on timing
      3. Oral caffeine 300 mg p.o. bid (useful if no iv access)
      4. Caffeine sodium benzoate 500 mg/2ml iv
         a. May be placed in 500 ml of Ringer's lactate if patient needs fluids.
         b. May be repeated in 1 to 2 hours.

5. Mechanism of action
   a. Induces cerebral vasoconstriction.
   b. Acts as a cerebral adenosine receptor antagonist.

C. Other Pharmacologic Interventions

1. Sumatriptan in doses of 6 mg subcutaneously with a repeat injection in 1 hour (maximum 12 mg in 24 hours) has a success rate of 50% to 70%
2. Cafergot (ergotamine tartrate 1 mg and caffeine 100 mg) has a reported success rate of 85% after a single dose
3. Theophylline 300 mg p.o. single-dose sustained-release tablet
4. Proposed mechanism
   a. All the preceding drugs cause decreases in cerebral blood flow by cerebrovascular vasoconstriction.
5. These options would probably not be suitable for patients with certain systemic diseases which could be adversely affected by these drugs' actions.
6. Despite reported success, studies are limited.

D. Saline Epidural

1. Place catheter in epidural space or possibly use existing catheter—caudal approach requires more volume.
2. Infuse preservative-free normal saline approximately 50 to 60 ml (90 ml if caudal).
3. May repeat procedure if initially ineffective.
4. The continuous infusion of 1 to 1.5 liters of lactated Ringers solution in 24 hours through an existing catheter as a prophylactic measure after accidental dural puncture with a large gauge needle has had limited success.
5. Mechanism of action
   a. Increased volume in epidural space transmits pressure to intrathecal space and bolsters sagging CSF pressure.
6. Seldom employed today unless epidural blood patch (EBP) is contraindicated.

E. Epidural Blood Patch

1. Recognized as the definitive treatment for postdural puncture headache
2. Method
   a. All procedures must be performed with meticulously sterile technique.
   b. Need not be performed at the level of the dural puncture. (A cervical dural puncture headache has been successfully treated with a lumbar EBP.) Spread of blood is primarily cephalad.
   c. When epidural needle is in place, draw 15 to 20 ml of the patient's blood and inject it slowly or until discomfort (greater success rate with the greater volume).

    d. If paresthesias are elicited during needle placement or injection, reposition needle.

    e. The patient may remain supine for about 30 minutes, though early ambulation is encouraged.

3. The HIV-positive patient

    a. There are theoretical concerns of providing a possible route of viral entry into the central nervous system.

    b. Successful treatment of HIV-positive patients with EBP and no untoward sequelae have been reported.

    c. General feeling is that EBP should be used only when conservative methods have truly failed.

4. The septic patient

    a. Better to avoid EPB and employ conservative measures, saline epidural

    b. Epidural Dextran-40 in volume of 20 to 30 ml, 10 ml/min, or an infusion of 100 ml at 3 ml/hr with appropriate monitoring has proved effective.

5. Prophylactic EBP

    a. More recent studies have found this to be effective in the majority of cases.

    b. If a catheter is in place this is definitely worth considering before removal, especially if the placement was difficult. (Catheter end and procedure must be kept sterile.)

    c. May give prophylactic dose of antibiotics prior to procedure.

RECOMMENDED READING

Abouleish E. Epidural blood patch for the treatment of post-lumbar puncture cephalgia. *Anesthesiology* 1978;49:291–292.

Bevacqua BK, Slucky AV. Epidural blood patch in a patient with HIV infection. *Anesthesiology* 1991; 74:953.

Carbaat PAT, van Crevel H. Lumbar puncture headache: Controlled study on the preventive effect of 24 hours' bed rest. *Lancet* 1981;2:1133–1135.

Carp H, Singh PJ, Vadhera R, Jayaram A. Effects of the serotonin-receptor agonist sumatriptan on post-dural puncture headache: Report of six cases. *Anesth Analg* 1994;79:180–182.

Gibbons JJ. Post-dural puncture headache in the HIV-positive patient. *Anesthesiology* 1991;74:953–954.

Schwalbe SS, Schiffmiller MW, Marx GF. Theophylline for post-dural puncture headache. *Anesthesiology* 1991;75:A1082.

Sechzer P, Abel L. Postspinal analgesia headache treated with caffeine: Evaluation with the demand method. Part I. *Curr Ther Res* 1978;24:307–312.

Stuart AL. Sumatriptan and other wet tap options. Lecture Notes. Scott and White Memorial Hospital, Texas A & M University College of Medicine, Temple, Texas.

Thornberry EA, Thomas TA. Posture and post-spinal headache: A controlled trial in 80 obstetric patients. *Br J Anaesth* 1988;60:195–197.

The Pain Clinic Manual, Second Edition,
edited by Stephen E. Abram and J. David Haddox.
Lippincott Williams & Wilkins,
Philadelphia, © 2000

28

Central Pain Syndromes

Kenneth A. Follett

*K. A. Follett: Division of Neurosurgery, The University of Iowa Hospitals
and Clinics, Iowa City, Iowa 52242.*

I. CENTRAL ("DEAFFERENTATION") PAIN

Central ("deafferentation") pain is one of the most difficult pain syndromes to treat effectively. No existing treatments are uniformly successful, and the pathophysiology is understood poorly, which limits development and application of new treatments. The goal of therapy is pain "management"; it is unrealistic to anticipate pain "cure." Like many other chronic pain problems, adequate treatment of central pain usually requires that therapy be individualized. It may be managed most effectively using a multidisciplinary approach.

A. Pathogenesis
  1. Central pain arises following a partial or complete injury within the nervous system (spinal cord, brain stem, brain).
  2. Traumatic, vascular, inflammatory, neoplastic, and developmental abnormalities may give rise to central pain syndromes.
  3. The pathophysiologic mechanisms of central pain are not understood fully. Following deafferentation, synaptic connections remodel and neurotransmitter levels change within the CNS. These structural and neurochemical alterations may occur at the level of the spinal cord and/or brain. These CNS changes give rise to spontaneous and ectopic neuronal activity and abnormal excitability of central neurons to activation of peripheral receptors.

B. Characteristics
  1. Central pain, which is neuropathic, must be distinguished from nociceptive pain.
  2. Nociceptive pain reflects normal activation of nociceptors outside the CNS. In contrast, deafferentation pain reflects abnormal neuronal activity within the central nervous system.
  3. The structural and neurochemical changes that occur within the CNS after deafferentation account for the stereotypical qualities of central

pain (which can be similar to those observed in neuropathic pain of peripheral origin).

    a. Steady pain (aching, burning, tingling) may represent ongoing spontaneous activity in central neurons.

    b. Intermittent pain (lancinating, shooting, shocking, stabbing) may represent ectopic neuronal activity.

    c. Evoked pain (allodynia, hyperpathia) may reflect abnormal excitability of central neurons to normal peripheral receptor activation.

4. Pain may be felt in an anesthetic body area because of the deafferentation.

5. The onset of pain is delayed typically until several months following the CNS injury.

II. GENERAL APPROACH TO MANAGEMENT

A. Diagnosis

1. The underlying etiology of central pain is apparent in most cases through history alone (e.g., trauma, stroke, multiple sclerosis).

2. The physical examination may reveal neurologic abnormalities (motor or sensory loss, spasticity) but may be normal in some instances (e.g., lacunar stroke with no residual sensory or motor loss). Allodynia and/or hyperpathia may be present.

3. Be alert for complicating abnormalities that may generate superimposed chronic pain (e.g., painful spasticity after stroke or spinal cord injury, myofascial syndromes after trauma). These associated problems, rather than the underlying deafferentation, may be responsible for the pain for which the patient seeks treatment.

4. Radiographic studies may be used to confirm the diagnosis (e.g., CT or MRI for stroke, MRI for spinal cord pathology, myelography or MRI for root avulsion).

B. Treatment

1. Medical therapy is the primary means of treatment. Medications used generally for treating neuropathic pain can be beneficial. These agents may reduce abnormal neuronal activity. Be familiar with side effects of medications and monitor patients closely for side effects. Start with small doses, increase gradually to minimize intolerance, particularly in elderly individuals.

    a. Anticonvulsants may be especially useful for lancinating pain (e.g., carbamazepine 400 to 1200 mg/day, phenytoin 200 to 600 mg/day). The efficacy of gabapentin (may need 1800 to 2700 mg/day) is less certain, but it is generally better tolerated. Other anticonvulsants may prove useful occasionally. In general, the doses should be increased slowly until a therapeutic effect is achieved or side effects occur. Monitoring of blood levels is unnecessary unless toxicity develops or doses approach the high end of the recommended ranges.

    b. Antidepressants may be particularly useful for constant, dysesthetic pain. Tricyclic antidepressants in small to moderate doses (e.g., amitriptyline, 75 to 100 mg/day) should be tried initially. High doses are generally no more effective than smaller ones. Other classes of antidepressants (e.g., selective serotonin reuptake inhibitors) may be useful, but their efficacies are less certain.

    c. Miscellaneous medications

       (1) Analgesics (e.g., NSAIDs, aspirin, acetaminophen, opiates)

       (2) Baclofen (important for patients in whom spasticity may cause or contribute to pain)

       (3) Clonidine

       (4) Clonazepam

       (5) Mexiletine

2. Adjuvant therapies used for management of other chronic pain syndromes may be useful in selected instances (e.g., physical rehabilitation, TENS, cognitive and behavioral programs, acupuncture).

3. Surgical management may be considered if (a) pain has a clearly defined etiology, (b) pain intensity interferes with daily activities or employment, (c) pain duration is severe enough that spontaneous resolution is unlikely (greater than 6 to 12 months), (d) more conservative therapies have failed, (e) psychologic evaluation reveals no substantial confounding factors, and (f) expectations of surgical treatment are clear to physicians and patients.

    a. Surgical procedures have moderate success rates at best but may be useful in selected instances.

    b. Many procedures (e.g., deep brain stimulation, intracranial ablative procedures) require special expertise in the surgical management of chronic pain.

    c. Augmentative procedures include spinal cord stimulation (SCS), deep brain stimulation (DBS, not FDA approved for use within the United States at this time), and intraspinal or intraventricular drug administration. The overall success rate of spinal cord stimulation is low, but a trial of SCS is simple and safe (used primarily for pain of spinal origin, such as phantom limb pain). Intraspinal drug infusion therapy provides partial pain relief in approximately 65% of patients with deafferentation pain, but the long-term effectiveness is not established. The long-term efficacy of DBS is not well established but is generally 50% or less.

    d. Ablative procedures are used rarely and are performed typically at centers with special expertise in the surgical management of intractable pain. Ablative procedures include dorsal root entry zone (DREZ) lesion, cordotomy (open or percutaneous), mesencephalic tractotomy, and thalamotomy. Cingulotomy is reported to attenuate neuropathic pain of nonmalignant origin, but it is used rarely and typically only for patients with cancer-related pain.

e. In general, the simple augmentative procedures (spinal cord stimulation and spinal drug infusion therapy) should be tried prior to ablative procedures. Central pain arises from neuronal injury and may worsen following further destruction of neural tissues. The major exception to this rule is that DREZ lesioning can be considered early in patients with phantom-limb pain and "end zone" pain following spinal cord injury.

f. The efficacies of specific surgical procedures are influenced by the characteristics of the pain.

   (1) Stimulation procedures (SCS, DBS) are most effective for steady, dysesthetic pain and have little or no effect on lancinating or evoked pain.

   (2) Ablative procedures may have little effect on steady pain but can attenuate lancinating or evoked pain.

III. SPECIFIC PAIN SYNDROMES

A. Pain of Spinal Origin

   1. General characteristics

      a. Most cases (2/3) result from trauma.

      b. Pain may occur in patients with complete or incomplete spinal injuries.

      c. Most patients (2/3) have steady pain; the rest have steady pain with superimposed paroxysmal (lancinating) pain.

      d. Pain may occur in a bandlike distribution at the level of sensory loss ("end zone" or "border zone" pain), or it may be diffuse or patchy below the level of the lesion, or may be felt as "visceral" pain (pelvic or perirectal).

      e. Allodynia and hyperpathia are common (in areas of preserved sensation).

      f. Posttraumatic syringomyelia may be present. This possibility can be evaluated with MRI or myelography if necessary. The syrinx can enlarge and result in symptom progression (although its role in pain generation is unknown).

   2. Treatment

      a. Nonsurgical therapy is the mainstay of treatment.

      b. Surgical therapies have low success rates in general (exception: DREZ).

         (1) Spinal cord stimulation (more effective in patients with partial spinal cord injuries with sparing of some sensory function) has a low overall success rate but a trial is simple and safe.

      (2) Spinal drug infusion therapy may be beneficial, but the long-term success rate is not established. Patency of the spinal canal should be evaluated (MRI or myelography) prior to consideration of this therapy.

      (3) Deep brain stimulation may provide long-term pain relief but appears to be effective in fewer than 40% of patients.

      (4) Rhizotomy is of limited use but may control radicular allodynia/hyperpathia.

      (5) Cordotomy may be useful for managing lancinating pain and allodynia/hyperpathia below C-5 level (29% complete pain relief, 43% partial pain relief over long-term follow-up).

      (6) DREZ lesioning may provide pain relief in as many as 70% of patients with border zone pain at the level of spinal cord injury or pain associated with brachial or lumbosacral plexus root avulsion. (Root avulsion can be confirmed with MRI or myelography.) These are among the best indications for surgery for chronic neuropathic pain.

B. Postamputation Pain

  1. Stump pain

    a. General characteristics

      (1) Stump pain is not the same as phantom-limb pain. Stump pain is felt in the remaining portion of the amputated limb, not in the absent portion of the limb.

      (2) It may be diffuse or focal.

      (3) It may occur in conjunction with phantom-limb pain.

      (4) It may be caused by a neuroma in the stump.

    b. Treatment

      (1) Therapy is usually nonsurgical.

      (2) Stump revision may be beneficial if pain is related to a specific stump abnormality (e.g., infection, bone spur), but revision as a measure to treat pain in the absence of specific pathology is not useful.

      (3) Pain/paresthesias related to a neuroma (pain produced by palpation at a discrete site on the stump) may improve following resection of the neuroma.

      (4) Surgical procedures have low success rates. In contrast to phantom-limb pain, spinal cord stimulation does not improve stump pain. Spinal drug infusion therapies may be useful.

  2. Phantom-limb pain

    a. General characteristics

      (1) Pain is present in an absent portion of the extremity (unlike stump pain).

   (2) Pain usually develops shortly after amputation. It may resolve spontaneously (usually within 1 year).

   (3) Pain can be steady and/or intermittent, burning, aching, or cramping. The phantom limb may be perceived as being in a state of painful dystonic posturing.

  b. Treatment

   (1) Nonsurgical therapy should be tried initially, but surgical treatment may be more useful in this disorder than for other central pain syndromes.

   (2) Sympathectomy may relieve causalgic pain.

   (3) Either spinal cord stimulation (trial is simple, safe) or DREZ lesion is the surgical procedure of choice (up to 67% of patients report improvement after DREZ). Other surgical procedures have low long-term success rates.

 3. Poststroke pain

  a. General characteristics

   (1) "Thalamic pain" is a misnomer because lesions in other areas of the brain can produce pain.

   (2) Pain usually arises in a delayed fashion.

   (3) The most common etiology is ischemic supratentorial stroke, but pain may occur after hemorrhagic supratentoral stroke or after brain stem stroke (especially lateral medullary or "Wallenberg's" syndrome).

   (4) Pain is present typically in a body area with stroke-related sensory loss. (Sensory loss may be minimal.)

   (5) Pain may be steady and/or intermittent.

   (6) Hyperpathia and allodynia are common.

  b. Treatment

   (1) Therapy is usually nonsurgical.

   (2) Surgical treatments that have been advocated include mesencephalic tractotomy, medial thalamotomy, or deep brain stimulation, but these procedures have relatively low long-term success rates.

IV. SUMMARY

The primary method of controlling central pain is through nonsurgical means. Surgical procedures have relatively low long-term success rates. Simple augmentative procedures (spinal cord stimulation and intraspinal drug infusion) are low-risk procedures and may warrant consideration if more conservative measures do not provide adequate pain relief. Concern about lesioning neural tissues to treat pain that arises from neural injury (with the attendant risk of causing additional postsurgical dysesthetic pain) has reduced enthusiasm for ablative procedures. Given the relatively low long-term success rates of ablative surgery and their potential complications, they should not be offered to patients indiscriminately, but they may be considered in carefully selected cases and performed by surgeons with special expertise in ablative surgery for pain management.

RECOMMENDED READING

Levy RM, Lamb S, Adams JE. Treatment of chronic pain by deep brain stimulation: Long-term follow-up and review of the literature. *Neurosurgery* 1987;21:885–893.

Loeser JD. Pain after amputation: Phantom limb and stump pain. In: JJ Bonica, ed. *The Management of Pain*. Philadelphia: Lea and Febiger; 1990:244–256.

Nashold BS, Friedman AH, Sampson JH, Nashold JRB, El-Naggar AO. Dorsal root entry zone lesions for pain. In: JR Yeomans, ed. *Neurological Surgery*. Philadelphia: WB Saunders; 1996:3452–3462.

Tasker RR. Pain resulting from central nervous system pathology (central pain). In: Bonica JJ, ed. *The Management of Pain*. Philadelphia: Lea and Febiger; 1990:264–283.

Tasker RR, DeCarvalho GTC, Dolan EJ. Intractable pain of spinal cord origin: Clinical features and implications for surgery. *J Neurosurg* 1992;77:373–378.

The Pain Clinic Manual, Second Edition,
edited by Stephen E. Abram and J. David Haddox.
Lippincott Williams & Wilkins,
Philadelphia, © 2000

29

Management of Painful Medical Diseases

John W. Luckwitz

J. W. Luckwitz: Mountain West Anesthesia, Salt Lake City, Utah 84117

I. INTRODUCTION

Management of chronic pain associated with medical illnesses presents some difficult challenges. Certain diseases are associated with long-standing persistent nociceptive stimulation, and drug tolerance is a common problem. Acute exacerbations of the disease may cause intense nociception, which, coupled with underlying tolerance, creates very high analgesic dose requirements. Pre-existing substance abuse further complicates management. Coordination of pain management with care by the physician managing the underlying disease is essential, since specific treatment for disease exacerbation is often a critical element of pain control.

II. PANCREATITIS

A. General Features

    1. May occur as an acute or chronic disease process.

    2. Pain management is a key feature in the treatment plan.

    3. Acute pancreatitis can often be diagnosed with a elevated serum amylase. Many other disorders must be included in the differential diagnosis.

    4. Chronic pancreatitis often presents with abnormal physical examination findings and normal laboratory results.

    5. Multidisciplinary pain management is necessary

        a. Behavioral modification, including cessation of alcohol abuse, is essential to treatment success.

        b. Coping strategies and lifestyle changes are often more beneficial than medications for patient management.

B. Clinical Features

    1. Acute pancreatitis

        a. Abdominal pain is a major feature.

(1) Poorly localized, continuous, steady, or boring in character

(2) Usually in the epigastrium and left upper quadrant, often with radiation to the back.

(3). The time of onset of pain to peak intensity ranges from minutes to hours.

b. Other symptoms

(1) Nausea, vomiting, abdominal distension, and decreased bowel sounds

(2) Tachycardia and hypotension often occur in the acute phase.

(3) Twenty percent of patients will develop pulmonary findings, including atelectasis, pleural effusion, basilar rales, or adult respiratory distress syndrome (ARDS).

c. Disease course

(1) In 85% of patients, the disease is self-limited.

(2) Ten percent mortality occurs during acute attacks despite aggressive medical management.

2. Chronic pancreatitis

a. Pain is predominant symptom.

(1) May be relatively constant or may occur as low-grade pain with superimposed recurrent acute attacks.

(2) Other, less common pain manifestations include bone pain from intramedullary fat necrosis and tender lower-extremity nodules from subcutaneous fat necrosis.

(3) Physical examination often reveals less abdominal tenderness than would be expected from patient complaints.

C. Pathogenesis

1. Major causes

a. Alcohol is the most common cause in the United States.

b. Biliary tract disease

c. Trauma

(1) Postoperative

(2) Nonsurgical, especially blunt trauma

d. Drugs

e. Infections

f. Connective tissue disease

g. Mechanical

h. Familial

2. Mechanisms of action

a. Proteolytic enzymes cause autodigestion of the pancreas and adjacent tissues.

b. Active enzymes cause digestion of cellular membranes, causing vascular damage, hemorrhage, fat necrosis, cellular injury, and further release of proteolytic enzymes.

c. Mechanism of action of most causative agents not yet identified.

D. Diagnosis
  1. Laboratory findings
     a. Serum amylase levels exceeding 200 Somogyi units per 100 ml usually establish the diagnosis of acute pancreatitis.
     b. The degree of amylase elevation does not correlate with the severity of disease.
     c. Elevation of amylase levels greater than 7 days usually indicates severe disease.
     d. Chronic pancreatitis is often not associated with elevated serum amylase.
     e. Other abnormal studies with acute pancreatitis include increased leukocyte count, increased hematocrit from hemoconcentration, hyperglycemia, hypocalcemia, and hyperlipidemia with gallstone pancreatitis.
     f. Roentgenograms
        (1) Acute—nonspecific ileus or localized gas collections in loops of bowel overlying the pancreas
        (2) Chronic—diffuse stippled pancreatic calcifications
  2. Differential diagnosis
     a. Acute bowel obstruction
     b. Perforated viscus
     c. Acute cholecystitis
     d. Dissecting abdominal aortic aneurysm
     e. Mesenteric artery occlusion
     f. Nephrolithiasis
     g. Myocardial infarction
     h. Diabetic ketoacidosis
     i. Pneumonia
E. Complications of Acute/Chronic Pancreatitis
  1. Pancreatic pseudocyst formation
  2. Pancreatic abscess
  3. Common bile duct obstruction
  4. Diabetes mellitus
  5. Exocrine insufficiency
F. Treatment
  1. Objectives
     a. Pain control
     b. Behavioral modification and patient education
     c. Decreased pancreatic stimulation and secretion
     d. Supportive medical care
  2. Acute pancreatitis
     a. Decrease pancreatic secretion
        (1) No oral alimentation

(2) Intravenous fluids

(3) NG suction when indicated

(4) Bedrest

b. Surgical intervention during acute stage associated with increased morbidity and mortality

c. Pain control

    (1) Nonsteroidal antiinflammatory drugs have theoretical risk of hemorrhagic pancreatitis.

    (2) Narcotic analgesics for acute phase are often indicated.

        (a) Meperidine is particularly poor choice because of low potency and toxic metabolite.

        (b) Patient-controlled analgesia (PCA) with morphine, hydromorphone

    (3) Continuous thoracic or lumbar epidural anesthetic infusion usually effective during acute phase.

    (4) Percutaneous intrapleural catheter. Useful mainly in patients requiring chest tubes resulting in significant chest pain.

    (5) Celiac plexus blockade with local anesthetic with or without steroid

        (a) Used in conjunction with conservative therapy

        (b) Should decrease opioid requirement.

        (c) Immediate risks include intravascular, epidural, or intrathecal injection.

        (d) The most common side effects include hypotension and diarrhea.

        (e) Retroperitoneal abscess can occur; may be greater risk if steroids are used.

d. Parenteral nutrition for protracted pancreatitis

e. Antibiotic therapy for infection

f. Patient education

    (1) Identification of inciting factors

    (2) Avoidance of alcohol, fatty foods

3. Chronic pancreatitis

a. Pain control—medications

    (1) Chronic opioid maintenance—controversial

        (a) Long-acting opioid (e.g., methadone or sustained-release morphine preferred over short-acting opioids such as oxycodone)

        (b) Potent, short-acting opioids appropriate for acute exacerbations

    (2) Try to achieve a stable, nonescalating dose.

    (3) Opioid abuse is a real concern among patients with alcohol abuse history.

    b. Nonneurolytic celiac plexus block
      (1) Celiac plexus blockade with local anesthetic may provide weeks or months of pain relief.
    c. Neurolysis of the celiac plexus
      (1) Should be considered only in patients with transient but excellent relief with local anesthetic blockade.
      (2) Temporary relief from local anesthetic block is not a good predictor for long-term benefit from neurolytic block.
      (3) Patients with a history of alcohol abuse are less likely to have good response; reduction in opioid use unlikely; continued pain complaints likely.
      (4) Either phenol or ethyl alcohol may be used.
      (5) Neurolytic agents may cause disruption of normal anatomy, making subsequent surgical interventions more difficult.
      (6) There is the potential for deafferentation pain after neurolysis.
      (7) Visceral deafferentation may lead to masking of a subsequent intraabdominal crisis (e.g., perforated ulcer).

III. SICKLE CELL DISEASE
  A. General Features
    1. Chronic medical condition with frequent acute painful crises
    2. High opioid requirements, frequent pain exacerbations common
      a. Many health care providers are uncomfortable with high long-term opioid needs.
    3. Multiple organ dysfunction affects opioid pharmacokinetics.
  B. Etiology
    1. Results from structural abnormality of B globin.
    2. Hb S is caused by a single amino acid replacement at position 6 of B globin.
    3. Sickle cell disease results from homozygous state Hb S S polypeptide chain (valine instead of glutamic acid).
  C. Prevalence
    1. Increased incidence in blacks of African or Afro-American heritage but also found in persons of Mediterranean, Saudi Arabian, and Indian ancestry.
    2. Incidence of homozygosity for Hb S S in blacks in the United States equals 1 in 400 births.
  D. Pathophysiology
    1. Polymerization of Hb S molecules inside erythrocytes results in chronic compensated hemolytic anemia, chronic progressive tissue damage, and intermittent acute painful crisis.
    2. Polymerization of Hb S occurs in deoxygenated conformation.
      a. Increased oxygen demand—fever, infection, exercise
      b. Decreased oxygen supply—hypoxia
      c. Decreased tissue blood flow—dehydration, hypothermia

E. Diagnosis
  1. Screening tests evaluate sickling tendency by adding antioxidants to erythrocytes.
  2. Hemoglobin electrophoresis is a definitive exam.
F. Pain Management
  1. Acute painful crisis
    a. Vasoocclusive crises occur at multiple sites, causing cerebrovascular accidents, acute chest syndrome (occlusion of pulmonary vessels), hepatic crisis, priapism, acute renal papillary infarction, and bone infarction.
    b. May present difficult differential diagnosis (acute appendicitis, bowel obstruction, septic arthritis, pneumonia, pulmonary infarction).
  2. Chronic pain resulting from recurrent vasoocclusive crisis.
    a. Refractory skin ulcers of the lower extremity
    b. Orthopedic sources
      (1) Degenerative arthritis
      (2) Aseptic necrosis of the hip (from infarction of the femoral head)
      (3) Vertebral compression fractures
G. Treatment
  1. Acute painful vasoocclusive crisis
    a. Hospitalization often required
    b. Supportive care, including IV hydration, supplemental oxygen, and antibiotics if secondary infection
    c. Patient controlled analgesia (PCA) becoming standard of care over intermittent parenteral (IV, IM, SQ) routes
    d. Demerol is a particularly poor opioid choice because of low potency and toxic metabolite, especially in patients with associated renal impairment and dehydration
  2. Chronic pain
    a. Mild pain may be managed with acetaminophen, NSAIDs.
    b. NSAIDs have risk of causing renal failure in patients with renal dysfunction.
    c. Opioid tolerance is common.
IV. HIV DISEASE
  A. General Features
    1. Infection with the human immunodeficiency virus covers a broad spectrum, ranging from asymptomatic infection to full-blown acquired immunodeficiency syndrome (AIDS).
    2. HIV patients may develop pain from multiple causes, and life-threatening opportunistic infections must first be ruled out before instituting pain management strategies.
    3. Approach to pain management in the HIV patient is similar to that in the cancer patient.

      a. Multidisciplinary approach ideal

      b. Underlying psychologic issues such as guilt, depression, and fear may interfere with normal coping strategies.

B. Clinical Features of Pain

  1. Incidence

      a. Prevalence of persistent pain in HIV disease ranges from 40% to 60%.

      b. Frequency and intensity of pain associated with HIV disease are higher with more advanced disease.

      c. Several distinct pain syndromes may occur simultaneously.

      d. One study indicates that 85% of HIV patients were receiving inadequate analgesic therapy.

         (1) Risk factors for undertreatment

            (a) Female sex

            (b) Low level of education

            (c) History of IV drug abuse

  2. Etiology of pain in HIV disease

      a. Direct effect from HIV disease

      b. Opportunistic infections

      c. Malignancies

      d. Medications, chemotherapy, or invasive procedures

  3. Clinical presentation

      a. Abdominal pain

         (1) Biliary tract disorders—sclerosing cholangitis, acalculous cholecystitis, infection (CMV, cryptosporidium), or cholelithiasis

         (2) Pancreatitis—often caused by pentamidine or didanosine

         (3) Bowel obstruction—non-Hodgkin's lymphoma or Kaposi's sarcoma

         (4) Idiopathic (nonspecific) abdominal pain

      b. Neuropathic pain

         (1) Distal asymmetrical polyneuropathy

            (a) HIV

            (b) Vitamin deficiency (B_2, B_6, B_{12})

            (c) Medication induced

         (2) Acute demyelinating polyneuropathy—Guillain Barré

         (3) Chronic relapsing inflammatory demyelinating polyneuropathy

         (4) Mononeuritis multiplex

         (5) Autonomic neuropathy

         (6) CMV-related polyradiculopathy

         (7) Postherpetic neuralgia

      c. Oropharyngeal and esophageal pain

         (1) Recurrent aphthous ulcers—candida, CMV, HSV, or medication induced

(2) Ulcerative esophagitis

(3) May cause significant anorexia and dysphagia, resulting in weight loss.

d. HIV-related headaches

(1) HIV encephalitis

(2) CNS lymphoma

(3) Cryptococcal meningitis—most common opportunistic infection causing headaches in HIV patients

(4) AZT-induced headaches

e. Herpes zoster

f. Back pain—osteomyelitis, disc herniation, facet arthropathy

g. Arthralgias

C. Treatment of Pain in HIV Patients

  1. Unique considerations to HIV disease

    a. Diarrhea or malabsorption may alter oral drug pharmacokinetics.

    b. Dysphagia may limit oral administration.

    c. Guilt and depression have an even greater impact than other chronic pain syndromes.

  2. General treatment strategies

    a. Multidisciplinary approach involving pain physician, psychologist, physical therapist, and hematologist most effective

    b. Basic principles of cancer pain management should be followed (WHO analgesic ladder).

      (1) Mild to moderate pain may often be managed with NSAIDs or acetaminophen.

      (2) Moderate to severe pain is generally treated with opioids.

      (3) Time-contingent dosing of long-acting opioids is generally preferred over prn short-acting opioids.

      (4) Judicious use of adjuvant agents may decrease opioid side effects and improve treatment efficacy.

  3. Specific agents

    a. Acetaminophen—risk of hepatotoxicity, masking of fever

    b. NSAIDs—gastrointestinal upset, risk of bleeding diathesis, renal and hepatotoxicity

    c. Tramadol

      (1) Careful use required in patients with CNS irritability

      (2) Increased blood levels in patients on TCAs, SSRIs, opioids

        (a) High blood levels associated with seizures

    d. Transdermal fentanyl—good choice for patients unable to tolerate oral medications or for patients noncompliant secondary to cognitive impairment

    e. Oral transmucosal fentanyl—quick-onset opioid for breakthrough pain

    f. Adjuvant medications

      (1) Antidepressants

          (a) Tricyclic antidepressants—improve sleep, antihyperalgesic in neuropathic pain states

          (b) Serotonin reuptake inhibitors—possibly less effect on neuropathic pain but often better tolerated as antidepressants

      (2) Anticonvulsants

          (a) Carbamazepine—good choice for intermittent lancinating neuropathic pain

          (b) Gabapentin—newer anticonvulsant with favorable side effect profile, good results with neuropathic pain

      (3) Sodium channel blockers

          (a) Systemic lidocaine

          (b) Oral mexiletine

      (4) Topical local anesthetics—EMLA cream, iontophoretic local anesthetic

      (5) Alpha-2 agonists

      (6) NMDA antagonists for neuropathic pain, central hyperalgesia—ketamine, amantadine, dextromethorphan

      (7) Gamma-aminobutyric acid (GABA) agonists

   4. Other treatment modalities

     a. TENS unit

     b. Neural blockade

        (1) Somatic or sympathetic nerve blocks

          (a) Celiac plexus blockade for chronic pancreatis

          (b) Sympathetic, intercostal or nerve root blocks for acute herpes zoster

        (2) Cryoanalgesia

        (3) Radiofrequency neurolysis

        (4) Neurolytic blocks using alcohol or phenol

     c. Implantable epidural or intrathecal opioid infusion systems*

     d. Spinal cord stimulators or peripheral nerve stimulators*

     e. Neurodestructive surgical procedures—rhizotomy, cordotomy, myelotomy, and celiac plexus surgical ablation

RECOMMENDED READING

Breitbart W, Rosenfeld B, et al. The undertreatment of pain in ambulatory AIDS patients. *Pain* 1996; 65:243–249,

Hanowell ST, Kennedy SF, MacNamara TE, et al. Celiac plexus block: Diagnostic and therapeutic applications in abdominal pain. *South Med J* 1980;73:1330–1332.

Lefkowitz M. Pain management in the AIDS patient. *J Florida Med Assoc* 1996;83(10):701–704.

O'Neill W, Sherrard J. Pain in human immunodeficiency viral disease: a review. *Pain* 1993;54:3–14.

Tassonyi E, Kun M, Rozsa I, et al. Epidural block in the treatment of acute pancreatitis. *Reg Anesth* 1981;6:8–12.

---

*Risk of infection of implantable systems in immunocompromised patients is considerable.

The Pain Clinic Manual, Second Edition,
edited by Stephen E. Abram and J. David Haddox.
Lippincott Williams & Wilkins,
Philadelphia, © 2000

30

Chronic Pain in Children

Doralina L. Anghelescu

*D. L. Anghelescu: Department of Anesthesiology,
St. Jude Children's Research Hospital, Memphis, Tennessee 38101.*

Chronic pain in children has been historically underappreciated and undertreated. Management of pediatric chronic pain involves a spectrum of therapeutic approaches delivered by a multidisciplinary team that includes pediatricians, psychologists, physical therapists, and anesthesiologists.

I. PEDIATRIC CANCER PAIN
  A. The Problem
    1. Moderate to severe pain is experienced by most children with malignancies at some point during the course of the disease.
    2. In the selected population of the National Cancer Institute, including children with advanced cancer undergoing aggressive chemotherapy and radiation protocols, 50% of inpatients and 25% of outpatients were found to experience some degree of pain. In defining goals, one should consider
      a. Pain control
      b. Functional improvement
      c. Quality of life
    3. Pain as a presenting symptom has been found in 62% of the children with newly diagnosed malignancy.
      a. Important initial symptoms of cancer often present for a significant period of time before the diagnosis is established.
      b. Potential indicator of a serious disease, persistent pain requires careful evaluation in children.
  B. Types of Cancer
    1. Leukemia, lymphoma, primary brain tumors, and sarcomas (Ewing's sarcoma, soft-tissue sarcoma, osteosarcoma) are the most frequently diagnosed cancers in children.
    2. Carcinomas are rare in children.

3. Many of these tumors are quite sensitive to chemotherapy or radiation therapy. Initiation of aggressive treatment strategies produces rapid tumor regression in the vast majority of newly diagnosed pediatric malignancies. A median duration of pain of 10 days was found to follow the initiation of cancer treatment.

C. Etiology
   1. Pain caused by malignancy
      a. As opposed to the adult cancer pain, which is caused by the tumor itself in 60% to 70% of cases, a minority of children have tumor-related pain.
      b. Tumor-related pain was found to be due to
         (1) Bone invasion
         (2) Soft-tissue invasion
         (3) Cord compression
         (4) Multiple concomitant causes
   2. Treatment-related pain
      a. Therapy-related pain was consistently found to be the predominant etiology of pain in children with cancer.
      b. Treatment-related pain represented two-thirds of the pain experienced by inpatients and more than 80% of pain experienced by outpatients (excluding procedure-related pain), and included the following:
         (1) Severe oral mucositis (after chemotherapy or total body irradiation)
         (2) Postoperative pain
         (3) Neuropathic pain (vincristine-related peripheral neuropathy, phantom-limb pain)
         (4) Prolonged postdural puncture headache
         (5) Abdominal pain from protracted chemotherapy-induced vomiting
         (6) Radiation dermatitis
         (7) Infection
      c. The high incidence of treatment-related pain in the pediatric population reflects
         (1) The aggressiveness of most pediatric cancer treatment protocols
         (2) The high long-term disease-free survival rates
   3. Pain unrelated to malignancy or treatment
      a. Preexisting painful conditions
      b. Trauma
D. Evaluation of Cancer Pain in Children
   1. Evaluate the location, nature, and intensity of pain. The characteristics of the pain can be suggestive of the etiology. Burning, shooting, tingling as descriptors of pain indicate pain of neuropathic origin.

2. Assess the etiology of pain. Effective treatment will be directed to the cause and mechanism of pain.

3. Anticipate the duration of pain. Tumor-associated pain at the initial diagnosis of cancer will be rapidly responsive to anticancer therapy. Terminally ill children often require invasive methods for long-term pain management.

4. Review previous therapeutic modalities and individual response to therapy.

5. Self-reported pain should be relied upon as the gold standard for pain assessment. In evaluating the younger, preverbal children or infants, clinicians must rely on behavioral assessment and physiologic assessment to detect and estimate the pain.

E. Therapeutic Strategies

1. Specific cancer treatment should be thought of as a primary means of controlling cancer pain. Chemotherapy and radiation therapy, as well as nonspecific treatment, such as corticosteroids (beneficial in decreasing pain caused by cerebral edema associated with brain tumors), should be considered as initial therapeutic choices.

2. Nonpharmacologic modalities include the following:

   a. Physical therapy: heat, cold, massage

   b. Transcutaneous electrical nerve stimulation

   c. Cognitive/behavioral measures: relaxation, guided imagery, hypnosis, activities therapy, art or music therapy

   d. Individual or family counseling

3. Pharmacologic management

   a. Analgesic management of pediatric cancer pain is based on the analgesic ladder suggested by the World Health Organization for the treatment of cancer pain in adults.

   b. The algorithm involves progression from the use of acetaminophen and nonsteroidal antiinflammatory agents for mild pain, to weak opioids (e.g., such as codeine for moderate pain) and strong opioids (e.g., morphine or methadone for severe pain).

   c. Important principles in the use of analgesics for cancer pain include the following:

      (1) The oral route of administration is preferable whenever possible because it is easily accepted by most children, it is the most convenient, and it provides adequate pain control in 90% to 95% of children with cancer-related pain.

      (2) Pain medication should be titrated around the clock rather than only as needed. Regular administration results in an even level of pain control and avoids the discomfort and anxiety experienced with breakthrough pain.

      (3) Side effects must be anticipated and treated aggressively. Children may not report side effects such as constipation, dysphoria,

and pruritus unless asked specifically. Antiemetics, stool softeners, promotility agents, and antihistamines for itching should be considered.

(4) The therapeutic plan should be individualized, based on the patient's unique condition.

d. Adjunctive medications include tricyclic antidepressants, anticonvulsants, and sodium-channel blockers.

(1) Tricyclic antidepressants are useful in the treatment of children with neuropathic pain resulting from nerve damage or vincristine-related peripheral neuropathy. Adequate sleep at night can be ensured by administering the tricyclic dose an hour before bedtime. The analgesic and sedative effects are achieved at lower than standard antidepressant doses. Imipramine has been used most widely in pediatric patients, whereas amitriptyline has been the first choice for treatment of pain in adults. Starting doses for imipramine are 0.2 to 0.4 mg/kg. The dose may be increased by 50% every 2 to 3 days up to 1 to 3 mg/kg. Common side effects include anticholinergic effects such as dry mouth and somnolence; less common side effects are disorientation, urinary retention, constipation, and heart block.

(2) Anticonvulsants are used for neuropathic pain, as a second line of therapy after tricyclic antidepressants, because of higher risk of side effects. Carbamazepine and phenytoin have sodium-channel blockade as their major mechanism of action. Gabapentin, a new anticonvulsant, is an analog of g-aminobutyric acid and has few drug interactions and a better side effect profile.

e. Regional anesthetic techniques should be viewed as an extension of the World Health Organization algorithm in pediatric patients with terminal malignancy. Among children dying of terminal malignancy, about 3% will need neuraxial infusions or neurolytic blocks to control pain.

(1) Indications for epidural or subarachnoid infusions of local anesthetics and/or opioids in the pediatric cancer patients are

(a) Limiting side effects of parenteral opioids, such as nausea, clouded sensorium, or respiratory depression

(b) Opioid resistance—massive opioid requirement is defined as more than 3 mg/kg/hr of morphine equivalent, or approximately 100 times the average infusion rates required for postoperative analgesia.

(c) Neuropathic pain produced by involvement of spinal nerve roots, large peripheral nerves, or spinal cord compression by the tumor.

(d) Analgesia required for repeated procedures.

f. Guidelines to manage opioid resistance in children with terminal malignancy include the following:
   (1) Nerve involvement as the cause of rapidly escalating opioid use
   (2) High-dose steroid therapy, radiotherapy, or palliative surgical decompression
   (3) Regional anesthetic infusions, which can provide adequate analgesia when escalation of parenteral opioids is limited by side effects.

   Complications of long-term epidural or subarachnoid infusions in children with terminal malignancy are
   (a) Local anesthetic toxicity—reaching the upper limit of safety. In this case, the use of an esther-type local anesthetic like 2-chloroprocaine (faster metabolism and less likelihood of causing systemic toxicity) or replacement of an epidural catheter with a subarachnoid catheter should be considered.
   (b) Motor dysfunction
   (c) Bladder dysfunction—possibly requiring bladder catheterization
   (d) Postdural puncture headache
   (e) Respiratory depression
   (f) Infection
g. Neurolytic blocks using phenol or alcohol can be considered for intractable localized pain, if the associated neurologic deficits are considered an acceptable price to achieve pain control. Celiac plexus block with alcohol, under radiographic guidance, can be useful for refractory upper abdominal visceral pain.
h. Neurosurgical approaches can be classified as
   (1) Neurostimulatory (dorsal column stimulation, deep brain stimulation)
   (2) Neurodestructive (cordotomy, rhizotomy, dorsal root entry zone lesions, sympathectomy)

   In choosing such invasive methods for pain control, one should consider the overall prognosis and expected longevity.

II. COMPLEX REGIONAL PAIN SYNDROMES IN CHILDREN
  A. Definition
    1. To satisfy a diagnosis of complex regional pain syndrome (CRPS) type I (reflex sympathetic dystrophy), the clinical findings include regional pain, sensory changes (allodynia and hyperalgesia), abnormalities of temperature, abnormal sudomotor activity, edema, and abnormal skin color, all occurring after a noxious event.
    2. Chronic regional pain syndrome type II (causalgia) includes all the preceding features in addition to an identifiable peripheral nerve lesion.

3. The diagnosis of CRPS is precluded by the existence of any known pathology that would otherwise account for the clinical picture found in the distal part of an extremity but outside of the territory of an injured nerve.

B. Particularities of CRPS in Children

Despite similar clinical features to CRPS in adults, the syndrome demonstrates some important differences in children:

1. CRPS in children is much more responsive to conservative treatment. Children are more likely to respond favorably to a single regional or sympathetic block. Whereas the pediatric literature emphasizes vigorous physical therapy and psychologic treatment, the adult literature supports the aggressive use of sympathetic blocks.

2. Only a few children with CRPS develop the severe debilitating form requiring aggressive invasive treatment.

3. Cognitive, behavioral, and psychologic strategies are particularly useful for pediatric patients with CRPS.

4. There is a strong association between CRPS in children and family dysfunction.

5. The radiographic findings typically seen in advanced CRPS in adults are only rarely seen in children. Plain radiography and bone-scanning should be part of the work-up—not to make the diagnosis, but to rule out other conditions (e.g., fracture, infection, tumors).

6. Believed to have been underdiagnosed or undiagnosed in the past, CRPS is becoming increasingly recognized in the pediatric population. The interval from onset of symptoms to the time of diagnosis of CRPS averages 12 months. Early diagnosis and treatment is crucial in determining the response to therapy.

C. Clinical Diagnosis of CRPS in Children

1. Chronic pain with neuropathic descriptors: burning, allodynia, dysesthesia, hyperalgesia to cold—persistent and out of proportion to the initial injury

2. Objective signs of sympathetic dysfunction: coldness (at least 3°C), cyanosis, mottling, hyperhidrosis (increased sweating), edema

3. Exclusion of other orthopedic, rheumatologic, or neurologic diagnoses

D. Etiology of CRPS in Children

1. Is identifiable in the vast majority of cases.

   a. In about two-thirds of cases the initiating injury is vague and apparently minor, such as a sprain, a twist, or a minor soft-tissue injury.

   b. In about half of the cases, the injury is sustained during a supervised sports activity: ballet, gymnastics, ice skating, swimming.

   c. Not infrequently there is a history of having had the extremity immobilized for variable periods of time before referral to a pain clinic.

    d. Affected children are predominantly girls. The lower extremity is involved more often than the upper extremity.

    e. The onset of CRPS can sometimes follow a surgical procedure.

  2. In rare cases there are no obvious initiating events.

E. Psychologic Aspects of CRPS in Children

  1. Profound emotional and behavioral changes can follow the onset of CRPS in children.

  2. There is no valid evidence in the adult or pediatric literature to substantiate the fact that certain personality traits predispose to develop CRPS.

  3. When compared with patients with chronic back pain or persistent local neuropathy, patients with CRPS do not display a unique pattern of psychologic dysfunction. A survey of childhood trauma found that physical abuse, emotional abuse, and sexual abuse were evenly distributed among those three groups.

  4. The severity of symptoms can be amplified by

    a. Family stress factors such as sibling rivalry, marital conflict, or divorce

    b. Pressure of academics or sports

F. Treatment Algorithm

Treatment is based on a multidisciplinary team approach, including behavioral medicine, physical therapy, and anesthesia.

  1. Step one: physical therapy, transcutaneous electrical stimulation, and cognitive and behavioral pain management techniques

    a. Physical therapy is the mainstay of treatment for CRPS in children. For patients with severe symptoms who cannot tolerate touch or passive movement of the affected extremity, the program can start with desensitization to tactile stimuli, use of heat and whirlpool, followed by passive and active range-of-motion exercises, and progressive strengthening and physical conditioning exercises. In this phase it is essential to educate the patient and the family about the nonprotective nature of neuropathic pain.

    b. A trial of transcutaneous electrical nerve stimulation includes use of variable frequencies. It is important to be considered early in the course of physical therapy, since it is safe and often efficient.

    c. Behavioral management of pain includes

      (1) Relaxation training, with or without temperature or electromyographic biofeedback

      (2) Cognitive/behavioral therapy to improve skills in the management of stressful situations

      (3) Interventions in the behavioral patterns of the family

  2. Step two: Add nonsteroidal antiinflammatory drugs and tricyclic antidepressants.

    a. Tricyclic antidepressant drugs have been shown to be efficacious for several types of neuropathic pain and can be particularly beneficial in children exhibiting
      (1) Symptoms suggestive of depression (poor appetite, loss of energy, and loss of interest)
      (2) Disturbed sleep pattern
    b. Amitriptyline, doxepin, or desipramine can be started at 0.1 to 0.2 mg/kg orally, at bedtime. The dosage can be advanced to 0.5 to 1 mg/kg/day, as limited by side effects.

3. Step three: trial of sympathetic blocks
    a. An early trial of a sympathetic block with a local anesthetic may be justified if
      (1) The intensity of pain prevents successful progress of the physical therapy program.
      (2) There is evidence of worsening dysfunction of the limb despite conservative strategies.
    b. Blocks in children are performed under general anesthesia for younger patients or conscious sedation for older children.
    c. Continuous techniques are preferred to multiple blocks in children, to limit the number of anxiety-producing procedures and exposure to radiation. After an initial diagnostic block, an indwelling catheter can be placed in the lumbar epidural space, lumbar paravertebral area, or brachial plexus (axillary approach), and maintained for 7 to 10 days, to facilitate aggressive physical therapy. A 20-gauge catheter can be placed through an 18-gauge Tuohy needle in the lumbar paravertebral area under radiologic guidance, for blockage of the lumbar sympathetic chain.
    d. The lumbar epidural catheter has the advantage of easier placement, without the need of radiologic guidance, but has the disadvantage of possible sensory or motor dysfunction interfering with physical therapy requirements.
    e. An alternative to the indwelling catheter is the use of an intravenous regional sympathetic block with bretylium.
    f. A typical infusion via a lumbar epidural catheter is bupivacaine 0.1%, at a rate of 0.15 to 0.25 ml/kg/hr. Walking with assistance can be permitted.
    g. For severely affected patients, an initial bolus of bupivacaine 0.25%, 0.5 ml/kg can be administered to permit initiation of passive mobilization.
    h. Stellate ganglion blockade (paratracheal approach) for upper-extremity CRPS in children is done with bupivacaine 0.25%, 0.2 ml/kg injected slowly, following a negative test dose of lidocaine 1% in 0.1-ml increments to a total test dose of 0.05 ml/kg.

        i. Chemical (phenol), radiofrequency, or operative sympathectomy can be considered as a last resort if more conservative approaches have failed. It is rare that such invasive treatment of CRPS in children is required.

    4. Step four: trial of one or more of the following medications:
        a. Alpha-and beta-adrenergic antagonists
        b. Anticonvulsants
        c. Calcium-channel blockers
        d. Steroids

G. Outcome
    1. Outcome of CRPS in children is superior to that in the adult population.
    2. More than half of the pediatric patients respond to a combined approach of
        a. Physical therapy
        b. Transcutaneous electrical nerve stimulation
        c. Cognitive and behavioral management
    3. The use of early sympathetic block is usually unnecessary. The goal of such blocks is to enable or facilitate participation in the physical therapy programs.

III. FIBROMYALGIA IN CHILDREN
A. Diagnostic Criteria
Fibromyalgia is a chronic pain syndrome characterized by the following:
    1. Widespread chronic muscular pain
        a. Above the waist
        b. Below the waist
        c. In the left side of the body
        d. In the right side of the body
    2. Lasting for a period of at least 3 months
    3. Pain in 11 of 18 tender point sites (nine pairs) on digital palpation:
        a. Occiput: bilateral, at the suboccipital muscle insertion
        b. Low cervical: bilateral, at the anterior aspect of the intertransverse spaces at C-5–7
        c. Trapezius: bilateral, at the midpoint of the upper border
        d. Supraspinous: bilateral, at origins above the medial border of the scapular spine
        e. Second rib: bilateral, upper surfaces, lateral to the costochondral junctions
        f. Lateral epicondyle: bilateral, 2 cm distal to the epicondyles
        g. Gluteal: bilateral, in upper outer quadrants of buttocks
        h. Greater trochanter: bilateral, posterior to the trochanteric preeminence
        i. Knee: bilateral, at the medial fat pad proximal to the joint line

B. Associated Symptoms
1. Fatigue
2. Stiffness—diffuse joint stiffness, common in the morning
3. Sleep disorders
   a. Nonrestorative sleep
   b. Non-REM sleep abnormalities
4. Migraine or tension headaches
5. Irritable bowel syndrome—episodes of constipation alternating with cramping and diarrhea

C. Physical Exam
1. Palpation of the trigger points produces a dull, aching or burning pain in referral areas remote from the trigger point, not corresponding to segmental or dermatomal distribution.
2. Affected muscles may feel tight and ropelike.
3. Trigger points may twitch or fasciculate in response to pressure or percussion of the affected muscle.

D. Psychologic Aspects
1. The frequency of depression is increased compared with normal controls but does not differ significantly from the frequency of depression in other chronic pain patients. Indicators of depression in children are
   a. Altered sleep pattern
   b. Decreased appetite
   c. Loss of interest in previously enjoyed activities
2. Most children presenting with fibromyalgia have experienced a major family crisis: marital discord or divorce, sibling rivalry, death of a member of the family.

E. Therapeutic Strategies
1. There is no single completely effective treatment for fibromyalgia.
2. Nonpharmacologic therapies
   a. Physical therapy is the most important aspect of treatment
      (1) Cardiovascular fitness training
      (2) Muscle stretching and toning
      (3) Walking and swimming
      (4) Heat and massage
   b. Cognitive and behavioral strategies
      (1) Electromyographic biofeedback
      (2) Relaxation techniques
      (3) Guided imagery
      (4) Self-hypnosis
   c. Psychologic counseling
   d. Encouraging the child to return to school and avoid isolation is essential.
3. Pharmacologic approaches

  a. Tricyclic antidepressants
    (1) The choice of antidepressant is based on the side effect profile.
    (2) Amitriptyline
      (a) Beneficial in about one-third of patients with fibromyalgia
      (b) Sedating effect useful in patients with sleep disturbances
    (3) Desipramine has the least anticholinergic and sedative effects.
    (4) Start with a low dose and titrate upward over several weeks.
  b. Nonsteroidal antiinflammatory drugs
IV. RECURRENT ABDOMINAL PAIN SYNDROME
  A. Definition
  Recurrent abdominal pain syndrome (RAPS) is defined as nonprogressive abdominal pain that occurs at least once a month for 3 consecutive months and includes pain-free intervals.
  B. Incidence and Etiology
    1. Recurrent abdominal pain occurs in as many as one in seven school-aged children, with a slight female predominance.
    2. An organic cause is identified in about 10% of these children
      a. Gastrointestinal origin: inflammatory bowel disease, ulcer disease, hepatitis
      b. Genitourinary origin: recurrent infections, lower tract obstruction, vulvovaginitis
    3. A psychologic cause is associated with RAPS in 10% of the cases
      a. Conversion reactions
      b. Somatoform disorders
    4. Pain is referred to as dysfunctional in 80% of the children with RAPS
      a. Specific dysfunctional pain is most commonly caused by lactose malabsorbtion, and less frequently by sorbitol or fructose intolerance.
      b. If the cause remains unknown, the syndrome is considered idiopathic.
      c. Causal mechanisms include
        (1) Abnormal intestinal muscular activity (dysmotility)
        (2) Autonomic dysfunction
        (3) Endogenous opioid system
        (4) Irritable bowel syndrome
        (5) Nonulcer dyspepsia, with *Helicobacter pylori* infection
  C. Clinical Picture
    1. Typically, the pain is localized in the periumbilical area. The further the pain is from the umbilicus, the more likely it is to be organic.
    2. The pain usually lasts less than 1 hour and almost always less than 3 hours. Pain that occurs at night is not suggestive of RAPS.
    3. Associated symptoms
      a. Nausea

        b. Vomiting

        c. Perspiration

        d. Flushing

        e. Palpitations

        f. Constipation

  D. Treatment

     1. Reassurance regarding the self-limited and non-life-threatening character of the pain syndrome is important for the child and the family.

     2. Dietary intervention to change bowel habits by increased dietary fiber is often beneficial.

     3. Behavioral pain management techniques are useful by empowering the children with stress reduction and coping strategies.

     4. Pharmacologic approaches

        a. Tricyclic antidepressants

        b. Acetaminophen or nonsteroidal antiinflammatory drugs may be appropriate during episodes of exacerbation of symptoms.

RECOMMENDED READING

Berde C, Ablin A, Glazer J, et al. Report of the subcommittee on disease-related pain in childhood cancer. *Pediatrics* 1990;86(5):818–825.

Collins J, Grier H, Kinney H, Berde C. Control of severe pain in children with terminal malignancy. *J Pediatr* 1995;126(4):653–657.

Collins J, Grier H, Sethna N, Wilder R, Berde C. Regional anesthesia for pain associated with terminal pediatric malignancy. *Pain* 1996;165:63–69.

Lynch M. Psychological aspects of reflex sympathetic dystrophy: A review of the adult and pediatric literature. *Pain* 1992;49:337–347.

Miser A, Dothage J, Wesley R, Miser J. The prevalence of pain in a pediatric and young adult cancer population. *Pain* 1987;29:73–83.

Miser A, McCalla J, Dothage J, Wesley M, Miser J. Pain as a presenting symptom in children and young adults with newly diagnosed malignancy. *Pain* 1987;29:85–90.

Stanton-Hicks M, Baron R, Boas R, et al. Complex regional pain syndromes: Guidelines for therapy. *Clin J Pain* 1998;14(2):155–167.

Wilder R. The management of chronic pain in the child. In: Ashburn R, ed. *Management of Chronic Pain.* New York: Churchill Livingstone, 1998: 635–649.

Wilder R, Berde C, Wolohan M, Vieyra M, Masek B, Micheli L. Reflex sympathetic dystrophy in children. *J Bone Joint Surg* 1992;74-A(6):910–919.

The Pain Clinic Manual, Second Edition,
edited by Stephen E. Abram and J. David Haddox.
Lippincott Williams & Wilkins,
Philadelphia, © 2000

31

Substance Abuse and Addiction

Doralina L. Anghelescu and Margaret Charsley

*D. L. Anghelescu: Department of Anesthesiology, St. Jude Children's Hospital,
Memphis, Tennessee 38101.
M. Charsley: Department of Anesthesiology and Critical Care Medicine, University of
New Mexico, Health Sciences Center—School of Medicine, Albuquerque, New Mexico 87131.*

I. DEFINITIONS

The Committee on Pain of the American Society of Addiction Medicine recognizes the following definitions as appropriate and clinically useful when assessing the use of opioids in the context of pain treatment.

A. Physical Dependence

    1. A physiologic state in which abrupt cessation of the opioid, or administration of an opioid antagonist, results in a withdrawal syndrome

    2. An expected occurrence in any individual who uses opioids continuously

    3. It does not, in and of itself, imply addiction.

B. Tolerance

    1. Neuroadaptation to the effects of chronically administered opioids, indicated by the need for increasing the dose or more frequent doses to maintain drug effect.

    2. Tolerance may occur both to the analgesic effects and to unwanted side effects, such as respiratory depression, sedation, or nausea.

    3. The occurrence of tolerance is variable and does not, in and of itself, imply addiction.

C. Addiction

    1. True addiction is a psychologic and behavioral disorder.

    2. Addiction in the context of pain treatment with opioids is characterized by a persistent pattern of dysfunctional opioid use that may involve any or all of the following:

        a. Adverse consequences associated with the use of opioids

        b. Loss of control over the use of opioids

            (1) Compulsive drug use, craving for an opioid

            (2) The need to use the opioid for effects other than pain relief

       c. Preoccupation with obtaining opioids despite the presence of adequate analgesia

    3. Drug-seeking behavior is an indicator of addictive disease.

       a. Requesting medication from multiple providers

       b. Repeated episodes of prescription loss

       c. Multiple requests for early refills

II. PREVALENCE

The prevalence of addictive disease is no greater in patients with chronic pain than in the general population. It is estimated that between 3% and 19% of chronic pain patients suffer an addictive disorder, which parallels the life time prevalence rates of addictive disease in the general population (6.1% to 16.7%).

III. DIFFERENTIAL DIAGNOSIS

  A. Pseudoaddiction

    1. Defined as a behavioral pattern similar to opioid addiction, characterized by overwhelming and compulsive interest in the acquisition and use of opioids

    2. Unlike true addiction, pseudoaddiction is an iatrogenic syndrome caused by the undermedication of pain. Drug-seeking behavior arises when a patient fails to obtain adequate pain relief because of inadequate dose or excessive dosing intervals. It resolves when pain is adequately treated.

  B. Therapeutic Dependence

    1. Drug-seeking behavior is manifested in a patient receiving good pain relief to ensure adequate medication supply.

    2. This behavior is based on the fear of reemergence of pain and on the emergence of withdrawal symptoms.

IV. FACTORS PREDICTIVE OF ADDICTION

  A. Strong Predictors for the Presence of Addictive Disease in Chronic Pain Patients

    1. The patient believes he/she is addicted.

    2. Progressive increase in dose or frequency

    3. Route of administration preference

    4. Prescription drugs obtained from nonmedical source

    5. Sale of controlled drugs

    6. Forging of prescriptions

    7. Injection of oral formulations

    8. Excessive use of alcohol or use of street drugs

    9. Deterioration of family, social, or workplace function

    10. Frequent loss of medications

    11. Stealing or borrowing of drugs from others

  B. Weaker Predictors for Addictive Disease

    1. Drug hoarding during periods of reduced symptoms

    2. Request for specific drugs

3. Openly (as opposed to covertly) obtaining drugs from other medical sources
4. Unapproved use of drug to treat other symptoms

C. Clinical Assessment
1. Assess functional status changes as a result of opioid administration. Should produce
   a. Reduction in reported pain levels
   b. Improved function in recreational, social, vocational activities
2. Signs of opioid addiction should be evaluated at each visit. (See preceding lists.)

V. PATIENT MANAGEMENT

Once the issue of substance abuse or addiction has been identified for a particular patient, further pain management must reflect this information. The patient may be aware or unaware of his or her condition. Whichever the situation, a frank and open discussion of the implications of substance abuse or addiction on the pain treatment program may be necessary.

A. General Treatment Plan
1. Maximize aggressive pain management with nonopioid and nonpharmacologic interventions such as nerve blocks, TENS, physical therapy, heat and cold, massage, relaxation, imagery, behavioral therapy, hypnosis, acupuncture, surgical procedures.
2. Assess the patient's cognitive level, quality of life, willingness to cooperate, presence or absence of psychologic or behavioral disorders, history of prior drug treatment programs, and so on. (May need to enlist the help of a psychologist or addictionologist.)
3. Decide if the patient needs to enter an addiction treatment program, preferably one experienced in the care of patients with pain, or if a drug taper can be managed on an outpatient basis.
   a. About 25% of the previous daily dose is required to prevent withdrawal.
   b. One schedule is reduction of the dose by 25% every 2 to 3 days.
   c. Refer to formal outpatient drug treatment program, psychotherapy, or 12-step recovery meetings.
4. If all other options are exhausted consideration of opioid management may be appropriate and can be achieved if clear goals are defined and agreed upon.

B. Opioid Use
1. The goal of treatment must be clear and realistic. The patient may have to accept that the elimination of all pain is impossible. Addiction constricts a person's life, whereas appropriate treatment improves it. Goals may be defined as follows:
   a. Palliation of pain
   b. Improvement in the patient's quality of life

    c. Increase in the patient's level of functioning (e.g., ability to work, to complete activities of daily living, etc.)

  2. Educate the patient regarding the potential for narcotics such as morphine to produce hyperalgesia with chronic use and the possible need for occasional controlled withdrawal (i.e., "drug holidays").

  3. Impress upon the patient the implications of opioid prescribing for the physician and the pain management clinic (i.e., state and federal monitoring, physician accountability, etc.) and the need for a written contract between the patient and the physician or clinic.

C. Patient Responsibilities

  1. The patient agrees to allow the clinic access to all prior records.

  2. Only one physician should prescribe all psychotropic medications and should be notified in advance of acute needs (e.g., dental work or surgery).

  3. If possible, only one pharmacy should dispense medications.

  4. No changes in drug doses without prior discussion with contracting physician.

  5. The patient will be allowed no early refills, no replacement of prescription if stolen, lost, "dropped in the toilet," "eaten by the dog," and so on.

  6. The patient must call in a timely fashion for refills (i.e., 3 days before running out, not late on a Friday just a few minutes before the clinic closes).

  7. Obtain any recommended consultations.

  8. Abstain from alcohol and illegal drug use.

  9. Consent to random urine or blood screens when asked.

  10. The patient must agree to bring unused medications to each clinic visit.

D. Physician Responsibilities

  1. Selection of the best opioid for the patient

    a. Avoid a power struggle with the patient. If possible, start with the drug that has worked in the past, thus promoting patient cooperation.

    b. Consider that if the drug contains acetaminophen, excessive doses (greater than 4 g/day) risk liver toxicity.

    c. Consider changing to a long-acting opioid. This provides a steady level of pain control and avoids peaks and valleys.

      (1) Morphine:MS Contin, Oramorph, Kadian

      (2) Oxycodone: Oxy-Contin

      (3) Transdermal fentanyl: Duragesic patches

      (4) Methadone

      (5) Levorphanol

       d. Advantages of methadone

         (1) Powerful analgesia

         (2) Less euphoric effect than morphine

         (3) Less street value than morphine

         (4) Very inexpensive

E. Selection of the Best Dose of Opioid for the Patient

    1. The aim is to settle on a dose that the patient thinks would be adequate. The goal is not to minimize the dose but to get to a steady-state level and assess over time whether the patient can use the medication in a controlled manner.

       a. Give the patient the benefit of the doubt. If the patient is using the drug for other than pain relief, his or her loss of control will soon become apparent.

       b. Prescribe the drug in pharmacologically meaningful doses at appropriate intervals. Use frequent assessments to guide dose titration.

       c. Initially calculate the weekly dose and prescribe the medication 1 week at a time. The patient is responsible for regulating use. If he or she needs less one day, some will be left over for another day when there is more pain or the patient has been more active. Patients are in control within the confines of the weekly dose.

       d. Some changes may be required to find the optimal treatment regimen and drug.

       e. When prescribing long-acting opioids, some short-acting opioids may be given for breakthrough pain or when there is increased activity.

       f. Regularly assess the need for breakthrough dosing and adjust the dose of the long-acting opioid accordingly.

       g. Be flexible in unusual circumstances. Some situations, such as travel or acute injury, require unusual responses but will need to be verified.

F. Visits

    1. Initially weekly, then monthly. Same for prescription writing.

    2. Document why the patient is on the drug and the contractual agreement. Then at each visit document the following:

       a. Efficacy (i.e., extent of analgesia)

       b. Side effects such as impaired thinking, somnolence, constipation, nausea

       c. Functional status; ability to work, increase in activity, etc.

       d. Compliance with the agreement and any "drug-seeking" behaviors

       e. Reasons for any changes in drug or dose

G. Other Issues
   1. Tolerance
      a. Patients do not usually develop rapid tolerance to the pain-relieving effects of opioids.
      b. If they do, consider changing to a different opioid. Some patients on large doses of morphine can get good relief with fairly minimal doses of fentanyl.
      c. Consider a "drug holiday."
      d. Evaluate other medications that the patient is on concurrently, because these may affect blood levels of the opioids and give the appearance of tolerance.
      e. Methadone is metabolized at a rapid rate in patients who are taking antiseizure medications that enhance liver metabolism. Some antibiotics also alter metabolism.
   2. Noncompliance
      a. If after a reasonable period the patient is noncompliant with the agreement and violates the written contract, it may be necessary to discontinue narcotic therapy or terminate the physician/patient relationship.
      b. The opioid therapy may be gradually reduced and discontinued.
      c. The patient may need to be referred to an addiction specialist or enter an inpatient detoxification/drug rehabilitation program.
      d. Document the patient's noncompliance and all discussions regarding discontinuation of therapy or treatment.
      e. Consider medicolegal aspects. Different states have different laws regarding physician/patient relationships.
      f. Inform the referring physician.
H. The Addicted Patient
   1. Beware of opioid pseudoaddiction.
   2. Addicts in recovery must be approached differently from other patients.
      a. Some addiction medicine specialists feel there should be strict avoidance of all psychotropic medications for these patients.
      b. Others recommend controlled access to the medications combined with intensified relapse prevention.
      c. Physician and patient should anticipate the possibility that opioid cravings may be induced and that there may be an increased risk of relapse to drug abuse.
      d. Seek consultation from an addiction medicine specialist.
      e. Patients should increase their recovery activities (e.g., attend more 12-step meetings, increase frequency of psychotherapy).
      f. Patients who are physically dependent on opioids should not be given pure antagonists (naloxone or naltrexone) or mixed agonists/antagonists (e.g., butorphanol nasal spray, pentazocine, bupre-

norphine, and nalbuphine) because they will precipitate acute withdrawal.

RECOMMENDED READING

Compton P, Darakjian J, Miotto K. Screening for addiction in patients with chronic pain and "problematic" substance use: Evaluation of a pilot assessment tool. *J Pain Symptom Manage* 1998;16:355–362.

Schneider JP, Addiction medicine and chronic pain. AAPM 1997 review course in pain medicine. Scottsdale, AZ.

Weissman, D. Is it pain or is it addiction? *Cancer Pain Update* 1997; 44:3–4.

Weissman D. Is it pain or is it addiction? Part 2: Management. *Cancer Pain Update* 1997;45:3–4.

Weissman DE, Haddox JD. Opioid pseudoaddiction: An iatrogenic syndrome. *Pain* 1989;36:363–366.

Wesson DR, Ling W, Smith DE, Prescription of opioids for treatment of pain in patients with addictive disease. *J Pain Symptom Manage* 1993;8: 289–296.

PART V

Cancer Pain Management

The Pain Clinic Manual, Second Edition,
edited by Stephen E. Abram and J. David Haddox.
Lippincott Williams & Wilkins,
Philadelphia, © 2000

32

Oncologic Pain Management

Richard B. Patt

R. B. Patt: The Patt Center for Cancer Pain and Wellness, Houston, Texas 77030.

After incurability, cancer patients have ranked pain as the most fearful aspect of their illness, and of the range of symptoms associated with cancer, pain has been reported to be the most distressing. Inadequately controlled pain, especially when chronic, combined with the impact of cancer is associated with profound alterations in nearly all aspects of wellness. Increasing interest in the management of pain in the setting of oncologic disease is partly related to a recognition that optimal pain management may hasten a return to normalcy in each of the at-risk domains of personhood (i.e., functional, physiologic, spiritual, psychologic, economic, vocational, and even survivorship). Thus, rather than adopting a unidimensional view that considers pain intensity as the ultimate outcome, the concept of total pain has been invoked to more broadly capture the degree to which pain interferes with determinants of quality of life and various functional domains (e.g., activity, mood, rest, nutrition, posture, sexuality). In addition to an increased focus on pain as a determinant of quality of life, there is an increasing understanding that adequacy of pain control may directly and indirectly influence the outcome of cancer treatment and the likelihood of survival. Arguments for a linkage between pain and mortality include a recognition that uncontrolled pain detracts from overall performance status, which in turn influences compliance with recommendations for demanding cytotoxic therapies as well as candidacy for investigational therapies. In addition, basic science studies of the influence of pain on immune function and limited clinical trials suggest more direct linkages. Of the many negatives associated with a diagnosis of cancer, pain is one that not only need not be endured, but that, when controlled, makes other privations more manageable.

I. EPIDEMIOLOGY AND CURRENT STATUS
    A. Epidemiology of Cancer
        1. Cancer is a highly prevalent disorder.
            a. In the United States alone, an estimated 1.04 million new cases of cancer were diagnosed in 1990, and of the 6.35 million annual new cases worldwide, half were diagnosed in developing nations.

       b. Cancer is the second most common cause of death in the United States, accounting for an estimated 510,000 deaths annually.

  2. Despite advocacy for aggressive treatment and new treatment methods, outcome remains poor.

       a. Despite declaration of a war on cancer, the overall 5-year survival rate in the United States is about 50%, essentially unchanged over the last four decades.

       b. The overall 5-year survival rate worldwide is less than one-third, accounting for one of every 10 deaths and an annual mortality of about 4.3 million.

       c. Outcome is disproportionately poor in developing nations. Because of poor physician access, early detection is infrequent and patients commonly present to health care providers with advanced and incurable disease.

B. Epidemiology of Cancer Pain

  1. Despite the high mortality of cancer, many patients undergo intensive treatment, hoping to achieve a cure, to extend survival, or to improve quality of life.

       a. Ironically, pain and disability are common outcomes of aggressive antineoplastic therapy. Most treatments aimed at eradicating diseased cells almost inevitably result in injury to neighboring healthy tissue in the process. Neural structures and soft tissue are most vulnerable. Pain may occur with or without a survival benefit and may persist indefinitely. Examples of posttreatment pains follow.

       b. Even when cure is not achieved, intensive treatment may prolong survival, often for years, or, as in the case of lymphoma, breast, or prostate cancer, even decades. Thus over the course of a lingering illness many of today's patients and even survivors will experience pain and other symptoms that need treatment.

  2. Overall, about two-thirds of cancer patients experience pain that is sufficient to warrant treatment. Of those receiving active treatment for early or intermediate-stage disease, 15% to 25% experience significant pain.

       a. Pain is present in up to 90% of individuals with advanced cancer.

  3. Fortunately, most of the estimated 1.1 million Americans treated for cancer pain annually can achieve adequate, durable relief when established guidelines are followed. Seventy percent to 90% of patients report favorable outcomes with relatively low-tech, noninvasive pharmacologic therapies. A high proportion of remaining patients can achieve comfort with the judicious application of anesthetic and neurosurgical approaches.

C. Barriers to Optimal Pain Treatment

  1. It is curious, indeed tragic, that despite the availability of straightforward, cost-effective therapies, cancer pain remains undertreated.

2. The factors contributing to undertreatment are complex but well documented. Undertreatment is usually conceived of as relating to knowledge deficits, beliefs, and attitudes maintained by (a) health care providers, (b) patients and family members, and (c) regulators and health care delivery systems. Representative barriers are listed in Table 32-1.

TABLE 32-1. *Barriers to effective cancer pain management*

A. Health care provider–related barriers
  1. Lack of education and knowledge about the assessment and management of pain, especially with regard to the pharmacology of chronically administered opioids and management of opioid mediated side effects
  2. Lack of education and knowledge about the assessment and management of refractory pain, especially with regard to alternatives such as adjuvant analgesics (antidepressants, anticonvulsants, etc.), parenteral routes, and other treatment modalities
  3. Lack of education and knowledge about the actual risks of analgesic therapy, especially with regard to addiction (failure to distinguish among addiction, physical dependence, and tolerance) and respiratory depression
  4. Belief that pain is an inevitable feature of advanced cancer that cannot be effectively managed
  5. Belief that the use of opioids in doses sufficient to manage pain is comparable to euthanasia, or that opioids should be reserved for dying patients
  6. Belief that patient reports of pain are unreliable
  7. Reluctance to utilize triplicate prescriptions (added cost, added effort, fear of reprisal from regulatory agencies, and inherent restrictions such as limits on quantity prescribed and telephone refills). Resultant over reliance on less restricted but less effective medications
  8. Possible lack of time, energy, or motivation to make frequent changes often required to maintain control of pain or may not recognize patients' reluctance to spontaneously discuss pain, and so do not initiate inquiries

B. Cultural or health care system–related barriers
  1. War on drugs that fails to distinguish among illicit and medical use, and has resulted in restrictive limits on prescribing and failure of pharmacies to stock strong opioids
  2. Lack of information in medical school curricula and residency training programs on pain management and inadequate availability of reference material on the management of chronic pain. Failure of texts to distinguish between recommendations for the management of acute versus those for the management of chronic pain
  3. Acute disease-oriented health care model engenders lack of accountability for control of chronic symptoms, failure of coordination as patients move from one care setting to another (hospital, home, nursing home, etc.), and fragmentation of care due to involvement of multiple specialists
  4. Lack of recognition of pain management or palliative care as legitimate medical subspecialty interests and inadequate resources for procedurally based (anesthetic, neurosurgical) pain management. Resultant failure of some insurers to provide hospice benefits and to favorably consider reimbursement aimed specifically at comfort

continued

TABLE 32-1. *Continued*

C. Patient and family-related barriers
   1. Belief that pain inevitably accompanies cancer and cannot be managed or that painkillers must be withheld until late in the disease process
   2. Belief that opioids are inevitably associated with serious side effects, make people incoherent or "high," and lead to addiction. Reluctance to take opioids because of their association with serious illness and fears that their use may either hasten death or signify that their disease is incurable
   3. War on drugs: pressure from family and friends, as well as the government and media campaigns, not to take opioids under any circumstances
   4. Reluctance to discuss pain with health care provider. Desire to be perceived as a "good patient," concern not to be perceived as drug seeking, concern that complaints of pain will not be regarded as signs of a weak character or an insult to health care providers. Fear that patients will "use up" the doctor's time, which would be otherwise devoted to controlling the cancer, or that they would be acknowledging that the cancer is progressing or has returned.

   3. The most prevalent underlying issues relate to an inadequate understanding of the pharmacology of the opioid drugs and exaggerated fears of addiction. Thus workable solutions relate less to developing new drugs or technology; instead they involve improving the utilization of currently available techniques.

II. ASSESSMENT
   A. General Features (See Tables 32-2 and 32-3)
      1. Although an assessment that is limited to cancer pain can be performed rapidly, it should be integrated with a more complete history and physical examination.
      2. A broad-based approach helps identify features that may exert important influences on decision making and outcome.
      3. Assessment also serves to orient the patient, family, and referring physician to what can realistically be accomplished. It should serve an educational function, and, because prognosis for controlling pain is usually good, should be reassuring to the patient.
      4. A detailed, unhurried, and compassionate approach to assessment is essential to ensure optimal outcome.
   B. Operationally, assessment can be regarded as pertaining to the person, disease, pain, and interactions between these factors. These are discussed later under the headings "Oncologic History," "Psychosocial History," and "Pain History."
   C. Assessment is best supplemented by an appropriate standardized pain questionnaire. Although increasingly advocated, unfortunately these are rarely used in most clinical practices.

TABLE 32-2. *General principles of pain management in the cancer patient: assessment*

- Assess the patient carefully prior to initiating treatment. A careful history and directed physical examination (especially of the painful region and neurologic and musculoskeletal systems) are essential.
- Assess pain in a global context. Elicit past medical history, oncologic and social history, and presence of other distressing symptoms. Seek history of alcohol or drug abuse.
- Listen to and believe the patient's reports of pain and other symptoms, as well as the observations of the patient's relations.
- Ask explicitly about the presence and nature of pain and other symptoms. Pertinent information is often not otherwise volunteered.
- Seek the presence of multiple complaints of pain. When multiple complaints exist, they should each be evaluated as discrete, independent entities, as well as in their wider context. When appropriate, prioritize complaints based on how distressing they are, as well as their treatability.
- Assess the characteristics of each pain complaint: chronicity, location and referral or radiation, severity (best, worst, average, current), quality, temporal features, associated symptoms, aggravating and relieving factors.
- Assess pain complaints globally: in addition to pertinent physical aspects, assessment and ultimately management should address emotional, psychological, environmental, and spiritual factors that influence pain and well-being.
- Determine beneficial and adverse effects for each analgesic in current use, as well as those taken in the past. Determine to what degree trials of other agents have been adequate and thorough.
- Determine to what degree pain and other symptoms are distressing and interfere with activities that are important to the patient.
- Consider the use of a simple validated written instrument that can be rapidly completed to document self-report (e.g., Brief Pain Inventory or Memorial Pain Assessment Card).
- Teach and encourage the consistent use of a simple verbal tool to monitor pain intensity (e.g., 0–10, none–slight–moderate–severe).
- Develop a problem list based on data obtained during assessment.
- Based on the initial evaluation, develop a provisional diagnosis for the cause and type of each pain.
- Formulate a treatment plan that includes primary recommendations for each targeted symptom, with contingencies for titration or alternate interventions.
- Obtain and personally review needed diagnostic tests.
- Document findings and recommendations in medical record, and communicate with the patient and family and the referring and other treating physicians.

1. Minimally, a pain-intensity rating should be used consistently from visit to visit. It is important to select a method that you and the patient feel comfortable with.

   a. Pain intensity is best elicited as severity over the last week: at best, at worst, on average, and right now.

   b. Most clinicians prefer to rate pain intensity on a 0 to 10 scale or 0 to 5 scale, with 0 corresponding to an absence of pain and the

TABLE 32-3. *General principles of pain management in the cancer patient: reassessment*

- Reassess at appropriate, individualized intervals, to gauge response to interventions and to monitor for disease progression and the development of new symptoms.
- Reassess at frequent intervals after initial evaluation and after commencing new drugs or performing an intervention (e.g., nerve block.).
- Use preestablished verbal tools to assess pain intensity longitudinally (e.g., 0–10, none–slight–moderate–severe).
- When reassessing, ask about efficacy and side effects of current treatment regimen.
- When reassessing, routinely inquire about bowel habit, nausea, and alertness.
- Be alert to findings consistent with epidural spinal cord compression and other neurologic syndromes. Pertinent information is often not otherwise volunteered.
- Review problem list and progress made in treating each distressing symptom.
- Encourage patients to focus on whether symptoms have improved, rather than on whether they've been entirely eliminated.
- Determine overall satisfaction with treatment.
- Document findings and recommendations in medical record, and communicate changes in condition and modifications in treatment regimen with referring and other treating physicians.

highest number representing the worst pain the patient can imagine. Alternatively, a categorical scale (mild–moderate–severe–intolerable) can be utilized.

   c. Pain intensity and pain relief are distinct concepts. The former usually best guides drug titration, whereas patients tend to be more interested in the latter. Despite a high intensity, patients may be very satisfied if current severity represents a significant improvement.

2. Specific assessment tools

   a. The Brief Pain Inventory (BPI) and the Memorial Pain Assessment Card (MPAC) are the best-accepted standardized questionnaires. They were both specifically designed and validated for patients with cancer pain and are easy to administer, even in the presence of pain and distress.

   b. The BPI requires an average of 15 minutes, and can be self-administered or used as an adjunct to the interview. It includes several questions about the characteristics of the pain, including its origin, prior treatments, and the efficacy of prior treatments. In addition, it incorporates two valuable features of the McGill Pain Questionnaire: a graphic representation of the location of pain and groups of qualitative descriptors. Severity of pain (at best, at worst, on average) and perceived level of interference with normal function (enjoyment of life, work, mood, sleep, general activity, walking, relations with others) are quantified with visual analog scales. A short form is available for follow-up evaluations.

    c. The MPAC is simple, efficient, and valid, and can be completed by experienced patients in less than 20 seconds. It consists of a two-sided 8.5- × 11-inch card folded to create four separate measures, and features a set of descriptive adjectives and scales for measuring pain intensity, pain relief, and mood.

    d. The Edmonton Staging System for Cancer Pain is performed by the health care provider rather than the patient. It is different in that it was developed to prognosticate the likelihood of providing effective pharmacologic relief from cancer pain. Patients are staged with an alphanumeric code, similar to that used to characterize the clinicohistologic status of tumors. Five features (neuropathic pain, incident- or movement-related pain, recent history of tolerance to opioids, psychologic distress, and a history of alcohol or drug abuse) correlate with a poor outcome for treatment with analgesics, whereas neither the dose of opioid nor the presence of cognitive function predicts outcome.

D. History

  1. Preassessment: When appropriate, prior to the interview the assessment is preceded by a review of medical records (including the results of laboratory and radiologic studies), the result of questionnaires, and discussion with health care providers already caring for the patient. (These may include the referring physician, primary care provider, oncologists, and even the responsible adult caring for the patient at home.)

      Rationale: Provides orientation to the nature of the patient's problems and background, which the patient may be unfamiliar with or may be unwilling to discuss. Particularly useful to define the oncologic history, likely sources of pain, and probable prognosis. Discussion with health care providers who have known the patient over time may provide insights not apparent in the medical record.

  2. Introduction: Consciously take a moment to introduce yourself and describe the reason for the interview and its format.

      Rationale: Assessment is always a two-way street. Be aware that patients are constantly assessing their health care providers' values, style, knowledge, and goals. Developing an effective method of initiating contact with the patient is an important first step to gaining their confidence.

  3. Psychosocial history: Includes the patient's marital and residential status; employment history; educational, religious, cultural, and ethnic background; and history of drug or alcohol abuse. The health and capabilities of the spouse or significant other should be reviewed, along with the patient's functional status, including ability to complete activities of daily living, recreational activities, nature of active networks of support, and beliefs about pain and disease.

Rationale: Although the psychosocial history is traditionally obtained further along, obtaining this information on the front end signals an interest in the whole person, helping to develop rapport early on. Exploring the patient's resources and values will provide clues as to what sorts of treatments will be acceptable and appropriate. A history of problems with substance abuse suggests the need for additional consultation or support early on.

4. Medical history (exclusive of oncologic history): Elicits the presence of coexisting systemic disease, exercise tolerance, allergies to medications, medication use, and prior surgery.

Rationale: May disclose nononcologic causes of pain (e.g., arthritis, lumbar strain, diabetes) and data that may influence treatment recommendations (e.g., drug/drug or drug/disease interactions). Avoiding too early a discussion of the oncologic history that may produce distress can interfere with the rest of the history.

5. Review of systems. See Table 32-4.

Rationale: This is an extremely important part of the history that is too often overlooked. Cancer is a multisymptomatic disease. Even when the presenting complaint is pain, the overriding goal is to achieve and maintain the best quality of life possible. Seeking the presence of other symptoms is pertinent because failure of pain control is typically related to the development of new symptoms (side effects) or exacerbation of preexisting symptoms. As is true with pain, patients may not volunteer complaints related to other symptoms, assuming they are inevitable. Many symptoms previously regarded as irremediable can now be effectively treated.

6. Oncologic history: Includes history of prior cancer illnesses, family history of cancer, diagnosis and evolution of disease, metastatic status,

TABLE 32-4. *Review of systems*

Systemic/constitutional	Neurologic	Gastrointestinal
Anorexia	Sedation	Dysphagia
Weight loss	Confusion	Nausea
Cachexia	Hallucinations	Vomiting
Fatigue/weakness	Headache	Dehydration
Insomnia	Motor weakness	Constipation
Respiratory	Altered sensation	Diarrhea
Dyspnea	Incontinence	Dry, sore mouth
Cough	Genitourinary	Psychologic
Hiccough	Hesitancy	Irritability
Integument	Urgency	Anxiety
Decubitus	Loss of libido	Depression
Ulcerations	Impotence	Dementia

prior antineoplastic therapies and outcome (including side effects), and the patient's understanding of disease process and prognosis.

Rationale: A history of cancer or of cancer in a close family member may influence the patient's attitude about his or her present illness and attendant pain. Witnessing the painful death of a loved one, as was once extremely common, may generate fear, anxiety, and hopelessness on the part of the survivor. The tempo of disease progression and response to therapies predict optimism and frustration. The histopathologic diagnosis, extent of spread, and prior treatments help determine whether further antitumor therapy is feasible and is likely to be associated with meaningful results. Knowledge of prior treatments and their temporal relationship to pain may suggest a treatment-related pain syndrome. Improvements in pain around the time of chemotherapy may suggest a steroid-responsive syndrome if corticosteroids were a part of the chemotherapy or were given as an antiemetic. Invasive therapies such as neurolysis are more reasonable in the context of a poor prognosis, and finally the patient's understanding of the prognosis and reaction to it help determine how treatment recommendations are best framed.

7. Pain history. See Table 32-5.
   a. History of premorbid chronic pain (predating the cancer diagnosis). Patients with premorbid chronic pain often demonstrate learned pain behavior, predicting a treatment challenge.
   b. History of drug or alcohol abuse. Patients with a prior history of drug or alcohol abuse also present potential management problems.

TABLE 32-5. *Elements of a comprehensive pain history*

- Premorbid chronic pain
- Premorbid drug or alcohol use
- Pain catalogue (number and locations)
- For each pain
  - Onset and evolution
  - Site and radiation
  - Pattern (constant, intermittent, predictable, etc.)
  - Intensity (best, worst, average, current): 0–10 scale
  - Quality
  - Exacerbating factors
  - Relieving factors
  - How the pain interferes
  - Neurologic and motor abnormalities
  - Vasomotor changes
  - Other associated factors
  - Current analgesics (use, efficacy, and side effects)
  - Prior analgesics (use, efficacy, and side effects)

Although the provision of medications with abuse potential may rekindle addictive behavior, in the absence of ongoing abuse, problems are more likely to be related to undertreatment, either because of provider reluctance to prescribe as they might for others or because of the patient's refusal of treatment out of fear of readdiction or, when involved in a recovery group, fear of being stigmatized. Nevertheless, a history of drug abuse warrants consideration of involving other disciplines such as psychology, psychiatry, and social work.

c. Pain inventory. Although a single complaint may be prominent, most patients with cancer pain have multiple sites of discomfort. The importance of the pain inventory lies in the recognition that each pain may be explained by a different mechanism and thus may respond to alternative treatment measures.

d. Other features of the pain history. The evolution of the pain, its site, and the presence of referred or radiating pain help determine anatomic origin. The quality of pain, as intimated by the patient's choice of descriptors (e.g., sharp, burning, dull, agonizing), provides useful information about its underlying mechanism and thus suggests specific treatment. Patients usually accustomed to thinking that pain is pain understandably need to be coached to apply these distinctions. The temporal pattern of pain helps determine the need for around-the-clock analgesics, prn administration, or, as is usually indicated, a combination of both. Pain intensity helps determine what broad classes of analgesics (i.e., NSAIDs, so-called weak or potent opioids) are most appropriate and how aggressive a titration schedule is warranted. Exacerbating and palliative factors may suggest the underlying mechanism as well as simple interventions, such as a brace or walker. Determining how the pain interferes with various aspects of the patient's life helps evaluate associated distress and how urgent it is to provide relief. Neurologic and vasomotor changes help pinpoint the mechanism and source of the pain and may alert the clinician to impending or ongoing spinal cord compression, plexopathy, or leptomeningeal carcinomatosis. A careful history of analgesic use, focusing especially on efficacy and side effects, influences therapeutic decision making. A careful history will help determine whether medication trials have been adequate, whether side effects may be related to a dose or schedule inappropriate to a particular patient, and whether a so-called allergy just represents the occurrence of a normal side effect.

E. Physical examination.
  1. General considerations: Like a careful history, the physical examination is a relatively noninvasive, cost-effective, and time-conservative means of obtaining information. Examining patients with advanced illness is challenging to the clinician, as well as to the patient, because when patients are debilitated, even a thorough examination can be demanding of their limited resources. A basic physical examination, though, is important, especially in home-bound patients whose access to routine medical care may be limited. Studies have demonstrated that it is common for the pain assessment to first disclose new metastases, new neurologic findings, infections, and oncologic emergencies, any one of which may require treatment.
  2. The physical examination should include a determination of weight and vital signs, a thorough examination of the site of pain, surrounding sites (to check for referred pain), sites of known tumor invasion, a complete musculoskeletal and neurologic examination, and auscultation of the heart and lungs and examination of the lymphatic system. The examination should be conducted with the patient in a hospital gown. Since this exchange of garments is depersonalizing and may be intimidating, meaningful exchange should be postponed until the patient is fully clothed.
  3. Findings, particularly on examination of the neurologic and musculoskeletal systems, may be difficult to interpret when acute pain is present.
     Signs of simple nononcologic causes of pain such as trigger points (myofascial pain, muscle contraction headache) and positive straight leg raising (sciatica) should not be overlooked.
  4. Compression of the spinal cord and major nerve plexuses frequently presents with pain as the first sign, and examination may reveal subtle neurologic signs that support such a diagnosis. When integrated with data obtained from the history, findings of pain and neurologic deficit may alert the clinician to the need for an urgent diagnostic work-up to exclude the presence of spinal cord compression, leptomeningeal metastases, and intracranial hypertension, which are oncologic emergencies that require rapid specialist consultation and intervention.
  5. More subtle findings may suggest the presence of neuropathic pain that will require treatment with adjuvant analgesics in addition to opioids.
III. TREATMENT
  A. General Strategies
    1. All efforts at managing cancer pain can be conceived of as pertaining to one of three general strategic approaches: (a) eliminating or modifying the source of pain (e.g., surgery, radiotherapy, chemotherapy), (b) modifying the interpretation of the pain message at the level

of the CNS (i.e., analgesics), (c) interrupting or modifying the pain signal en route from the periphery to the central nervous system (CNS) (i.e., neural blockade).

2. Of the preceding approaches, modifying the source of pain with antineoplastic therapy, when feasible, is generally the most desirable modality. Because of its overall favorable risk-to-benefit ratio, modifying pain perception with analgesics is most commonly applied. Finally, interrupting pain transmission with neural blockade is indicated in specific settings, usually when more conservative modalities have failed.

B. Antineoplastic Therapy
1. These therapies, which may be curative or palliative in their intent and which can be administered singly or in combination, tend to be highly acceptable to patients and their families because in addition to the potential for symptomatic relief, they may slow or halt the progress of the underlying disease. Antineoplastic treatment, however, has limitations and potential side effects, and as with all other medical treatments must be subjected to a risk/benefit analysis and require informed consent. Even with ongoing cancer treatment, concomitant treatment with analgesics is usually indicated while awaiting tumor response. Even when the goal of cancer cure has been abandoned, further antitumor therapy should be considered when new symptoms develop or a change in pain therapy is planned.

2. Surgical therapy: Surgery for pain relief is usually considered only when it has a reasonable likelihood of affecting cure or major palliation. In the case of an early diagnosis that precedes the development of distant metastases, surgical excision may be curative, in which case there is a high likelihood that pain control will be achieved as well. Even with successful surgical treatment of the cancer, however, pain may persist due to tumor-mediated damage to neighboring nerves and other adjacent structures. In addition, new pain may result from tissue damage incurred during surgery or positioning. Well-recognized postsurgical pain syndromes that occur with a relatively high degree of frequency include postthoracotomy, postmastectomy, postradical neck surgery, postamputation, and postnephrectomy pain.

3. Radiation therapy: Although often curative, radiation therapy is the most common antineoplastic modality used for palliation of pain and related symptoms (e.g., bleeding, ulceration, dyspnea, symptoms associated with obstruction or any space-occupying lesion). Various treatment schedules are undertaken, depending on the circumstances (radiosensitivity, prognosis, performance status, etc.), but when treatment is palliative in intent, especially for pain, there is a growing trend toward treating

in a limited number of sessions (hypofractionation), which is often more practical for patients who primarily need symptomatic relief. Radiation therapy is a particular consideration for the treatment of painful bone metastases.

4. Chemotherapy: In the absence of the potential for cure or remission, systemic chemotherapy is less frequently implemented specifically as a means to control pain. Dramatic and durable reductions in pain are commonplace in the setting of a biologic response to hormonal and chemotherapy, as is common with prostate cancer, lymphoma, and multiple myeloma, although when compared with radiation therapy, relief may be slow to accrue.

C. Pharmacotherapy

Pharmacologic management, of which the mainstay of treatment is the opioid analgesics, is considered the first line of therapy for patients with cancer pain (Table 32-6). An estimated 70% to 90% of patients can be rendered relatively free of pain when straightforward guideline-based principles of pharmacologic management are applied in a thorough, careful manner. The World Health Organization's three-step ladder approach to cancer pain management relies exclusively on the administration of oral agents (Fig. 32-1) and is usually effective. Noninvasive routes (e.g., oral, transdermal, transmucosal) should be maintained as long as possible for reasons that include simplicity, maintenance of independence and mobility, convenience, and cost. Treatment has been markedly simplified by the introduction of controlled-release preparations of oral opioids (e.g., MS Contin, Oramorph, Kadian Oxycontin) and novel, noninvasive approaches (e.g., transdermal fentanyl, oral transmucosal fentanyl citrate), and most important, the widespread acceptance of guideline-based therapies, as summarized later. Pharmacotherapy is effective in adults and children and across different cultures. The analgesia associated with systemically administered medications is titratable and suitable for pain that is multifocal and/or progressive, as exists in most patients with cancer pain. Effects and side effects are reversible, and widespread implementation does not depend on sophisticated technology or scarce resources. As a result of the preceding features, most teaching about cancer pain and its management should focus on the proper use of such analgesics. Although pain can be managed in most patients with oral agents alone, even through the terminal stages of illness, a small but important number of patients require alternative forms of therapy. The role of more interventional forms of analgesia, ranging from parenteral analgesics to neural blockade and CNS opioid therapy, is discussed later.

1. Assessment (see Tables 32-2 and 32-3). As has been emphasized, assessment forms the basis for subsequent treatment and should include

TABLE 32-6. *General principles of pain management in the cancer patient: management*

- Develop and apply an algorhythmic approach to each pain problem, always being prepared to modify care plans based on individual features of a patient's presentation and response.
- When feasible, treat pain by attempting to modify its cause, usually with antineoplastic therapy. Institute concurrent symptomatic treatment with analgesics while awaiting therapeutic response, which may be delayed.
- Select specific drugs for specific reasons.
- Keep the treatment regimen simple whenever possible. Avoid polypharmacy unless indicated for specific reasons. Review drug regimen regularly and consider discontinuing agents that are of questionable value. They can always be restarted.
- Maintain exquisite familiarity with a core group of drugs that are frequently used. Ensure ready access to reliable information on less frequently prescribed drugs.
- Be knowledgeable about the range of side effects associated with prescribed drugs. When considering drugs with similar primary effects, be aware of the opportunity to exploit "side effects" (secondary effects) that may be beneficial in a given patient (e.g., nighttime use of a sedating antidepressant for neuropathic pain in a patient with concomitant insomnia).
- Start new drugs in low doses and be prepared to titrate dose upward rapidly once a therapeutic response and the presence or absence of side effects has been established.
- Avoid starting multiple drugs simultaneously, both to minimize the risk of drug interactions and to avoid uncertainty about which agent is responsible for changes.
- Always express a generic willingness to help the patient and family. Ask explicitly what they want or need. Be aware that it may be not a prescription, but advice or just an empathetic listener. Never say or imply "nothing more can be done."
- Consider nonpharmacologic therapies, both invasive (antineoplastic, anesthetic, neurosurgical, orthopedic) and noninvasive (behavioral, counseling, psychiatric), when appropriate.
- Discuss treatment decisions with patient and family members. When appropriate, present options in the context of their alternatives and relative risk and benefit. Always try to provide clear recommendations based on your knowledge of the patient and the merits of each treatment option.
- Provide education to patients and their families or significant others regarding all aspects of treatment. When appropriate, involve the family in establishing realistic goals. Seek its help in maintaining compliance with treatment recommendations. Interact with family members in a supportive manner that communicates concern about their well-being and a willingness to ease their distress.
- Encourage patients to understand their illness and their treatments and to maintain and carry with them a list of medications they take. When appropriate, provide instructions on the use of pain diaries.
- Discuss advanced directives when appropriate.

an evaluation of both physiologic determinants (the pain syndrome, the neoplastic process, associated symptoms, intercurrent medical conditions) and psychosocial determinants (beliefs, cultural milieu, economic status, family interactions). A problem list and a set of realistic goals

The WHO Analgesic Ladder

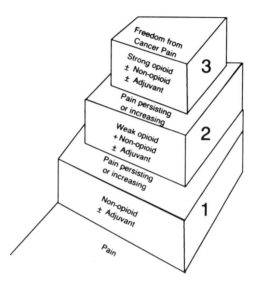

(WHO, 1986)

FIG. 32-1. World Health Organization–advocated ladder approach toward cancer pain relief that relies primarily on pain intensity and, to a lesser extent, pain mechanism as determinants of therapy. (World Health Organization. *Cancer Pain Relief.* Geneva: WHO; 1986. Used by permission.)

that are acceptable to the patient, family, and physician should be established, along with a treatment plan and contingencies. Treatment should be directed toward relief of total pain, which includes consideration of all aspects of function (e.g., disturbance of sleep, appetite, mood, activity, posture, and sexuality), and attention to both physical and emotional, psychologic, and spiritual aspects of suffering. Recommendations should include an explicit plan for reevaluation.

2. Nonsteroidal antiinflammatory drugs (NSAIDs)

   a. Consider the regular (around-the-clock) administration of an NSAID as the sole treatment for mild pain or an NSAID combined with an opioid analgesic for moderate to severe pain. Although potentially effective in all settings, NSAIDs are particularly effective for pain of inflammatory and bony metastatic origin, in virtue of interference with prostaglandin (PG) synthesis.

      Despite their apparent heterogeneity, the NSAIDs are, in most respects, clinically indistinguishable.

b. There is little evidence from controlled trials to suggest important medically based distinctions between NSAIDs. Thus decision making is somewhat arbitrary. Considerations include the patient's prior favorable or unfavorable experience, clinician experience, cost, schedule, and minor differences in toxicity.

c. Potential benefits need to be balanced against potential toxicity (e.g., GI, GU, CNS, hematologic, and masking of fever), considerations that are especially pertinent in the context of recent antitumor therapy and advanced age. Consider avoiding NSAIDs altogether or instituting prophylaxis in patients predisposed to developing gastropathy or bleeding diathesis. If gastrointestinal prophylaxis is indicated, misoprostol appears to be most effective. The nonacetylated salicylates (sodium salicylate, choline magnesium trisalicylate) are associated with a favorable toxicity profile, in that they fail to interfere with platelet aggregation, are rarely associated with GI bleeding, and are well tolerated in asthmatic patients. A parenteral formulation of ketorolac has been shown to be equianalgesic to low doses of morphine in some settings but is associated with the same range of potential side effects as oral NSAIDs. A new oral NSAID, bromfenac sodium (Duract), was recently shown to provide analgesia that is comparable to treatment with oxycodone-acetaminophen. As a result of just under a dozen reports of liver failure resulting in death or the need for transplant, bromfenac sodium was withdrawn less than a year after its release. Currently, ketorolac is recommended only for short-term use.

d. In contrast to opioid therapy, the NSAIDs are associated with a ceiling effect, above which dose escalations produce toxicity but no greater analgesia. The ceiling dose for a given drug differs from patient to patient, thus still allowing some potential for dose titration. Regular (as opposed to intermittent) use promotes both anti-inflammatory and analgesic effects.

e. When efficacy is poor, the clinician may consider rotating to another NSAID, usually from a distinct biochemical class. Although evidence from controlled trials is insufficient to support this practice, it is clear that, for a given patient, clinical response differs among various agents (interindividual variability), and recent evidence indicates that various classes of NSAIDs may exert their anti-PG effects on different subtypes of cyclooxygenase (cox-1 and cox-2), the enzyme primarily responsible for PG degradation. Preliminary research on cox-2 inhibitors suggests similar efficacy to traditional NSAIDs with little or no risk of side effects.

3. Opioids: The opioids mediate analgesia predominantly by effects on subcellular receptors at the level of the spinal cord and brain that when activated produce a complex series of events resulting in modification of the interpretation of the peripheral signals associated with tissue injury. When properly applied, adequate analgesia is achieved in most cases with minimal toxicity.

4. Analgesic conventionally used to treat moderate pain (so-called weak opioids)

   a. When NSAIDs provide insufficient relief, are contraindicated, or are poorly tolerated, or when pain is severe at presentation, the addition or substitution of a so-called weak opioid (i.e., codeine, hydrocodone, dihydrocodeine, oxycodone preparations) is recommended as an analgesic of intermediate potency. Almost exclusively formulated as combination products, these agents are weak only insofar as the inclusion of aspirin, acetaminophen, or ibuprofen results in a ceiling dose above which the incidence of toxicity increases. Thus the nomenclature opioids conventionally used to treat moderate pain are now endorsed over weak opioids in recognition of the fact that, when equianalgesic dosing is applied, the potency of the opioid per se is not a clinically important distinguishing feature of this class of drugs. For example, a sole entity preparation of oxycodone is now available that, when prescribed in sufficient doses, is effective for even severe pain, since the ceiling effect imposed by the aspirin/acetaminophen is absent. Likewise, fentanyl, although up to 100 times more potent than parenteral morphine, is rendered clinically useful by utilizing a dosing schedule in a microgram rather than a milligram range.

   b. Although the weak opioids are appropriate for mild or intermittent pain, practitioners often rely excessively on these agents, frequently long after their efficacy is lost, in an ill-advised attempt to avoid prescribing more potent opioids that are also more highly regulated.

   c. Common agents

      (1) Propoxyphene is rarely appropriate for the management of cancer pain because of its low potency.

      (2) Codeine is considerably emetogenic and constipating relative to its analgesic potency, and is used less frequently than in the past.

      (3) Hydrocodone and, less frequently dihydrocodeine preparations (e.g., Vicodin, LorTAB, Synalgos DC), are probably most commonly prescribed because they are stronger than codeine and have the perceived advantage of not requiring triplicate prescriptions (DEA Class C-III versus C-II). The potency

of hydrocodone and dihydrocodeine is between that of codeine and oxycodone. Neither is available as a single-entity preparation; both are formulated with various doses of opioid and coanalgesic. The clinician must be cautious not to exceed the usual recommended dose of aspirin or acetaminophen (4 to 5 g/day) as requirements increase.

(4) Oxycodone, now available not only as a combination product (e.g., Percocet, Percodan) but also as a sole-entity preparation (e.g., Roxycodone) and in a slow-release formulation (Oxycontin), is the most potent in this class—considerably more potent than codeine and possibly the most useful drug in this class.

5. Opioids conventionally used to treat severe pain (so-called potent opioids)

a. When combinations of codeinelike drugs and NSAIDs provide insufficient analgesia or when pain is severe at presentation, therapy should progress to include more potent opioid analgesics in a "ladder" fashion (see Fig. 32-1).

b. Morphine, hydromorphone, transdermal fentanyl, and oxycodone are appropriate first line agents for the institution of basal analgesia (Tables 32-7 and 32-8). Of these, only morphine has been shown to elaborate active metabolites. A small proportion of patients using morphine chronically may experience refractory sedation or nausea as a consequence of M-6 glucoronide accumulation, which may improve with rotation to an alternate opioid.

c. Methadone, although inexpensive, and to a lesser extent levorphanol are usually reserved for special circumstances because their half-lives are long and unpredictable, introducing the potential for accumulation, especially in the presence of advanced age and altered renal function. Recent evidence suggests that in addition to its opioid effects, methadone may antagonize NMDA receptors, providing an additional rationale for its use for refractory pain.

d. Less potent analgesics should not be summarily excluded, since NSAIDs may provide additive or synergistic analgesia, and codeinelike preparations may be useful for breakthrough or incident pain.

e. Opioids should initially be introduced in low doses because the early development of side effects will negatively influence compliance but should be rapidly titrated to effect.

6. Individualization: Pharmacologic therapy should be individualized in light of the specific characteristics and needs of each patient. Dose response and side effects vary widely based on various physiologic

TABLE 32-7. *Comparison of "potent" opioid agonists used in cancer pain management*

Generic name	Trade name	Route	Equivalent dose*	Duration (avg. range)
Morphine	Various	I.M.	10 mg	3–4 hr
	MSIR	Oral	20–30 mg	3–4 hr
	Various	Rectal	5 mg	4 hr
Controlled–	MS Contin	Oral	30 mg	12–8 hr
release	Oramorph	Oral	30 mg	12–8 hr
morphine	Kadian	Oral	30 mg	24–12 hr
Hydromorphone	Dilaudid	Oral	7.5 mg	3–4 hr
		I.M.	1.5 mg	3–4 hr
Oxymorphone	Numorphan	I.M.	1 mg	3–6 hr
		Rectal	5–10 mg	4–6 hr
Meperidine	Demerol	Oral	300 mg	3–6 hr
		I.M.	75 mg	3–4 hr
Heroin	Diamorphine	I.M.	5 mg	4–5 hr
		Oral	60 mg	
Methadone**	Dolophine	I.M.	20 mg	4–8 hr
		Oral	10 mg	4–8 hr
Levorphanol	Levodromoran	I.M.	2 mg	4–8 hr
		Oral	2 mg	4–8 hr
Oxycodone	Various	Oral	30 mg	3–6 hr
Controlled release	Oxycontin	Oral	30 mg	12 hr
Transdermal fentanyl	Duragesic	TD	Table 6	72 hr

*Compared with 10 mg parenteral morphine.
**Potency appears to be greater than reflected here. Slow titration is essential.

and behavioral factors, and effective doses often dramatically exceed guidelines recommended in standard texts (e.g., morphine, 10 mg I.M., 30 mg p.o.), which are for the most part derived from experience with acute or postoperative pain in opioid-naive individuals.

7. Dosing guidelines: The correct dose of an opioid for the management of cancer pain is that which effectively relieves pain without inducing unacceptable side effects. The starting dose is gradually and steadily titrated upward until either pain control is achieved or a troublesome side effect occurs. If the former ensues before adequate pain relief is established, the side effects should be treated aggressively in an algorithmic fashion. Other strategies that can be employed (e.g., opioid rotation, anesthetic interventions) are cited later.

8. Side effects
   a. Constipation and miosis are the only two opioid-mediated effects to which tolerance appears never to significantly develop. Opioid-induced constipation is sufficiently common that it should almost universally be treated prophylactically. Usually a combined mild

TABLE 32-8. *Dosage equivalency
for transdermal fentanyl*

Hourly dose based on 24 hour morphine equivalents		
Oral morphine* (mg/24 hr)	IM morphine† (mg/24 hr)	Transdermal fentanyl (μg/hr)
45–134	8–22	25
135–224	23–37	50
225–314	38–52	75
315–404	53–67	100
405–494	68–82	125
495–584	83–97	150
585–674	98–112	175
675–764	113–127	200
765–854	128–142	225
855–944	143–157	250
945–1034	158–172	275
1035–1124	173–187	300

Adapted from a package insert. By permission of Janssen Pharmaceutica.

*Conversion from oral morphine: Based on a *conservative* analgesic activity ratio of 60 mg oral morphine to 10 mg IM morphine (6:1 oral/parenteral conversion ratio rather than the widely accepted 3:1 ratio). As a result, converting from oral morphine to transdermal fentanyl using this chart, although generally quite safe, may result in underdosing of up to half of patients who will then require rapid upward titration to achieve analgesia.

†Conversion from IV or IM morphine: An analgesic activity ratio of 10 mg IM morphine to 100 μg IV fentanyl was used to derive the equivalence of parenteral morphine to transdermal fentanyl. *These recommendations tend to be reliable.*

laxative and softener (e.g., Senekot-S) is prescribed when opioid therapy commences, along with instructions for a sliding-scale regimen that provides progressively stronger cathartics until a regular bowel habit ensues. An osmotic agent (e.g., lactulose) is the usual second-line agent of choice for refractory constipation. The evaluating clinician should remain alert for the presence of bowel obstruction, as well as fecal impaction, which may present as spurious diarrhea due to the leakage of liquid stool around a distal fecal plug. Impaction is confirmed by manual rectal examination, and its occurrence leaves no other alternative than manual disimpaction, which is time-consuming, is unpleasant, and usually requires strong analgesics. Finally, unrecognized constipation can contribute to nausea and vomiting.

b. Opioid-mediated nausea and sedation occur in up to half of patients first exposed to an opioid and after dose increases. These symptoms usually resolve spontaneously with continued use, so patients should be reassured and encouraged to adhere to their prescribed regimen. If patients are not routinely apprised of these features, they will mistake side effects for allergy.

(1) For nausea and/or vomiting, a major tranquilizer (e.g., prochlorperazine, chlorpromazine) administered orally or rectally is the usual first-line agent of choice, especially when cost is a consideration. A properistaltic agent (e.g., metaclopramide) is appropriate when gastric stasis is suggested by nausea, bloating, and early satiety. Scopolamine is particularly useful for nausea that is vertiginous in nature (i.e., amplified by ambulation). Commonly used as an adjunct to emetic chemotherapies, ondansetron (Zofran) can be considered for refractory nausea, but is usually avoided due to cost. Dronabinol, an oral agent containing active elements of marijuana, and corticosteroids are other alternatives for refractory nausea. Sedation that fails to improve with time can often be managed effectively with a psychostimulant such as methylphenidate or dextroamphetamine.

(2) When side effects are refractory to pharmacoreversal, consideration should be given to a trial of a similar, alternative opioid analgesic because side effects are often idiosyncratic and may not be triggered by agents that are in other respects quite similar. Another strategy involves adding an adjuvant analgesic (see later), when appropriate, to produce an opioid-sparing effect. In patients with amenable pain syndromes, the presence of refractory side effects is an indication to consider other, more invasive therapeutic modalities (see later).

9. Follow-up: Once an acceptable drug regimen has been established, adequacy should be periodically reassessed. Patients are often reluctant to request more potent analgesics because of fear of addiction. Increased drug requirements related to progression of disease and the development of physical tolerance should be anticipated. Tolerance, which is most frequently manifested by decreased duration of analgesics, is now recognized to be a less frequent cause of dose escalation than disease progression.

10. Education, addiction potential: Patient and family education is an essential element of a successful pain relief program and is ideally accomplished through the combined efforts of physicians and nurses. Patients commonly maintain deeply rooted culturally reinforced fears of addiction. The distinction among addiction (psychologic dependence), physical dependence, and tolerance should be explained.

a. Tolerance, the need for increasing dosages over time to maintain a desired effect, and physical dependence (a state characterized by the onset of characteristic withdrawal symptoms when a drug is precipitously stopped or a specific antagonist is administered) are inevitable biophysiologic phenomena that should thus be regarded as a pharmacologic effects (see Table 32-9). They are unrelated to addiction and need not impede analgesic therapy. Since tolerance develops to most side effects as well as to analgesia, doses can usually be increased to counter tolerance; should opioid therapy become unnecessary, patients are generally able to discontinue use without problems when a gradual taper is instituted.

b. Addiction is a psychobehavioral phenomenon with possible genetic influences characterized by (a) overwhelming drug use, (b) nonmedical drug use, and (c) continued use despite the presence or threat of physiologic or psychologic harm. In contrast to tolerance and physical dependence, which are inevitable with chronic use, true addiction is an extremely rare outcome of medical therapy. The main exception involves patients with a previous history of drug abuse who pose significant risks of developing patterns of aberrant drug use.

TABLE 32-9. *Contemporary description of phenomena historically associated with addiction*

Phenomena	Etiology	Definition	Incidence	Management
Physical dependence	Physiologic, pharmacologic	Withdrawal if opioids abruptly stopped or naloxone administered	Almost invariable	Avoid by gradual taper
Tolerance*	Physiologic, pharmacologic	Increased dose required to achieve analgesia†	Almost invariable	Reestablish analgesia with upward titration
Addiction (psychologic dependence)	Psychologic, questionable genetic influences	Nonmedical use despite harm	Rare (<1%)	Identify, multidisciplinary management
Withdrawal (abstinence syndrome)	Physiologic, pharmacologic	Characteristic signs and symptoms‡	Almost invariable	Avoid, reverse with opioids

*Although inevitable to some degree, current thinking posits these phenomena as considerably less severe than previously thought, recognizing instead that dose increases in cancer patients are most likely due to disease progression.

†Tolerance develops to most adverse effects as well, especially nausea and sedation, but slowly if at all to constipation and miosis.

‡Characteristic signs and symptoms include lacrimation, diaphoresis, rhinorrhea, pupillary dilation, gooseflesh, muscle tremor, nausea and vomiting, abdominal cramping, diarrhea, raised heart rate, respiratory rate and blood pressure, chills, hyperthermia, flushing, yawning, restlessness, irritability, anorexia, disturbed sleep, and generalized body aches.

11. Schedule: Based on a recognition that if analgesics are withheld until pain becomes severe, sympathetic arousal occurs and even potent analgesics may be ineffective, a time-contingent schedule for the administration of analgesics is generally preferred to symptom-contingent administration. With prolonged prn administration, patterns of anticipation and memory of pain become established and may contribute to suffering, even during periods of adequate analgesia. Around-the-clock administration of appropriate analgesics maintains more even therapeutic blood levels and decreases the likelihood of intolerable pain (Fig. 32-2).

12. Basal analgesia: Compliance and overall quality of analgesia are enhanced by the regular administration of long-acting opioid analgesics for basal pain control, supplemented by a short-acting opioid analgesic administered prn ("escape doses" or "rescue doses") for breakthrough and incident pain. In contemporary practice, preferred basal analgesics include controlled-release morphine and oxycodone preparations that are available in a wide range of doses but cannot be broken, crushed, or chewed and transdermal fentanyl. Transdermal fentanyl is best reserved for the management of relatively stable basal pain (see later). When these agents are poorly tolerated, methadone or levorphanol may be prescribed with careful monitoring to avoid accumulation.

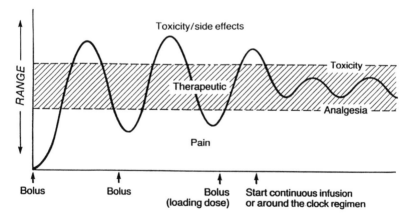

FIG. 32-2. Schematic graph depicting the potential for alternating bouts of toxicity and pain often associated with standard prn dosing. Note the transition to continuous infusion and reductions in peak and trough levels. Similar effect occurs with institution of controlled-release oral opioids or transdermal fentanyl administered around the clock. Problems may arise when, as a consequence of factors related to advanced illness (anorexia, cachexia, depression), the "therapeutic window" narrows, increasing the difficulty of achieving comfort without undesirable side effects, in which case strategies to "open" the window may be instituted (e.g., raising its threshold by treating side effects or lowering its threshold by reducing nociception with treatments like radiotherapy or neural blockade).

13. Escape (rescue) doses
    a. A drug of relatively high potency, short onset, and brief duration (e.g., immediate-release morphine, hydromorphone, or oxycodone) is selected for prn administration to manage exacerbations of pain. These agents should be prescribed at intervals based on their expected duration of action, usually every 2 to 4 hours, prn. Patients should be instructed to maintain careful records that accurately reflect their analgesic use. When breakthrough medications are utilized more than two or three times over a 12-hour period consistently, the dose of the basal, long-acting analgesic should be increased.
    b. If incident pain is a significant problem, patients should be instructed to take their prn (breakthrough) dose in anticipation of pain-provoking activity. A new formulation of oral transmucosal fentanyl citrate has been shown to produce meaningful relief of break-through pain within 5 minutes of initiating consumption, an onset that mimics IV administration, despite the noninvasive character of this therapy.

14. Adjuvant analgesics: Selected patients benefit from treatment with these agents. In general, these agents are mechanism-specific and should be utilized based on a specific indication (see later).

15. Oral and transdermal routes: When possible, analgesics should be administered orally or by a similarly noninvasive route (transdermal, rectal, oral transmucosal) to promote independence and mobility and for ease of titration. In the presence of a functional, intact GI system, once dose is adjusted to account for hepatic first-pass effect, oral administration provides analgesia that is as effective as parenteral (but not spinal) administration.

16. Alternate routes: When pain control is inadequate with oral analgesics or the oral route is contraindicated, consideration should be given to alternative means of drug delivery.
    a. Transdermal: Once treatment is established, transdermal fentanyl provides steady plasma levels of analgesic for 72 hours following a single application of a 25-, 50-, 75-, or 100- μ g/hr patch (see Table 32-7). The surface area of the patch is directly proportional to the administered dose of fentanyl. The system's rate-controlling membrane regulates drug release at a slower rate than average skin flux, thus ensuring that the delivery system, rather than the skin, is the main determinant of absorption. Of all the factors with the potential to influence the rate of absorption of transdermal fentanyl, temperature is most important. As a result, patients should be warned against applying such devices as heating pads. After the first administration and dose increases, a consistent, near-peak level is achieved only after 12 to 18 hours have

elapsed, after which steady state is maintained. Patients need to be cautioned that pain relief will accrue over the first day of treatment and should be provided with rescue doses of short-acting analgesics during this interval. In addition, as a result of the formation of a skin depot of drug, effects persist for 12 to 18 hours following removal of the patch, so that adverse effects may require prolonged treatment. Although the transdermal fentanyl system was originally studied in the perioperative setting, its current indications are limited to the management of chronic pain. Conversion schemes are conservative, so that up to half of patients dosed according to the product's package insert will require rapid upward titration. Because of the lag between dose and response, transdermal fentanyl analgesia is best suited for patients with relatively stable dose requirements and is particularly useful when the oral route is contraindicated. A small proportion of patients (5% to 10%) may require that their patches be changed every 60 or, rarely, 48 hours.

b. Rectal: The rectal route is reliable for short-term use, except in the presence of diarrhea, fibrosis, fistulas, or other anatomic abnormalities. Rectal administration is usually avoided in older children and in the presence of conditions that increase pain when patients are positioned for suppository insertion. Morphine and hydromorphone are available in rectal preparations, and oxymorphone hydrochloride (Numorphan) rectal suppositories provide 4 to 6 hours of potent analgesia. Rectal methadone has been shown to be safe and effective but must be compounded by a manufacturing pharmacist.

c. Other options include continuous subcutaneous or intravenous infusions of opioids by means of a portable pump, patient-controlled analgesia (intravenous or subcutaneous), and intrathecal or epidural opioids administered via an externalized catheter or internalized pump. New means of administering opioids are being explored and include mucous membrane (sublingual and transnasal), transdermal, and respiratory absorption.

17. Alternate drugs and drugs to avoid

a. The clinician should maintain familiarity with the pharmacologic profiles of a variety of opioids (see Tables 32-7 and 32-8) and should consider drug substitution when a patient exhibits tolerance to the analgesic effects or intolerance to the side effects of standard analgesics. When converting between drugs or routes, half to two-thirds the calculated equianalgesic dose of the new drug is usually recommended as a starting dose, which is then titrated rapidly, as needed.

   b. The chronic administration of meperidine, especially by the oral route, is contraindicated. Administered chronically, all opioids may produce some degree of myoclonus, but the accumulation of normeperidine, a metabolite, may lead to frank seizure activity, especially when renal function is impaired.
   c. Agonist/antagonist and partial-agonist opioids should generally be avoided for a variety of reasons, the most important of which is the presence of a ceiling effect, or dose above which toxicity but not analgesia increases. With the usual exception of buprenorphine, these agents may precipitate withdrawal, and their administration complicates the eventual, usually inevitable transition to pure agonist agents. Pentazocine (Talwin), the only one of these agents widely available orally, is associated with a high incidence of hallucinations and confusion, and buprenorphine is not easily or reliably reversed by naloxone.
18. Alternative therapies: Adequate pain relief cannot always be achieved through pharmacologic means alone. Initial screening should identify patients in whom behavioral or psychologic modalities may be employed successfully. When comprehensive trials of pharmacologic therapy have failed, consideration should be given to alternative modalities, including additional antitumor therapy, neural blockade, CNS opioid therapy, neurosurgical options, and, rarely, electrical stimulation.

D. Adjuvant Analgesics
   1. In the context of cancer pain management the term *adjuvant analgesic* refers to a heterogeneous group of medications (a) observed to promote analgesia only in specific clinical settings that (b) were all originally developed for purposes other than relief of pain.
   2. Although a large variety of drugs are purported to possess adjuvant properties, only a limited number have been shown to reliably relieve pain in controlled or partially controlled trials.
   3. The most well-established adjuvants that are clinically useful for cancer pain include (a) corticosteroids; (b) selected, usually tricyclic, antidepressants; (c) anticonvulsants; (d) amphetamines; and, more rarely, (e) n-methyl d-aspartate antagonists; (f) alpha-adrenergic antagonists; (g) antihistamines; and (h) phenothiazines. It is important to note that (a) not every agent belonging to each component drug class appears to possess analgesic properties, (b) even those agents with confirmed analgesic properties are potentially efficacious and thus applicable only for specific types of pain derived from specific selected conditions, and (c) even then pain relief will not occur with certainty in all patients.
   4. Adjuvant analgesics differ from opioid analgesics in important conceptual ways.

a. Opioids are all-purpose analgesics in that, independent of the clinical setting, if administered in a high enough dose, some degree of pain relief is elicited. Although side effects may eclipse their utility in the setting of less-opioid-responsive conditions, a correlation still exists between analgesia and dose escalations. In contrast, responses to adjuvant analgesics are more binary in nature: depending on the nature of the clinical condition, treatment with adjuvants may or may not elicit pain relief.

b. A second fundamental difference relates to the dose/response relationship. Even in conditions where adjuvants are clearly effective, the nature of the dose/response relationship is fundamentally different from that of the opioids. For opioids the relationship between dose and response is usually relatively linear and, temporally, tightly linked. Although, depending on the pain's opioid responsivity, the slope of the line describing the dose/response relationship may be shallow or steep, the correlation between dose and analgesia is manifested with each administration. In contrast, even when an adjuvant reduces pain, there is no certainty that raising the dose will enhance analgesia, or that if analgesia improves, it will do so in a proportionate, timely, or replicable manner.

c. These features form the basis for the administration of adjuvants in the context of sequential trials. Unfortunately, these features often render adjuvant therapy impractical for cancer pain that is of an urgent nature or that occurs in the presence of a reduced life expectancy.

d. Adjuvants, though, are especially useful for the neuropathic pain that commonly occurs in treatment-related syndromes, especially in cancer survivors.

5. Specific agents
   a. Antidepressants
      (1) The operant mechanism for antidepressant-mediated analgesia presumably relates to increased circulating pools of norepinephrine and serotonin induced by reductions in the postsynaptic uptake of these neurotransmitters. That, in responders, analgesia is characteristically induced with doses generally considered insufficient to relieve depression argues for a direct, independent underlying mechanism of effect.
      (2) The most compelling indication for TCA therapy remains variants of neuropathic pain (e.g., postherpetic neuralgia, intercostal brachial neuralgia, plexopathy, phantom limb pain). The TCAs are usually regarded as first-line therapy for neuropathic pain that is relatively constant and unrelenting but that is not predominantly intermittent, lancinating, jabbing, or shocklike.

Neuropathic pain of the latter (paroxysmal) type may also be treated effectively with TCAs but is often first treated with an anticonvulsant. As noted, TCAs have also been used successfully in headache and other syndromes, and thus a trial in nearly any cancer pain syndrome that has not responded favorably to primary analgesics is justified.

(3) Amitriptyline and, to a lesser extent, imipramine remain the most extensively studied of these agents; as a result, they are the usual first choices of academically based pain specialists. Although usually relatively innocuous, side effects are especially prominent with these agents. Since amitriptyline and imipramine are, respectively, metabolized to nortriptyline and desipramine, agents with superior side effect profiles, many authorities, especially in private practice, advocate the latter two agents as drugs of first choice. Data from controlled clinical trials support the use of amitriptyline, nortriptyline, desipramine, imipramine, doxepin, maprotiline, and clomipramine. Trazadone, although sedating and thus potentially helpful for sleep disturbances, appears to be of limited value as an analgesic. Interestingly, despite their efficacy for depression and generally favorable side effect profiles, the newer selective serotonin reuptake inhibitors (SSRIs) such as fluoxetine (Prozac), paroxetine (Paxil), and sertraline (Zoloft) appear overall to be less effective for treating pain than the heterocyclic antidepressants. Obviously, in cases where pain is a secondary manifestation of depression, the SSRIs and other antidepressants, administered in therapeutic doses, may be beneficial.

(4) Usually amitriptyline, nortriptyline, or desipramine are started in doses of 10 to 25 mg nightly and are gradually titrated upward, usually to a range of 50 to 125 mg and occasionally higher until toxicity occurs or analgesia is established. Dry mouth, constipation, drowsiness, and dysphoria are the most prominent of a wide range of potential side effects, although more serious, usually anticholinergic side effects may occur (e.g., urinary retention, cardiac dysrhythmias). Unlike the side effects of opioid therapy, the development of tolerance is less robust and side effects are less readily reversible; as a result, if side effects are more prominent than analgesia, the offending agent is usually discontinued and an analog or a drug from another class is usually started. Although not as reliably analgesic as the TCAs, the newer SSRIs may be preferred for (a) the fragile elderly, (b) patients predisposed to

developing serious anticholinergic side effects, (c) patients who have failed multiple trials of tricyclics due to side effects, and (d) those for whom depression is a prominent comorbidity. Usual starting doses of the SSRIs are the same as those suggested for the management of depression (fluoxetine 20 mg, paroxetine 20 mg, sertraline 50 mg), administered as a single morning dose to take advantage of their propensity to mildly stimulate activity.

b. Anticonvulsants and baclofen

(1) Carbamazepine, phenytoin, valproate, clonazepam, and most recently gabapentin, alone or in combination with the TCAs, have been used successfully as drugs of first choice for neuropathic pain that resembles classic trigeminal neuralgia (i.e., predominantly paroxysmal, jabbing, shocklike pain) and as a second-line therapy for relatively steady, constant neuropathic pain when TCAs are poorly tolerated or have been ineffective or only partially effective.

(2) Anticonvulsants presumably relieve pain in these settings as a result of their ability to dampen ectopic foci of electrical activity and spontaneous discharge from injured nerves, in a manner analogous to their salutary effects in seizure disorders. Carbamazepine therapy has been most thoroughly documented, and thus, in the absence of contraindications, it is usually considered the drug of first choice. The most toxic of the anticonvulsants used to treat pain, carbamazepine is associated with idiosyncratic hepatoxicity (rare) and bone marrow depression (incidence of up to 2%), and thus is avoided in patients with liver metastases, in those with bone marrow depletion, or in those receiving cytotoxic therapy. Used chronically, carbamazepine therapy requires monitoring of CBC and liver function tests every 2 to 3 months. Ataxia, confusion, dizziness, and nausea are relatively common with upward-dose titration, and thus carbamazepine is also best avoided in the fragile elderly, especially combined with other psychotropic agents. Clonazepam in doses of 0.5 mg bid is often well tolerated in patients who have experienced or are at risk for side effects with carbamazepine, phenytoin, and valproate. Carbamazepine is usually started at 100 mg bid and titrated upward toward 300 to 400 mg qid while awaiting an analgesic response or toxicity. Failure of one anticonvulsant does not appear to predict outcome for trials of an alternate agent. Gabapentin is a new anticonvulsant that, according to anecdote, may be highly efficacious for neuropathic pain, especially when lancinating,

although controlled trials have not yet been reported. Although felbamate, another new anticonvulsant, is known to interact with NMDA receptors, its use is probably only rarely warranted due to concerns regarding the development of aplastic anemia. Although it is a GABA agonist and not an anticonvulsant, baclofen, with or without carbamazepine, has been reported to be effective for lancinating, ticlike neuropathic pain. Baclofen is usually started at a dose of 5 mg bid or tid and may be titrated up to 30 to 90 mg/day, as tolerated. The other main role for baclofen in pain management is as an intrathecal infusion for spasticity, due especially to spinal cord injury and multiple sclerosis.

c. Oral local anesthetics: Based on historic accounts of transient relief of pain after IV infusions of local anesthetics, oral (and rectal) analogs already in use as antiarrhythmics have been exploited for relief of neuropathic pain. Although oral tocainide and rectal flecainide have been used with some success, the agent of choice from this group, especially in the United States, is mexiletine, which is usually regarded as a second- or third-line agent for continuous or intermittent neuropathic pain disorders. The oral local anesthetics block sodium channels and presumably relieve pain by mechanisms similar to those invoked to explain anticonvulsant-mediated analgesia. Mexiletine is usually started in doses of 150 mg/day and is titrated upward to a maximum dose of 300 mg tid. Up to 40% of patients may discontinue therapy due to side effects, the most common of which are nausea and vomiting.

d. Psychostimulants (amphetamines). Although the most accepted use for amphetamines in palliative care is as a means to reverse opioid-mediated sedation, research suggests that dextroamphetamine and methylphenidate (Ritalin) possess analgesic properties as well, and are also excellent antidepressants. Arrhythmias are almost nonexistent, and instead of inducing anorexia, these agents typically have a paradoxic effect of increasing appetite by enhancing alertness. Nervousness and agitation are the most common adverse effects and usually respond to dose reductions. Agitated delirium occasionally occurs in patients with coexisting psychiatric disorders, brain metastases, and metabolic disturbances, all of which are relative contraindications to use. Methylphenidate is typically started in doses of 10 mg on awakening and 5 mg with the noontime meal, after which titration to effect is instituted. Because of its short half-life, patients are usually able to sleep well at night, especially if they have become more active as a result of increased alertness. Dextroamphetamine can be administered on a similar schedule, and an extended-release formulation is available for both agents.

e. Corticosteroids

(1) The efficacy of corticosteroids as treatment for acute pain resulting from raised intracranial pressure (IAP) and spinal cord compression is well established. In addition, these agents have been administered empirically for a variety of cancer pain syndromes with good results.

(2) Pain relief is presumably related to reduced peritumoral edema and inflammation with consequent relief of pressure and traction on nerves and other pain-sensitive structures, although beneficial effects on mood, appetite, and weight also may indirectly contribute to improved subjective pain reports.

(3) Improvements in pain are often rapid and dramatic, but usually depend on continued administration. Although results may be maintained in a proportion of patients, benefits are often short-lived, plateauing in a few weeks, presumably due to the replacement of edema by tumor growth in patients with aggressive disease.

(4) A trial of oral steroids may be beneficial in any patient with pain that appears to be predominantly due to spread of bulky tumor (e.g., selected patients with pelvic, rectal, esophageal, or hepatic tumor deposits or invasion of the brachial and lumbosacral plexus).

(5) Dexamethasone is the usual drug of choice because it possesses less potent mineralocorticoid effects. Although a variety of side effects and complications can occur as a result of even acute steroid administration (e.g., diabetes mellitus, psychosis), serious problems usually rise only from chronic use. As a result, when a trial produces beneficial results, it is reasonable to maintain use without tapering, in the presence of progressive cancer. Although most patients note improvements in mood when steroid therapy is commenced, a small proportion experience dysphoria and even florid psychosis. The optimal dose of steroids, both for oncologic emergencies (e.g., raised IAP, cord compression) and chronic pain, is not known. For the former, 100 mg IV dexamethasone is administered initially in some institutions, followed by IV maintenance. For the management of nonemergent pain, oral doses of 2 to 6 mg dexamethasone qid or tid are common.

f. N-methyl d-aspartate (NMDA) antagonists: The NMDA receptor has recently been described and implicated in the transmission of pain. Although research on various agents with antagonist activity at the NMDA receptor is under way, ketamine, a partial NMDA antagonist, is the only agent currently available that appears to mediate pain by this nonopioid mechanism. Long used as an IV anesthetic agent, subanesthetic doses have been administered for prolonged periods with fair success in a small number of patients with refractory neuropathic cancer pain. Because of side effects and the risk of complications, ketamine infusion should be regarded as a treatment of desperation reserved for rare use until additional experience has been reported.

g. Alpha-2-adrenergic antagonists: The centrally acting antihypertensive clonidine has been observed to promote analgesia for neuropathic pain when administered near the neuroaxis. Epidural administration has recently received FDA approval, and trials of intrathecal clonidine are under way. Hypotension during the initiation of treatment and rebound hypertension during withdrawal are the main risks of treatment.

h. Other purported adjuvants
   (1) Despite an absence of data from controlled trials, antihistamines, benzodiazepines, and antipsychotics have been used, mostly historically, in efforts to enhance analgesia. Although these agents have clear roles for primary indications other than pain (e.g., anxiolysis, antiemesis), with few exceptions they are not reliably associated with analgesia and thus should not be relied on as substitutes for opioid analgesics.
   (2) In contrast to other neuroleptics, methotrimeprazine reliably produces dose-related analgesia that is comparable to the analgesia opioid-mediated analgesia. Controlled trials have confirmed analgesia that is comparable to that achieved with parenteral morphine in postoperative, labor, and cancer pain. Its analgesic potency is similar or slightly less than that of parental morphine (equianalgesic ratio of 3:2), and, like morphine, it has no apparent ceiling effect. Methotrimeprazine is considerably more sedating and less emetogenic than morphine, and because of its propensity to produce orthostatic hypotension, treatment is usually reserved for nonambulatory patients. Disadvantages include the lack of an oral preparation, limited availability, and high cost. Methotrimeprazine is an excellent option when a potent nonopioid is required in a bedbound patient, especially when sedative effects are desired.
   (3) Although clinical lore has perpetuated the hypothesis that the butyrophenones have utility as primary or adjuvant analgesics, these beliefs have been confirmed neither by controlled trials nor by survey data. Proponents advocate trials for rectal tenesmus,

bladder tenesmus, neuropathic pain, and whenever suffering or psychologic distress are prominent.

(4) A careful review of the literature reveals insufficient evidence to support the contention that the benzodiazepines have meaningful analgesic properties in most clinical circumstances. Although treatment with the benzodiazepines may reduce complaints of pain, this appears to be an indirect effect related to their psychotropic properties rather than true analgesia. Thus the use of benzodiazepines should be discouraged except in extremely specific settings. Clinical experience suggests a potential role for short-term use to manage acute muscle spasm, use as an anxiolytic when stress appears to influence reports of pain, and use for lancinating neuropathic pain as a part of sequential trials, in which case clonazepam and alprazolam are the agents of choice. They should probably not be considered as first-line choices even for the preceding indications, since potential benefits are often eclipsed by the potential for the development of cognitive impairment, physical and psychologic dependence, worsening depression, risk of overdose, and other side effects.

E. Anesthetic Interventions
  1. Indications and risk-to-benefit ratio
    a. General considerations
      (1) Pharmacologic management calls for upward-dose titration of opioids until either adequate comfort is achieved or unacceptable side effects supervene, as well as for consideration of adjuvant analgesics. More invasive interventions are considered for the 10% to 30% of patients in whom adequate comfort or freedom from serious side effects cannot be maintained with pharmacotherapy.
      (2) Anesthetic procedures may be considered earlier in the case of a few select syndromes (e.g., celiac or hypogastric plexus block for abdominopelvic pain) associated with uniquely favorable risk-to-benefit ratios.
    b. Specific indications
      (1) Persistent intractable pain
      (2) Persistent intractable medication-mediated side effects
      (3) The threshold of pain or side effect severity at which anesthetic procedures are considered depends on the inherent risk-to-benefit ratio of a given procedure in a given patient.
    c. Other considerations
      (1) All medical treatment is inherently invasive, including the administration of high doses of opioids. The guiding principle

in considering an alternate treatment modality relates to balancing its risk-to-benefit ratio against that of other available options in the overall context of the specific clinical setting.

(2) The risk-to-benefit ratio of a given treatment modality or intervention is dynamic: For the same therapy it differs from patient to patient, and even in the same patient over time.

(3) As with other aspects of treatment, decision making for invasive procedures is a highly individualized process that depends on multiple factors.

(4) Individuals with advanced disease are often debilitated and physiologically, psychologically, and emotionally overwhelmed by their prognosis and symptoms. On this basis, every intervention, no matter how minor, must be weighed carefully against its cost in terms of inconvenience, recuperative time, energy, and cooperation demanded of the patient as well as the potentially devastating impact of a poor outcome. Every effort should be made to select a therapeutic option with a high likelihood of success that is not too demanding on patients' limited resources.

(5) Despite the fact that invasive procedures are often avoided in the presence of advanced disease in deference to their inherent risks and demands, they may still have an important role near the end of life, given that maintenance of comfort is the main focus in this setting.

(6) When patients are too unwell for an outpatient procedure or refuse hospitalization, care is even occasionally rendered at the bedside in the patient's home.

(7) Anesthetic versus neurosurgical procedures: With the exception of percutaneous cordotomy, which in expert hands may not be excessively demanding, anesthetic procedures are generally preferable to their neurosurgical counterparts in the presence of advanced disease.

(8) Relative roles of invasive procedures and pharmacotherapy

(a) Anesthetic procedures are not a panacea and are best regarded as occupying a role that complements drug therapy.

(b) Successful application may result in discontinuation of opioid drugs but is much more commonly associated with better pain control at lower doses (opioid-sparing effect).

(c) The complementary, as opposed to primary, role of anesthetic interventions is all the more apparent when viewed against the larger construct of palliative care, a philosophy of care that endeavors to control the protean symptoms of terminal illness, including pain, with quality of life as the end point.

2. Nerve blocks/neural blockade
   a. Definition: The injection of an anesthetic or destructive substance (neurolytic) near a nerve or nerve plexus in order to interrupt its function for a brief or extended period, respectively. In addition to chemical blockade (described earlier), the application of intense heat or freezing (i.e., radiofrequency thermocoagulation and cryotherapy) may be employed for similar purposes.
   b. When introducing the concept of a nerve block to patients, their understanding is often enhanced by invoking the analogy of a local anesthetic block administered for dental care as a familiar example.
3. Local anesthetic blocks
   a. Widely used for pain of nonneoplastic origin but less commonly indicated for cancer pain because effects are usually evanescent.
   b. Based on their intent, they are classified as diagnostic, prognostic, or therapeutic.
   c. Diagnostic local anesthetic blocks help characterize the underlying mechanism of pain (somatic, sympathetic, central, psychogenic, or mixed) and help define the anatomic pathways involved in pain transmission.
   d. Main indication is as a preliminary step toward more definitive therapy. Nevertheless, depending on the setting, the same diagnostic nerve block may be utilized for prognostic and therapeutic purposes.
   e. In general medicine and neurology, diagnostic blocks are underused tools.
   f. Prognostic local anesthetic blocks: Affect a rough simulation of the effects expected to accompany more prolonged interruption. They help determine the potential for a subsequent neurolytic block to relieve pain and provide an opportunity for the patient to experience side effects that may accompany neurolysis.
   g. Results often have good predictive value, but reliability is still incomplete.
   h. Therapeutic local anesthetic blocks: Intended to produce or contribute to lasting therapeutic effects. Although patients with persistent pain due to tumor progression usually require neurolysis, local anesthetic blocks may be therapeutic in some circumstances.
   i. Specific indications for local anesthetic blocks in with cancer pain
      (1) Diagnostic block
      (2) Prognostic block
      (3) Pain emergency
      (4) Muscle spasm (trigger point injection, peripheral block, etc.)

        (5) Herpes zoster (subcutaneous infiltration with steroid, sympathetic blockade)

        (6) Premorbid chronic pain

        (7) Treatment-related pain

        (8) Tumor-induced reflex sympathetic dystrophy

        (9) Continuous infusion for chronic pain

  j. Specific syndromes that may benefit from local block include

        (1) Trigger point injections into painful regions of muscle spasm may be used to treat pain of muscular origin (cramps, myalgia, myofascial pain), a more common cause of pain than previously thought (underrecognition due to inability of standard x-rays to document muscle injury, as well as the varied, sometimes vague, and usually nonneurologic constellation of symptoms).

        (2) Sympathetic or epidural blocks, administered in series for tumor-induced reflex sympathetic dystrophy (i.e., extremity pain of a causalgic and/or dysesthetic nature). Symptoms arising from tumor invasion of nervous structures (brachial or lumbosacral plexopathy) may respond to local anesthetic blockade of the stellate ganglion or lumbar sympathetic chain. Such conditions are relatively uncommon, as pain from involvement of these structures is usually mixed.

        (3) Sympathetic block or subcutaneous infiltration with steroids has an important, often overlooked role in the management of acute herpes zoster and early postherpetic neuralgia.

        (4) Peripheral blocks with steroids also have a potential role in painful postsurgical syndromes associated with nerve impingement (postthoracotomy, postmastectomy, and postradical neck dissection pain).

        (5) Severe acute pain due to vertebral compression fractures may benefit from epidural steroid injections.

        (6) Epidural, facet, or peripheral blocks with a local anesthetic and steroids can be considered for premorbid chronic pain conditions (arthritis, sciatica, etc.).

        (7) Local anesthetics can be administered via a catheter to provide respite from a pain emergency so that a more accurate assessment and long-term plan can be formulated. Catheter-based infusions are occasionally administered for longer intervals when ablation is not feasible.

4. Neurolytic (neurodestructive, neuroablative) block: Usually refers to chemical neurolysis (i.e., the injection of alcohol or phenol near a nerve or nerves for the purpose of destroying a portion of the targeted nerve to interrupt the transmission of impulses for a prolonged interval).

a. Alternate techniques used less frequently include
  (1) Surgical neuroablation: Sectioning of a nerve under direct vision
  (2) Cryoanalgesia: Preservation of underlying neural architecture may result in more selective destruction. Requires careful placement of probe and, ultimately, ice ball directly on targeted nerve. Unfortunately, duration of action is often unacceptably short. Often considered for patients with longer predicted life expectancy (e.g., postthoracotomy or postmastectomy syndrome).
  (3) Radiofrequency-generated thermal lesions: Effective technique, also requiring exquisitely exact placement. Since there is no drug spread, results may be more discrete and controllable than those achieved with chemical blockade. Because of the need for specialized equipment and training, chemical techniques still predominate.
b. Neuroablation is more often considered than are local blocks in these settings of pain due to cancer because in most circumstances pain is due to ongoing tissue injury induced by tumor growth and pain is expected to persist.
c. Specialized training, careful selection of the proper procedure, and attention to technical detail should limit incidence of side effects and unwanted neurologic deficit.
d. Pain-related indications: Neurolytic blockade is most applicable for pain that is
  (1) Well characterized: Patients with vague complaints are likely to be ill served because their clinical presentation interferes with selection of the proper procedure. Patients who "feel bad all over" or who volunteer that "I can't describe it, it just hurts" may be experiencing a symptom complex more consistent with suffering (a more general construct of spiritual, psychologic, social, and/or economic malaise) than nociceptive pain (an element of suffering).
  (2) Well localized
    (a) Most neurolytic procedures are especially efficacious for pain that is well localized. When extended to provide analgesic coverage for pain that is distributed over an extensive topography, blocks are generally more prone to failure or are associated with increased risks of undesirable neurologic deficit.
    (b) Exceptions
      (i) Sympathetic blockade (stellate ganglion, celiac, lumbar sympathetic, and hypogastric block) often provides topographic analgesia that is ample for the visceral pain syndromes, most of which tend to be vague in character and relatively diffuse.

(ii) Epidural neurolysis, although currently performed in a limited number of centers, can often be successfully employed to manage broad-based pain without inducing unwanted neurologic deficit, although this is still a prominent risk.

(iii) Chemical hypophysectomy: Although availability is even more restricted, transnasal alcohol neurolysis of the pituitary gland is applicable for widely disseminated bony metastatic pain.

(3) Somatic or visceral pain is more likely to respond beneficially to neural blockade than is neuropathic pain. Although less likely to be effective, ablative procedures may still be considered for intractable neuropathic pain but should ideally be performed proximal to the causative lesion, preceded by a careful trial of local anesthetic blocks.

(4) Pain that is not a component of a syndrome characterized by multifocal aches and pains

(a) Surveys of patients with advanced cancer pain demonstrate that pain is usually present in more than one area simultaneously. Patients with a single predominant source of pain may find that if it is eliminated by a block or other procedure, previously secondary complaints may increase in severity.

(b) Nevertheless, when a single source of pain is strongly dominant, a procedure that reduces the primary complaint is sometimes of value by permitting control of secondary symptoms with more conservative measures.

e. Patient-related indications: Main indication—severe, intractable pain of neoplastic origin that is expected to persist, usually in the presence of limited life expectancy.

(1) Avoid in settings associated with a likelihood that pain will resolve naturally or otherwise (e.g., compression fracture, during or just after a course of palliative radiotherapy or injection of a radioisotope such as strontium).

(2) If possible, avoid when applicable procedures are associated with significant risks of inducing an undesirable neurologic deficit (e.g., leg weakness in an ambulatory patient or bladder paresis in a patient without a permanent urinary catheter or pre-exisiting bladder diversion).

f. Outcomes

(1) Study methodologies: Few controlled trials have been performed. Most reports are descriptive and are limited by small, unstratified populations; no blinding or randomization; and no

controls for differences in technique. Reported outcomes vary, depending on the type of block, pain complaint, and underlying medical and neurologic condition.

(2) Efficacy: Large series report significant relief of pain in an average of 50% to 80% of well-selected patients, with the best results obtained with inclusion of patients who have access to repeated or multiple different blocks. When interpreting outcome, it is important to recognize the influence of patient selection, since anesthetic interventions are usually reserved for patient with refractory pain.

(3) Duration: Effects tend to average 6 months, an interval that is usually sufficient for most patients. Anecdotal reports of pain relief persisting in excess of 1 to 2 years, but frequently blocks need to be repeated more often than expected, as a result of disease progression or sheltering (the effect of tumor-limiting contact between injected drug and the targeted nerve).

(4) Complications: Overall, significant complications are reported in less than 5% of well-selected patients. Optimal results are ensured by the judicious use of fluoroscopic and computed tomography (CT) guidance to verify needle localization, as well as the application of simple adjuncts such as careful aspiration, the use of a nerve stimulator, the administration of test doses of local anesthetic, and eliciting paresthesias.

(5) Hazards

(a) Neurologic deficit: Nervous structures are affected indiscriminately, requiring careful patient selection and technical attention to relieve pain without producing unwanted motor or autonomic dysfunction.

Potential for undesired deficits can often be assessed in advance with prognostic local anesthetic blockade. Blockade of a purely sensory peripheral nerve will not result in motor deficit.

In some patients a degree of motor weakness will be well tolerated (e.g., patients already confined to bed with preexisting motor deficit and individuals with pain sufficiently severe to render an involved limb useless).

(b) Damage to nonneurologic tissue: Unwanted spread may damage neighboring structures (e.g., slough of skin, kidney infarction). Usually avoidable with radiologic guidance, with other tests, and by limited volume of injection.

(c) Impermanence

(i) Neither chemical, surgical, nor cryothermal ablation reliably produces permanent relief of pain because of axonal regrowth, central nervous system plasticity, and/or the development of deafferentation pain.

(ii) Procedures ideally reserved for patients with life expectancy unlikely to exceed duration of relief. In the event that effects are more short-lived than anticipated, procedure can be repeated at same site or more proximally.

(d) New pain: Neurolysis is followed by neuritis and dysesthesias in a variable proportion of cases (2% to 28%) that can at times be severe and difficult to manage.

5. Neurolytic drugs
   a. Commonly used: Ethyl alcohol (50% to 100%) and phenol in water or glycerin (5% to 12%)
      (1) Perineural injection of alcohol is followed immediately by severe burning pain along the targeted nerve's distribution, which lasts only about a minute before giving way to a warm, numb sensation. Pain on injection may be blunted—indeed, often eliminated—by the prior injection of a local anesthetic.
      (2) The injection of phenol may also be accompanied by discomfort but is more often associated with sensations of warmth and numbness.
   b. Infrequently used: Ammonium sulfate and chlorocrescol

6. Specific nerve block procedures: Nerve blocks can technically be performed at almost any site. Technical aspects of performing specific procedures are discussed elsewhere. Discussion of indications, results, and special considerations follows.
   a. Peripheral nerve blocks
      (1) Limited but important role. Described in isolated case reports and small series, making outcome difficult to characterize
      (2) Specific concerns include risk of
         (a) Neuritis
         (b) New pain due to deafferentation or neuritis
         (c) Failure due to overlapping distribution
         (d) Motor deficit (when mixed nerves are targeted)
         (e) Unintended damage to neighboring neurologic structures
         (f) Risk of unintended damage to neighboring nonneurologic structures
      (3) The potential for developing these problems can be minimized by careful patient selection and attention to technical details.
         (a) Since postinjection dysesthesias due to neuritis or deafferentation are most common after peripheral blocks, they should ideally be undertaken cautiously if at all in patients

with life expectancies in excess of 1 year, unless the original pain is so severe that new neuropathic pain would be unlikely to produce greater distress.

(b) It is important to ensure that a sufficient number of nerves are accurately blocked to cover the painful region.

(c) To avoid meaningful weakness, peripheral blocks should be limited to purely sensory nerves, except in patients in whom a degree of motor weakness will be well tolerated (e.g., those already confined to bed, those with preexisting motor deficit, or those with pain or disease sufficiently severe to render the involved part useless).

(d) The likelihood of producing significant motor weakness or autonomic disturbance can be roughly assessed in advance with local anesthetic blockade.

(e) The potential for damage to nontargeted structures can be minimized by using radiologic guidance and other safety techniques (e.g., aspiration).

b. Sympathetic nerve block

(1) Continues to have an extremely important role, predominantly for visceral pain, and less frequently for neuropathic (causalgic) pain involving a limb.

(2) Sympathetic block for causalgic pain is unique in that some patients derive lasting benefit from a series of local anesthetic injections. If prolonged relief does not result from repeated local anesthetic injections or the patient is too ill to undergo repeated procedures, a neurolytic block may be considered.

(3) Neurologic deficit is unlikely to arise after neurolytic block because fibers normally subserve neither somatic motor nor sensory functions.

(4) Postinjection dysesthesias (sympathalgias) are rare, and as a result sympathetic ablation is considered somewhat more liberally in some patients with extended life expectancy.

(5) Types of sympathetic blockade

(a) Stellate (cervicothoracic) ganglion: An option for sympathetically mediated pain involving the face, neck, upper extremity—more likely to be invoked for pain due to cancer therapies (postherpetic neuralgia, postmastectomy pain), and rarely for sympathetic component of Pancoast syndrome. Neurolytic block is undertaken cautiously if at all due to risk of spread to brachial plexus and other neighboring nerves, and then only with dilute (3%) phenol, under radiologic guidance.

      (b) Lumbar sympathetic chain: Considered for sympathetically mediated lower-extremity pain, and pain after nephrectomy, again relatively infrequently.

      (c) Celiac plexus and splanchnic nerve block: Considered for upper-abdominal visceral pain, especially pancreatic carcinoma; among the most well-accepted and frequently applied nerve blocks in the setting of cancer pain. Can be performed by numerous approaches (described elsewhere).

      (d) Superior hypogastric plexus: Recently introduced but widely accepted for visceral pain in the pelvis and rectum. Plexus is located just anterior to the sacral promontory. Minimal to no risk of incontinence or sensory and motor deficit. Fluoroscopy is required.

      (e) Ganglion impar: Recently introduced for perineal and genital pain that is mediated by the sympathetic nervous system. Aim is to block the termination of sympathetic chain in the presacral region. Minimal to no risk of incontinence or sensory and motor deficit. Fluoroscopy is required.

  c. Central (neuroaxial) nerve blocks

    (1) Subarachnoid (intrathecal) neurolysis

      (a) Less commonly employed since advent of intraspinal opioid therapy, but important indications remain, especially for localized chest wall and (in the presence of urinary diversion) perineal/saddle pain.

      (b) Pain relief is owed to chemical rhizotomy; may be performed at any level(s) distal to midcervical region, above which the risk of brain stem injury increases.

      (c) Requires considerable skill and specialized training to avoid unwanted neurologic deficits, but in good hands it is extremely safe in well-selected patients. Suitable for aged or debilitated patients, although positioning is awkward and uncomfortable.

      (d) Usually performed on outpatient basis with little need for radiologic guidance or special equipment.

      (e) Key factor for success is restricting the spread of the neurolytic agent to targeted roots by prudent patient selection, careful positioning, and use of hyperbaric phenol or hypobaric alcohol.

      (f) Rather than trying to extend a single block to cover a large area, repetition is preferred to obtain durable analgesia without unwarranted risks of undesired neurologic sequelae. Average duration of effect is 3 to 6 months and occasionally longer.

(g) Technique

   (i) The root corresponding to the epicenter of the painful region's segmental innervation is targeted where the root exits the cord, as opposed to the level of the vertebral interspace. It is best to extend the block slightly above and below the painful region, and if feasible, several needles are usually introduced at interspaces adjacent to the targeted root(s), especially when the area to be covered exceeds one or two dermatomes. Large-caliber spinal needle (20 or 22 gauge) is preferred to minimize turbulence and a jet effect, and a 20-gauge needle is required for phenol due to its viscosity.

   (ii) Phenol mixed with 7% to 12% glycerin is hyperbaric and thus sinks when introduced to CSF. The patient is positioned laterally with the painful side dependent, and, once CSF is obtained, is tilted 45° posteriorly to concentrate drug on posterior (sensory) root and minimize motor block.

   (iii) Absolute (dehydrated) ethyl alcohol is hypobaric, and thus floats when introduced to CSF; as a result, the opposite position (painful side up, anterior tilt) is adopted.

   (iv) After a neurologic exam and confirmation of CSF flow and positioning, drug is gently introduced through each needle in increments of 0.1 to 0.2 ml/min, interrupted by serial sensory and motor examinations. The patient is cautioned to describe the onset and location of sensations of new warmth, burning, or numbness that usually accompany drug instillation. Alcohol may produce short-lived burning dysesthesias, whereas phenol is more commonly associated with the onset of a warm sensation. The injectate should be limited to no more than about 1 ml/segment, but within these limits the clinician should endeavor to continue injecting even after pain is relieved, since the hypalgesic field often shrinks, especially with phenol. Clear needles and maintain immobility for 30 minutes.

(v) Saddle block is performed with 10% to 12% phenol in glycerin at the L-5–S-1 or L-4–L-5 interspace with the patient seated and leaning backward.

(2) Epidural (phenol) neurolysis

    (a) Performed less commonly than subarachnoid neurolysis, usually for pain that is distributed over a wider region.

    (b) To accommodate for the lesser intensity of neurolysis due to limited contact between the drug and targeted roots imposed by the dura, a catheter is usually placed for gradual neurolysis performed serially over several days. As a result, hospitalization and daily access to fluoroscopy are usually required.

    (c) Generally avoided in favor of subarachnoid block because of the above, as well as the unpredictability of epidural spread and the absence of control related to baricity and afforded by drop-by-drop titration.

7. Consideration of nerve blocks by region

  a. Head and neck pain

    (1) Despite the erosive, endophytic nature of many tumors, surprisingly, pain is usually effectively managed with analgesics.

    (2) When pain is present it may be quite severe because of a rich, overlapping innervation (cranial nerves V, VII, IX, X, and the upper cervical nerves) and because pain may be aggravated by simple, relatively involuntary activities (swallowing, eating, coughing, talking) that render physiologic splinting ineffective.

    (3) Blocks may be difficult or prone to poor outcome as a result of

      (a) Anatomic distortion (due to tumor growth, surgery, and radiotherapy)

      (b) "Sheltering" (reduced access to nerve due to tumor invasion or radiation or surgical fibrosis)

      (c) Overlap among sensory fields

      (d) Influence of cranial nerves on swallowing and control of breathing

    (4) In deference to the preceding, neurolytic blocks should ideally be preceded by local anesthetic injections, and fluoroscopic or CT guidance is indicated when blocking roots as they emerge from the base of the skull.

      (a) The trigeminal nerve (V) Gasserian ganglion may be blocked at foramen ovale for pain in more than one division. This procedure is performed much less frequently than in the past. It is technically difficult, may be uncomfortable for the patient, produces unilateral facial numbness, and may result in masseter muscle weakness as well as corneal anesthesia.

(b) Mandibular or maxillary block (branches I and II of V) are considered for pain that is limited to the distribution of a single branch. Performance is easier than blocking at the ganglion level. Maxillary block is considered for pain in the middle third of the face (maxilla, cheek, nasal cavity, hard palate, tonsilar fossa), and mandibular block for pain involving the jaw or anterior two-thirds of the tongue. A few cases of localized gangrene and skin slough have been reported, presumably due to thrombosis or spasm-induced necrosis.

(c) Blockade of the first division (ophthalmic nerve) is rarely employed in contemporary practice.

(d) It is preferable to block Gasserian ganglion prophylactically if tumor progression is anticipated beyond the field of single branch or when tumor growth or postsurgical changes limit access to the pterygoid fossa.

(e) When pain extends cervically or to the angle of the jaw, supplementary paravertebral blockade of second or third cervical nerve root may be necessary.

(f) Blockade of the glossopharyngeal and vagus nerves (IX and X) is considered for less-well-localized pain or pain near the base of the tongue, pharynx, or throat.

  (i) Performance is technically difficult, is demanding for the patient, and requires radiologic guidance.

  (ii) IX: Nasopharynx, eustachian tube, soft palate, uvula, tonsil, base of tongue, part of external auditory canal

  (iii) X: Larynx, contributing fibers to ear, external auditory canal, and tympanic membrane

  (iv) Bilateral destruction of IX and X not recommended because of potential interference with swallowing mechanisms and protective airway reflexes

  (v) Stellate (cervicothoracic) ganglion block (see later) may be considered for sympathetically mediated pain of the face, usually due to lesion of cervical plexus or herpes zoster.

  (vi) Phrenic nerve block may be considered for hiccoughs (singultus) that are refractory to more conservative therapies. Prior to neurolytic phrenic nerve block, prognostic block with local anesthetic is undertaken on the most affected side to evaluate ventilatory function. Resuscitation equipment must be immediately available.

(vii) When intractable craniocervical pain is not amenable to nerve block therapy, intraspinal or intraventricular opioid therapy may be considered. Numerous neurosurgical procedures have been devised to manage rostral pain but are of limited practical value because of invasiveness and high morbidity and mortality.

b. Upper-extremity pain

(1) General considerations: due to the high prevalence of breast cancer and primary and metastatic lung cancer, neoplastic pain involving the shoulder girdle and upper extremity is common. Initial treatment is with the liberal prescription of routine analgesics. Many patients present with pain that is at least in part neuropathic, particularly when there is involvement of the brachial plexus by tumor or radiation fibrosis, in which case adjuvant analgesic therapy should be maximized.

(2) Refractory pain is challenging because of the mixed motor and sensory nerve supply to the upper extremity and consequent risks of loss of function after denervation.

(3) Percutaneous cordotomy, a neurosurgical procedure that is relatively unique in that decrement in motor function is unlikely, may be considered, but it is less frequently successful for arm than trunk pain because the extension of the lesion needed to produce such rostral analgesia increases the risks of respiratory and neurologic dysfunction.

(4) Specific procedures

(a) Intraspinal or intraventricular opioids are very reasonable options in this setting, unless intractable pain is associated with a functionless limb, in which case blocks may be considered more liberally.

(b) In therapeutically useful strengths alcohol and phenol destroy nerve fibers indiscriminately, and thus nerves that transmit motor impulses to the limbs should not be targeted unless useful movement is already compromised and the limb is nonfunctional or minimally functional.

(c) Of chemical denervation procedures, cervical subarachnoid injections of phenol or alcohol are most likely to relieve pain while preserving motor function because the drug is ideally deposited preferentially on sensory rootlets. Although advanced training is required, radiologic guidance is usually not needed.

(d) Intraforaminal or paravertebral block of the individual spinal roots as they exit the vertebral column can be considered for very localized pain, but because of sensory overlap multiple nerves usually need to be blocked, and motor dysfunction should be anticipated. Radiologic guidance and test doses are essential to avoid subarachnoid or epidural spread.

(e) An axillary or supraclavicular approach to the brachial plexus is straightforward, but to achieve durable analgesia, motor paralysis is almost inevitable, and thus this should be reserved for patients with a functionless upper extremity. Lysis is usually preceded by a prognostic local anesthetic injection.

(f) Suprascapular block has been used to treat pain localized predominantly to the shoulder girdle. Since only limited muscle groups are weakened, treatment may be better tolerated.

(g) Stellate ganglion block can be considered for dysesthetic or burning upper-extremity pain. Historically, repeated local anesthetic injections have been preferred to neurolysis because of concerns regarding spread to the brachial plexus or laryngeal nerves, although fluoroscopically guided dilute phenol stellate neurolysis has recently been described and appears to be safe and reliable.

c. Thoracic and abdominal wall pain

(1) General considerations: a thorough evaluation is indicated to determine etiology, because pain is often referred from deeper visceral structures and may respond best to treatment directed specifically at its source (celiac plexus, splanchnic nerve, or even intrapleural block).

(2) Pain originating in thoracic or abdominal wall or parietal peritoneum can be treated with peripheral blocks (multiple intercostal or paravertebral blocks) or subarachnoid block.

(a) Intercostal block: Except after pneumonectomy, there is just under a 1% risk of pneumothorax, although radiologic guidance is still rarely necessary. Because of risks of postblock neuritis and failure due to overlap, subarachnoid block may be preferred.

(b) Paravertebral block: Blockade of somatic nerve roots as they emerge from the intravertebral foramen can be performed, although this is usually not preferred because of the risks of neuritis, pneumothorax, subarachnoid and epidural spread, and failure because of the need to block several contiguous nerves completely. Radiologic guidance and test doses are required.

        (c) Subarachnoid neurolysis: Chest wall pain is the most important indication for subarachnoid neurolysis. Treatment is quite safe at thoracic levels because targeted nerve roots are distant from the outflow to the limbs, bowel, and bladder. Complications are rare in experienced hands. Alcohol is usually preferred because patients are loathe to lie on their painful side, as is required for treatment with phenol.

        (d) Periosteal infiltration: Localized bony pain associated with rib metastases may respond to local infiltration around the bone with steroids and even dilute phenol. Although clinical experience is limited, treatment appears to be relatively innocuous.

   d. Abdominal pain

     (1) General considerations: The role of nerve blocks is relatively unique. Despite a distribution of pain that is usually diffuse and bilateral, neural blockade may be very effective and safe because the innervation of the abdominal viscera is conducted by the sympathetic nervous system, which when ablated provides pain relief over a wide distribution without numbness, motor weakness, or deafferentation pain. Pancreatic cancer in particular is associated with a high incidence of intractable pain. Pain of pancreatic cancer is characteristically a boring sensation in the midepigastrium with radiation to the back. Both parts of this symptom complex are usually amenable to celiac plexus or splanchnic nerve block.

     (2) Celiac plexus and splanchnic nerve block

        (a) The plexus contributes to the innervation of all intra-abdominal structures derived from embryonic foregut, including much of the gastrointestinal tract (distal esophagus, stomach, duodenum, small bowel, ascending and proximal transverse colon), pancreas, adrenal glands, spleen, liver, and biliary system.

        (b) One of the most effective and commonly utilized nerve blocks performed to provide prolonged relief of cancer pain. Efficacy averages about 80% with relief that endures an average of 3 to 6 months, and often until death.

        (c) Despite its location deep within the body, the proximity of major organs (aorta, vena cava, kidneys, pleura, etc.), and requirements for a large volume of neurolytic drug (up to 50 ml of 50% to 100% alcohol), complication rates are uniformly low (usually under 1%). Treatment requires radiologic control (fluoroscopy or CT).

(d) The plexus is a diffuse periaortic structure. Success depends on adequacy and uniformity of drug spread, especially anterior to the aorta (near the origin of the celiac artery), where the fibers are characteristically concentrated. Various techniques are utilized, none of which has been shown conclusively to be superior.

(e) Classic technique of Kappis: The patient is positioned prone, and 7-inch × 22-gauge needles are inserted bilaterally, four finger-breadth's on each side of the spine beneath the twelfth ribs and angled medially and upward so that their tips come to lie in the retroperitoneum beyond the anterolateral aspect of the L-1 vertebral body. Although probably still the most commonly used approach, recent studies suggest that ultimately it is best considered a splanchnic block, because as long as needle tips remain retrocrural, injectate only reaches the plexus indirectly via passage through the aortic hiatus. Monitored anesthesia care (MAC) or sedation is required to minimize discomfort, and fluoroscopy or CT scanning is mandatory for neurolysis.

(f) Transcrural approach: Similar to the preceding except that CT is utilized to facilitate passage of needles beyond the anterolateral margins of the body so that tips are advanced 1 to 3 additional centimeters, through the diaphragmatic crura, ensuring a more predictable anterior spread of injectate.

(g) A transaortic approach is undertaken by advancing the left-sided needle an additional few centimeters. The deliberate passage of a 20- or 22-gauge needle through both aortic walls is intended to maximize preaortic spread. A loss of resistance technique and contrast studies help avoid intramural injections and aortic dissection. Technique is similar in concept to translumbar aortography and is rarely associated with complications.

(h) Also intended to deposit drug preferentially in the pre-aortic region, a CT (or sonographically) guided anterior approach, similar to techniques used for biopsy, is gaining popularity. It is simple, quick, and better tolerated because patients need not assume a prone position and are spared the discomfort that occurs when needles transgress the periosteum. Interestingly, this approach does not appear to be associated with a significant incidence of infectious or bleeding complications despite potential for passage of needle through bowel and liver.

(i) Although intraoperative infiltration under direct vision at the time of laparotomy is associated with a good result, it is not widely practiced. Usually, 15 ml of absolute alcohol is deposited over a guiding finger placed on the aorta. Concerns relate to anatomic distortion due to phlegmon and tumor masses, the potential for causing aberrant spread due to disrupted tissue planes, and for causing aortic dissection.

(j) Classic splanchnic block uses a similar approach to that of Kappis, except that needle placement originates slightly closer to the midline; tips are directed toward the body of T-10, T-11, or T-12; and needle passage is arrested once the anterolateral margin of the vertebral body is reached. A smaller volume of injectate (10 to 15 ml/side) is typically used, and instead of backache, patients may experience transient pleuritic pain for the first few postprocedure days. Splanchnic block is preferred when subdiaphragmatic tumor burden or adenopathy interferes with approaches to the celiac axis or after failure of another approach.

(k) Some form of radiologic guidance is required for all of the preceding except intraoperative blockade. Fluoroscopy is usually considered adequate, except in the case of the anterior approach, which requires CT or sonography, and the posterior transcrural approach, which requires CT scanning. CT permits visualization of viscera and vascular structures and thus is especially useful in the presence of anatomic distortion due to organomegaly, bulky tumor, or postsurgical changes.

e. Pelvic and perineal pain
(1) Pelvic pain of visceral origin is typically diffuse and bilateral.
(2) Although only briefly mentioned in the literature, lumbar sympathetic block was used in the past for pelvic pain with moderate success.
(3) Superior hypogastric plexus block, modeled after presacral neurotomy, tends to be preferred today.
  (a) The plexus is a retroperitoneal structure located bilaterally at the level of sacral promontory, near the bifurcation of the common iliac vessels.
  (b) Main indications include visceral pelvic cancer pain emanating from the descending colon and rectum, vaginal fundus and bladder, prostate and prostatic urethra, testes, seminal vesicles, uterus, and ovary. In addition, treatment is often effective for burning tenesmus after rectal anastomosis and radiation injury to the pelvic viscera.

(c) The technique is analogous to lumbar sympathetic block, except needles are directed more caudally (anterolateral aspect of the lower third of L-5 or upper third of S-1).

(d) Radiologic guidance (usually fluoroscopy) is necessary.

(e) Studies have demonstrated 70% or greater reduction in pain overall in treated patients, generally with no serious complications.

(4) Ganglion impar (ganglion of Walther)

(a) The ganglion is a midline retroperitoneal structure located anterior to the vertebral column at level of sacrococcygeal junction. It marks the termination of the paired paravertebral sympathetic chains.

(b) Although anatomic references rarely describe this structure in detail, it provides sympathetic innervation of the anus and genitalia and thus is involved in the transmission of visceral pain from these structures.

(c) Neural blockade, which requires fluoroscopic guidance, can be performed with a local anesthetic to determine the relative presence of somatic versus visceral pain or phenol for moderate-duration relief of burning, sympathetically mediated perineal pain (e.g., due to tumor invasion or nerve injury after resection or distal anastomosis).

(d) Most experience is for the treatment of cancer pain. Results are usually favorable, and serious complications have not been reported, although the potential for accidental caudal spread and infection exists. The standard treatment with a bent spinal needle inserted between the anus and tip of the coccyx has been supplemented with anecdotal reports describing access directly through the sacrococcygeal cartilage.

f. Somatically mediated perineal pain: This entity is more vexing because the proximity of nerves transmitting motor strength to the lower extremities and innervating bowel and bladder render neuroablation hazardous due to significant risks of undesired neurologic deficit.

(1) Neurolytic subarachnoid saddle block: An extremely simple and effective treatment for perineal pain of mixed or somatic origin, this is an extremely useful approach when urinary function is not a concern due to urinary diversion. Although the risk of urinary incontinence is considerable, anal incontinence and leg weakness are extremely remote concerns, even when 10% to 12% hyperbaric phenol is used. A lumbar puncture is performed at the lowest level possible and, with the patient seated

and leaned backward to minimize spread to anterior motor roots, 1.0 to 1.5 ml phenol is instilled through a TB syringe in 0.1 to 0.2 ml increments. Radiologic guidance is not required, and patients who had been unable to experience warmth and comfort do so almost immediately. Slight overtreatment is usually indicated to avoid recrudescence of pain as the phenol's field of analgesia shrinks over the first posttreatment day. Despite the need for a 20-gauge needle due to phenol's viscosity, headaches are infrequent.

(2) Sacral root block: treatment can usually be rendered without affecting bladder function, although this is a modest risk that must be accepted, even after prognostic local anesthetic blockade. May be preferred over saddle block when pain is unilateral or involves the upper sacral dermatomes. See the next section, "Lower-Extremity Pain."

g. Lower-extremity pain

(1) General considerations: As with upper-extremity pain, the applicability of denervation procedures is limited by a mixed motor and sensory nerve supply. In addition, the proximity of nervous outflow to the bowel and bladder further limits the role of destructive nerve blocks.

(2) Peripheral blocks: Sciatic, femoral, and obturator blocks should be avoided except in rare circumstances when the lower extremity is severely and permanently weak and pain respects the distribution of a single nerve and is unlikely to spread. Even in these circumstances, neuritis is a concern.

(3) Sacral nerve root block at the posterior plate of the sacrum (see "Perineal Pain," earlier). Sacral root blocks can be considered for pelvic, rectal and posterior lower-extremity pain. Selective sacral root block (guided by preliminary local blocks) may preserve sphincter control because a single sacral nerve (usually one of the third or fourth) usually exerts dominant influence on bladder musculature and must be injured bilaterally to produce incontinence.

(4) Paravertebral psoas compartment or psoas sheath block: Although motor weakness should invariably accompany this procedure because of the mixed function of the plexus, psoas block has been reported to actually be associated with a low incidence of leg weakness. Radiologic guidance is required for 10% phenol ablation.

(5) Subarachnoid neurolysis (see earlier): Although extremely effective, this treatment should not be considered unless leg weakness would be well tolerated because the patient is confined to bed or the limb is rendered irreversibly weak due to

tumor invasion. Although baricity and position can be manipulated to minimize spread to motor fibers, a guarantee that sensory fibers will be entirely isolated is impossible. Since block is usually undertaken at the root (as opposed to vertebral) level, risks of incontinence are more modest.

(6) Intraspinal analgesia

    (a) Intraspinal anesthesia: Administration of local anesthetics into epidural or intrathecal/subarachnoid space well accepted, with long history for the management of acute pain (e.g., labor, surgery, postoperative) but generally not applicable for chronic cancer pain because of nonselective effects (i.e., analgesia is accompanied by motor weakness, sensory anesthesia, and sympathetic block [hypotension], precluding home use).

    (b) Intraspinal analgesia: Achieved by the epidural or intrathecal administration of an opioid. Despite shorter history, has become widely accepted worldwide, although further research is needed to determine specific indications and proper timing with regard to systemic administration. Analgesia is highly selective, with an absence of motor, sensory, and sympathetic effects, and thus it is easily adapted to home administration.

    (c) In contrast to nerve blocks, treatment is effective for multiple or generalized pains.

    (d) Basis: The introduction of minute quantities of opioids in close proximity to receptors (substantia gelatinosa of spinal cord) is associated with high local concentrations at target sites, with profound analgesia, often superior to systemic administration, and reduced side effects. Most implanters aim to place the catheter tip near the spinal pain generator to achieve the best coverage in case lipophilic opioids or local anesthetics are ever infused.

    (e) Other advantages: Nondestructive (reversible), titratable analgesia and side effects, availability of reliable, simple screening to predict efficacy.

    (f) Disadvantages: Requires an anesthesiologist or neurosurgeon familiar with screening, implantation, and maintenance; requires suitable family support and home care; increases reliance on high-tech therapies.

    (g) Screening: Accomplished on out- or inpatient basis by one of two methods:

        (i) Observation of response to "single shot" injection of IT morphine, usually at an arbitrary dose ranging from 0.5 to 2.0 mg, with an expected duration of

12 to 24 hours. Usually repeated at least once to help exclude placebo response.

(ii) Observation of response to infusion through a temporary (percutaneous) epidural catheter, usually in a starting dose range of 0.5 to 2.0 mg/hr. Maintained for a few days or weeks with the assistance of a home care agency. Percutaneous IT catheters, although useful for trials because they more closely mimic the fully implanted pump, are usually reserved for short-term use in hospitalized patients.

(iii) Both screening protocols are quick, simple procedures, usually associated with little discomfort and generally well tolerated even in ill patients. Because serious side effects are so infrequent in patients using opioids chronically, outpatient treatment has become well accepted.

(h) Maintenance therapy

Considered if screen demonstrates an acceptable ratio of analgesia to side effect. Various long-term infusion systems are now available. Since therapy is new, selection process is still evolving.

(i) Externalized catheter systems: Although patients and family members can be instructed in self-injection, these systems are generally combined with a leased portable ambulatory infusion device with PCA.

- In patients whose death is imminent, continued use of temporary percutaneous catheter is considered for treatment expected to last no longer than about a month. Extended use is discouraged because of the risk of catheter extrusion and spread of local infection to spine.

- Tunneled temporary catheter: Standard therapy is modified at the bedside by tunneling a portion of the distal catheter so that the exit site is further from the spine. So easy to accomplish (with local anesthetic, scalpel, and additional epidural needle) that this option should be considered whenever a catheter is required for more than a few days.

- Permanent implanted silastic catheters utilize modified Hickman/Broviac technology. Involves minor surgery by anesthesiologist or neurosurgeon, under local, monitored anesthesia care or general anesthesia.

- DuPen epidural catheter: Comes in a kit; after incision, a slender silastic catheter (with guidewire) is threaded into the epidural space through a 14-gauge Tuohy needle. A larger distal catheter is tunneled under the skin from the flank to the paravertebral incision, where it is joined to the proximal catheter over a stainless steel pin.
- Subcutaneous port: Similar to the DuPen device except that the distal tip is not externalized but is attached to a vascular access port that is placed in a subcutaneous pocket. System becomes externalized when attached to a portable pump. Approved only for epidural use in the United States

(ii) Fully implanted systems: These appear to be the most costly alternatives ($10,000 to $20,000, including professional and hospital fees). However, almost all costs are up front, and as a result of savings realized in ongoing home care, nursing, and pharmacy costs, systems are actually extremely cost-effective when used for patients with indolent disease and a life expectancy of 6 months or more. Pumps, which are shaped like a hockey puck, are implanted in the subcutaneous tissue over the flank and usually are refilled every 1 to 2 months.

(iii) Fully implanted fixed-rate pump: Pioneered by Infusaid (reservoir 50 ml) for intraarterial hepatic chemotherapy in colon cancer. Slightly less expensive than programmable system but inconvenient because alterations in dosing require that the reservoir be emptied and refilled with a newly concentrated drug preparation.

(iv) Medtronic Synchromed system: Consists of a fully implantable pump (18-ml capacity), catheter, and access to a specially programmed laptop computer outfitted with telemetry. Rate can be changed readily and may even be enhanced with preprogrammed boluses.

(v) Medtronic Algomed system: Still in FDA trials; a manually activated device consisting of a 50-ml plastic reservoir attached by tubing to a bulblike actuator device and an IT catheter. Contains a valve resembling those used for hydrocephalus shunts that, although allowing patients to self-inject up to 1 ml/hr, is usually activated two or three times daily. Promises to offer the advantage of PCA and lower cost.

(i) Pharmacology: This is a rapidly changing area as a result of new drug development and approval.

    (i) Much of current practice involves off-label use of drugs approved for other indications or routes of administration. Caution is warranted when considering the use of such drugs to avoid neurotoxicity.

    (ii) The standard and most accepted starting regimen involves preservative-free morphine.

    (iii) Lipophilic drugs (fentanyl, sufentanil, methadone) are often used for refractory pain. Their effects tend to be localized, with better efficacy when the catheter tip is in proximity to the spinal level corresponding to the pain generator.

    (iv) The addition of dilute concentration of a local anesthetic (bupivacaine) is a widely recognized alternative for pain that is refractory to opioids administered alone, especially for neuropathic pain and pain associated with movement (incident pain). When titrated up from a low concentration, effects are usually well tolerated, with little numbness, motor weakness, and autonomic changes.

    (v) An epidural formulation of clonidine has recently been approved for the management of refractory neuropathic pain.

(j) Side effects and complications: Maintenance involves consideration of drug side effects as well as potential difficulties related to the implanted device (e. g., mechanical failure, infection, headache).

    (i) With regard to commencing therapy, opioid-naive patients are at high risk for side effects ranging from respiratory depression to nausea, vomiting, pruritus, urinary retention, and dysphoria, while serious side effects are extremely rare in the opioid-tolerant individual. However, if doses are increased to the usual range for systemic therapy, even opioid-tolerant patients may experience side effects as a consequence of systemic absorption, although these tend to be bothersome (e.g., constipation and sedation) rather than dangerous.

(7) Electrical stimulation

    (a) The gate control theory of pain and counterstimulation has been invoked to explain the potential for the application of electrical stimulation to influence pain.

    (b) From a pragmatic view, applications are predominantly for noncancer pain, although even in this setting indications are controversial.

    (c) Transcutaneous electrical nerve stimulation (TENS) involves the application of low-voltage electrical stimulation to the skin overlying the painful site or a pain generator. Treatment is applied by the means of portable power source (about the size of a beeper) that is attached to ECG electrodes and that is subject to some patient control. Treatment is noninvasive and inexpensive, with equipment usually leased through a physical therapy department. As confidence in drug therapies has increased, TENS tends often to be overlooked and is best used as an adjunct to other, more reliably effective modalities. Pain is rarely relieved entirely. Effect is probably partially placebo-dependent. Fifty percent of cancer patients may respond with reduced pain initially, but response rate decays over time. Despite low efficacy, TENS is innocuous and may enhance autonomy and sense of control.

    (d) Spinal cord stimulation (SCS): Involves the surgical implantation of a miniaturized series of epidural electrodes that are tunneled under skin and attached to a subcutaneous pacemaker-type battery.

        Role in cancer pain is just about nil. Systems are costly and prone to mechanical failure and migration. They require preoperative screening and surgery; are effective only for topographically fixed, localized pain, usually of a neuropathic nature; are minimally titratable; and are rarely associated with truly profound analgesia.

        Notwithstanding the preceding, they may have a role in posttreatment pain in survivors, because this tends to be neuropathic and confined to a specific area.

    (e) Deep brain stimulation: For pain, this has recently been re-relegated to experimental status in the United States, although approval for tremor Parkinsonism is forthcoming. Electrodes are placed through a burr hole under local anesthesia by a neurosurgeon. Stimulation of areas rich in opioid receptors (periaqueductal and periventricular gray matter) may produce profound analgesia that is usually naloxone-reversible and appears to be mediated by endogenous opioids. In contrast, stimulation of thalamic centers appears more effective for neuropathic pain in topographically discrete distributions and is resistant to naloxone. Remains a promising approach for intractable pain.

(8) Other neurosurgical approaches

  (a) Although a variety of neurosurgical procedures have been introduced with the intention of providing safe, effective, and reliable pain relief, most have been abandoned because of failure to adequately achieve these goals.

  (b) Consideration of even the most practical of these is limited, as experience with less invasive alternatives has increased, and access to experienced specialists is limited.

  (c) Percutaneous cordotomy, the most frequently utilized neurosurgical procedure performed to relieve cancer pain, is indicated for refractory unilateral pain below the level of the midtrunk. Under monitored anesthesia care a radiofrequency probe is advanced below the mastoid using fluoroscopic guidance, until stimulation confirms placement of its tip in the lateral spinothalamic tract. A thermal lesion is generated within the substance of the spinal cord, resulting in selective analgesia and thermoinsensitivity below the trunk on the contralateral side. Unlike its precursor, open thoracic cordotomy, and many other neurosurgical procedures, it is minimally demanding of the cancer patient, is associated with low risk and morbidity in experienced hands, and, because there is no incision, requires minimal recuperation. Duration of effect is usually limited to about 1 year, and burning, neuropathic pain may arise as relief recedes. As opposed to many ablative procedures, pain relief is often quite dramatic, and because proprioception, tactile sensation, and motor strength are usually preserved it is usually well tolerated. Bilateral or more extensive lesions (considered to produce higher levels of analgesia) are usually avoided because of an unacceptable incidence of ataxia, urinary incontinence, and even fatal sleep apnea (Ondine's Curse).

  (d) Midline myelotomy (commisurotomy) is an extensive operation and involves a laminectomy and midline incision of the spinal cord. It is only occasionally performed for intractable perineal or pelvic pain because of a moderate failure rate and significant incidence of serious neurologic complications.

(e) Transnasal pituitary ablation, usually with alcohol, is performed today in only a limited number of centers, but may be effective for pain due to widespread bony metastases, especially in patients with hormone-dependent cancer (breast and prostate). Under light general anesthesia a radiographically guided needle is inserted through the nose into the pituitary fossa, where a small quantity of alcohol is injected. Risks include blindness, diabetes insipidus, and panhypopituitarism, but pain relief is often dramatic.

(7) Behavioral pain management: Hypnosis, relaxation, biofeedback, sensory alteration, guided imagery, and cognitive strategies have been used with varying success in patients with cancer and pain. Behavioral intervention involves instruction in specific skills that, with practice, the patient can utilize independently or with supervision to enhance the effectiveness of intercurrent methods of pain relief. Their use is highly situation-specific. Because profound analgesia is an infrequent outcome, these modalities are usually regarded as adjuvants to drug therapy. One of their main draws is to enhance an individual's personal sense of control and mastery. Because these therapies require learning and practicing new skills, it is extremely important that the patient be highly motivated as well as able to concentrate.

IV. CONCLUSIONS

Cancer pain is comprised of a group of heterogeneous disorders characterized by variable natural histories and treatment responsivity, which thus demand a carefully individualized guideline-based approach to management. Durable, gratifying outcomes can be achieved but are dependent on a programmatic commitment, access to interdisciplinary management, communication and assessment skills, and attention to detail. The application of a cogent program of analgesic therapy is effective in 70% to 90% of patients over time. In addition, specific anesthetic procedures comprise an important category of complementary therapeutic options that, when carefully selected, promote improved outcome.

The Pain Clinic Manual, Second Edition,
edited by Stephen E. Abram and J. David Haddox.
Lippincott Williams & Wilkins,
Philadelphia, © 2000

33

Psychologic Assessment and Treatment of Patients with Cancer Pain

Antonio M. Goncalves

A. M. Goncalves: Cancer Research/Treatment Center, University of New Mexico, Health Sciences Center—School of Medicine, Albuquerque, New Mexico 87131.

I. BACKGROUND
  A. Inadequately controlled cancer pain has been a focus of attention for more than 20 years.
  B. Physical, psychologic, interpersonal, and spiritual well-being have been identified as "quality-of-life" issues for cancer patients.
  C. Cancer pain had been conceptualized as multidimensional, consisting of affective, behavioral, cognitive, and sensory aspects.
  D. Barriers to adequate cancer pain relief have been identified as follows:
     1. Societal and cultural views on the appropriate use of opioids
     2. Influence of government regulatory agencies (whether real or imagined)
     3. Deficits in knowledge concerning pharmacologic studies of cancer pain by health care providers
  E. In 1994 the Agency for Health Policy and Research (U.S. Department of Health and Human Services) published the Clinical Guidelines for the management of cancer pain.
  F. The guidelines recommend a multidisciplinary approach for the treatment of cancer pain, including a psychologic component.
II. EXPRESSION OF PAIN
  A. There is significant agreement in the discrimination of what is painful.
     1. Culture can impact its tolerance and expression.
     2. Ethnic groups differ in pain expression in the affective, cognitive, and behavioral dimensions.
  B. Pain has meaning. Cancer pain can mean to the patient that the disease is progressing and death may be imminent.
  C. Exacerbation of pain behaviors and demands for analgesics can rise from poorly controlled pain. If not appropriately addressed it can trigger mistrust between the patient and the health care team. This has been called *opioid pseudoaddiction.*

III. CANCER PAIN ASSESSMENT
  A. Cancer-related pain can be assessed at three levels: severity, characteristics, and impact.
    1. *Severity* can be assessed by simple subjective scales (visual analogue, numeric ratings, verbal descriptions, distress ratings).
    2. *Characteristics* refers to type of pain (quality, location, breakthrough, resistance to treatment).
    3. *Impact* focuses on
        a. Mood (anxiety, sleep, appetite, suicide ideation, depression)
        b. Functioning (work, sexuality, activity level)
        c. Social life (family relations, friendships)
        d. Symptoms (nausea, constipation, fatigue)
  B. More comprehensive pain assessments can also be done through the use of instruments developed on and for cancer patients, such as the Brief Pain Inventory.
IV. PSYCHIATRIC DIAGNOSIS AND SYMPTOMS IN CANCER PAIN PATIENTS
  A. A sample of 215 cancer patients at three different centers yielded the prevalences outlined in Table 33-1 (modified from Derogatis LR, et al.).
    1. Nearly 90% of the diagnoses were related to disease or treatment.
    2. Panic disorders, phobias, and to a lesser extent posttraumatic stress disorders can also be seen.
  B. Adjustment disorders with depression or anxiety with severe symptoms can be difficult to distinguish from major depression and other anxiety disorders.
    1. Medications, withdrawal symptoms (including those from alcohol), various medical conditions, weight loss, fatigue, insomnia, poor appetite, physical symptoms further complicate the diagnosis.
    2. Adequate cancer pain relief and taking a good history can be helpful in establishing a diagnosis.

TABLE 33-1. *Psychiatric diagnosis and symptoms in patients with cancer*

Normal responses to cancer	Psychiatric diagnosis	
53%	47%	
	Adjustment disorders (mood and anxiety)	68%
	Major depression	13%
	Organic mental disorder	8%
	Preexisting personality disorders	7%
	Preexisting anxiety disorders	4%

3. Mental disorders in cancer patients can be related to the illness, or there may be preexisting disorders exacerbated by the illness.

V. WORKING WITH CANCER PAIN PATIENTS

A. Establishment of rapport is important to avoid the perception that the pain is not accepted as real.

B. Although slightly more than half of cancer patients do not carry a psychiatric diagnosis, they may still benefit from psychologic services.

C. Patients with mild to moderate pain levels who are disease-free and motivated to learn new skills can often benefit from psychologic approaches to pain management. Opioid medications may prove of limited value for these patients.

D. Patients with major psychiatric disturbances do not benefit as much from psychologic approaches as those with reactive symptoms of depression or anxiety.

E. Adequate cancer-related pain relief reduces psychiatric symptoms.

VI. SUPPORT OF THE CANCER PAIN PATIENT AND FAMILY

A. Support is more useful when tailored to the needs of the patient and family.
   1. Emotional support (listening, sharing, providing positive feedback)
   2. Informational support (most useful coming from health professionals regarding treatment, health maintenance, expectations)
   3. Practical or instrumental support (helpful behaviors such as shopping, cooking, cleaning, taking the patient to doctors appointments)

B. The patient's environment may reinforce pain behaviors. It is useful to assess it. Sometimes family or couple therapy can be helpful.

C. The patient's cancer and pain affect the family:
   1. Communication or emotional difficulties
   2. Household management difficulties
   3. Role changes
   4. Financial pressures
   5. The caregiver may experience anticipatory grief, lack of social support, avoidance, guilt, depression, health problems.

VII. PSYCHOLOGIC TREATMENT INTERVENTIONS

A. The challenge
   1. It is difficult to isolate cancer pain from the disease process.
   2. It is not easy to find pain-free cancer patients and match them on diagnosis, stage, sex, age.
   3. Much of what is known is based on U.S. white female patient samples with breast cancer.

B. Although few clinical trials specifically focusing on psychologic treatment approaches for cancer pain have been done, there is considerable evidence that psychologic interventions:
   1. Improve general psychologic functioning (reduce distress and increase a sense of control).

      2. Assist with specific treatment side effects of cancer therapy.

      3. Appear to consistently help reduce pain through imagery or hypnosis.

      4. Can reduce pain through cognitive/behavioral techniques (although this body of work has been more specific to noncancer pain).

C. There is evidence of specific affective distress but no apparent evidence of global psychologic disturbance due to cancer pain.

D. Pain intensity and functional status do not appear to differentiate between depressed and nondepressed patients.

E. It is unclear whether pain follows distress or precedes it. However, at least for bone marrow transplant patients, distress related to treatment side effects accounted for pain more than any other factor.

F. Two main psychologic treatment approaches have been:

      1. Improving general functioning through the enhancement of coping skills and reduction of distress.

         a. Distraction

         b. Identification of problems and exploration of solutions

         c. Reframing (new ways to consider old problems)

         d. Challenge of cognitive distortions

         e. Education

         f. Audios, videos, humor, music, bibliotherapy

         g. Psychotherapy

      2. Ameliorating disease- or treatment-related symptoms such as anxiety, anticipatory nausea, pain. Methods can include:

         a. Counseling

         b. Hypnosis

         c. Modeling

         d. Operant conditioning

         e. Biofeedback

         f. Imagery

         g. Deep breathing and relaxation

         h. Progressive muscle relaxation

      3. The work of Spiegel and Fawzy has also generated intriguing data related to possible survival benefits of psychologic interventions.

G. Methods that have been effective in reducing cancer treatment–related pain

      1. Relaxation and deep breathing have

         a. Decreased pain and pain distress (patients' expectations play a role in the amount of relief)

         b. Decreased anxiety

         c. Decreased nausea and vomiting

         d. Improved mood, sleep, rest, food, and fluid intake

         e. Increased participation in treatment

         f. Improved sense of personal control

        g. Theoretical contraindications for their use: patients who are psychotic, have bradycardia or heart block, or are unaccustomed to relaxation and are fearful or inflexible. Some of these patients may benefit from progressive muscle relaxation.

    2. Imagery: How the mind is used can have important consequences in treatment outcomes.

        a. One issue is the challenge or problem, such as the pain.

        b. The other issues are beliefs, expectations, and hopes about the challenge or symptom, such as the pain.

        c. One first creates a mental image of a scene in which one is deeply relaxed. Changes are then suggested in the body that simulate the relaxed state.

VIII. CANCER PAIN, PSYCHOLOGIC RESPONSES, AND THE DISEASE CONTINUUM

  A. Diagnosis

    1. Pain may come from neoplastic processes that are acute, resolvable, and not life-threatening. Pain may also come from advanced cancer.

    2. Normal responses to cancer diagnosis

        a. Shock, denial, despair

        b. Emotional and/or physical symptoms to the diagnosis, such as anxiety, depression, insomnia, anorexia

        c. Adaptation to the diagnosis influenced by medical, patient, family, and societal variables.

    3. Ways of coping include

        a. Moving toward or away from social support

        b. Cognitive or behavioral escape or avoidance

    4. Crisis intervention may be appropriate.

  B. Treatments

    1. Cancer treatments can both relieve and introduce pain.

    2. Fears can include

        a. Uncertainty about the future

        b. Physical disability

        c. Pain

        d. Loss of work

    3. Side effects and psychologic reactions to them can be distressing.

        a. Nausea

        b. Pain

        c. Temporary mental status changes

        d. Hearing loss

        e. Hair loss

        f. Sexual dysfunction

        g. Burns

        h. Physical disfigurement

        i. Changes in taste of food

        j. Medical complications

    4. Cancer recurrence or relapse

        a. This can be viewed as a more intense diagnosis phase.

        b. Cancer pain may be more of a problem.

        c. The patient may view mortality as imminent.

        d. Withdrawal, depression, or denial may be present.

        e. Communication with the doctor may become more guarded because of limited options for treatment.

C. Advanced Disease

    1. Pain can come from advanced disease processes, and there is an expectation of pain increase with disease advance.

    2. Good pain control is essential, as fear of poorly controlled pain and suffering can increase suicide risk.

    3. Management of symptoms of distress, including psychologic interventions as appropriate, should be part of the treatment plan.

    4. Spiritual, religious, or existential issues may need to be addressed as appropriate.

    5. What patients want most is

        a. Freedom from pain

        b. Dignity

        c. Protection

        d. Truth

        e. Control

        f. Privacy

        g. Closeness

        h. Not being a burden to the family

    6. End-of-life tasks for the patient include coming to terms with one's finality, relationship completeness, and letting go.

IX. SUMMARY

The management of cancer pain can be complex. Cancer pain has been undertreated. The Clinical Guidelines for it have included psychologic modalities as part of the standard of care. In general, it can be said that although these modalities do not constitute the primary approach to cancer pain treatment, they can be helpful adjuncts. Whether used for specific cancer-related pain, treatment, side effects, distress reduction, or end-of-life issues, they can improve quality of life for patients, patients' families, and caregivers.

RECOMMENDED READING

Byock I. *Dying Well.* New York: Riverhead Books, 1997.

Clinical Guidelines for the Management of Cancer Pain (1994). Agency for Health Policy and Research. U.S. Department of Health and Human Services. AHCPR Publication No. 94–0592.

Daut RL, Cleeland CS, and Flanery RC. Development of the Wisconsin Brief Pain Questionnaire to Assess Pain in Cancer and other Diseases. *Pain* 1983;17:197–210.

Derogatis LR, Morrow GR, Fetting J, et al. The prevalence of psychiatric disorders among cancer patients. *JAMA* 1983;249:751–757.

Fawzy FI, Fawzy NW, Hyun CS, et al. Malignant melanoma: Effects of an early structured psychiatric intervention, coping, and affective state on recurrence and survival 6 years later. *Arch Gen Psychiatry* 1993;50:681–689.

Massie MJ, Holland, JC. The cancer patient in pain: Psychiatric complications and their management. *J Pain Sympt Manag* 1992;2:99–109.

Meyer TJ, Mark MM. Effects of psychosocial interventions with adult cancer patients: A meta-analysis of randomized experiments. *Health Psychol* 1995;14(2):101–108.

Spiegel D, Bloom, JR. Group therapy and hypnosis reduce metastatic breast carcinoma pain. *Psychosom Med* 1983;45:333–339.

Spiegel D, Bloom JR, Kraemer HC, Gottheil E. Effect psychosocial treatment on survival of patients with metastatic breast cancer. *Lancet* 1989;2:888–891.

Syrjala KL, Donaldson GW, Davis MW, Kippes ME, Carr JE. Relaxation and imagery and cognitive/behavioral training reduce pain during cancer treatment: A controlled clinical trial. *Pain* 1995;63:189–198.

Trill MD, Holland J. Cross cultural differences in the care of patients with cancer: A review. *Gen Hosp Psychiatry* 1993;15:21–30.

Weissman DE, Haddox JD. Clinical note. Opioid pseudoaddiction—an iatrogenic syndrome. *Pain* 1989;36:363–366.

The Pain Clinic Manual, Second Edition,
edited by Stephen E. Abram and J. David Haddox.
Lippincott Williams & Wilkins,
Philadelphia, © 2000

34

Palliative Care of the Terminally Ill Patient

Denice C. Sheehan and Walter B. Forman

*D. C. Sheehan: Division of Nursing, The Breen School of Nursing, Ursuline College,
Pepper Pike, Ohio 44124.
W. B. Forman: Department of Internal Medicine, University of New Mexico, Health Sciences
Center—School of Medicine, Albuquerque, New Mexico 87131.*

I. PALLIATIVE THERAPY

The medical advances of the twentieth century have extended the average life span, sometimes at the expense of the quality of that life. Death has become a taboo topic, rarely discussed and even less often seen. More people die in institutions than at home. Indeed, in 1992 the U.S. mortality statistics reported that 57% of deaths occurred in hospitals, and 17% died in nursing homes. The National Hospice Organization estimated that only approximately 17% of the people who died in 1995 received hospice services. It is also clear that most terminally ill people receive care at the end of life from health care professionals who are not specifically trained in palliative care. This chapter highlights issues and symptoms specific to terminally ill people and their families, many of whom have been or will be seen by pain specialists.

The care of people who have an illness that cannot be cured or whose life might be at an end is indeed a great challenge. Many of us see this as a personal failure to prevent death. Yet the literature suggests that, depending on one's training and acculturation, caring for the person at this stage of life can be very rewarding.

Caring for people at the end of life has always been part of nursing. However, in recent years the nursing curriculum has focused on acute and chronic illnesses with little attention to care at the end of life. Nurses are in a pivotal position to improve care at the end of life.

A. What is palliative care?
   1. As defined by Doyle, "the study and management of patients with active far advanced disease for whom the prognosis is limited and the focus of care is quality of life."
   2. Palliative care includes the whole person and the family. It integrates the physical, psychosocial, and spiritual components of care to enhance quality of life.

B. Where and when does palliative care begin?
  1. Usually a very difficult decision. It is seen by many as giving up hope for a cure. Others will view this stage as the time to move to the point where the focus of care is quality of life.
  2. Much can be done for and with individuals at this stage of life. Although this textbook is primarily aimed at the treatment of pain, the terminally ill person can have a multitude of other problems, such as anorexia, fatigue, insomnia, weakness, cough, and dyspnea.
  3. It is estimated that people will experience an average of 11 symptoms, and at any one moment in time have on average four or five different symptoms. To care for only one of these symptoms (e.g., pain) will not necessarily improve quality of life, which is the primary focus of care at this time of life. Thus in this chapter about the care of the terminally ill we will attempt to provide a framework for holistic care rather than only one problem.
C. Who is the focus of care?
  1. As can be imagined, the multiple issues involved require the input of more than just the patient. The focus of care is the patient.
  2. However, the "family" unit is the group that the care professional must consider early in the course of treatment.
     a. This group is defined by the particular setting.
        (1) It might be the traditional unit, such as the patient, spouse, children, and grandchildren.
        (2) It may be any other association as determined by the patient.
     b. The family member who lives across the country and who wants to take charge of the situation has surprised all of us. It is important that the patient be the one who takes charge.
        (1) If that person becomes disabled during the course of the illness to the point of being unable to make treatment decisions, then a surrogate will be the decision maker.
        (2) It is infinitely better that the surrogate be appointed early in the course of care. Otherwise one faces the possibility of a struggle for control of decisions.
        (3) This person, known as the power of attorney for health care, is identified using an advance directive or a similar type of legal document. For continuity of care these issues must be addressed early in the course in order to have a seamless structure for the health care professional, the family, and the person who is facing the end of life.
D. Who are the professionals involved in this care?
   The need for multiple areas of expertise is obvious. To deliver the quality of care that is the backbone of palliative care a team approach is used. The basic team consists at a minimum of four members—a physician, a nurse,

a social worker, and a counselor. These individuals initially assess the patient and family unit. This information with all members of the team in attendance is used to formulate a plan of care.

1. The team
    a. The hospice medical director
        (1) This physician is responsible for a variety of medically related topics.
        (2) The most important issue in this role is communication with the medical community and working with the team members.
    b. The nurse
        (1) This person is critical to the team.
        (2) Often the nurse is involved with a multitude of problems that are part of the dying experience for the family as well as the patient.
    c. The social worker
        (1) Counsels the patient and family about financial issues, community referral, and the like.
        (2) Must be able to prepare the psychosocial assessment concerning the approach to home care for this family unit.
        (3) Bereavement counseling might also be part of the role for this person.
    d. The chaplain
        (1) The challenge of this role is the need to meet the family in their own spiritual belief system.
        (2) Since a nonmedical person occupies this position, a consumer approach is also brought to the team.
    e. The primary care physician
        (1) This is the physician who refers the individual patient to the hospice program.
            (a) Some physicians refer the patient, as in other types of medical situations, and anticipate that the hospice medical director will render treatment decisions.
            (b) Others remain the primary physician for the patient and work with the team to provide end-of-life care.
        (2) Although this role might be daunting for the primary care physician, it can be very useful and rewarding.
E. What issues must be addressed?
    1. Symptom management
        a. The symptom management model is used here because it is the model that all health care workers are trained to employ. The symptoms discussed in this chapter are commonly noted in other disease processes. However, it is important to recall that symptoms may be attributed to the specific disease process, therapy,

debilitation, poor nutritional status, or causes unrelated to the terminal illness.

   b. A prospective study of 1000 patients reported that pain was the most common symptom among advanced cancer patients, followed by fatigue, weakness, and anorexia. The most common symptoms were also the most severe. The number of symptoms ranged from 1 to 27, with a median of 11, and did not differ significantly by gender or by the primary cancer site.

   c. Earlier studies on a palliative care unit reported pain (99%), dyspnea (46%), and confusion (39%) during the last week of life.

   d. The consequences of unrelieved symptoms impact quality of life by impairing mobility, which results in depression, sleep disturbances, reduced social activities, malnutrition, cognitive dysfunction, polypharmacy, gait disturbances, and falls.

II. PAIN

Pain occurs in about 80% of people entered into a hospice program. We refer the reader to the multiple issues already covered in this volume. In particular, we recommend rereading the chapters that deal with pain assessment, cancer pain (Table 34-1), and the chapter on psychologic strategies for treating pain. When a person enters into the care of a hospice team, the issues for pain relief also change. We suggest that the following are most important:

   A. The person and family have many psychosocial issues to attend during this portion of their lives.

   B. A simplified method of pain relief is critical.
      1. The oral route is the preferred choice.
      2. This route is easy to administer, allows the patient access to pain relief without numerous appointments, and is cost-effective.

TABLE 34-1. *The "stepladder" treatment of cancer pain*

---

1. Mild pain (2–4/10 on self-assessment scale)
   Aspirin
   Acetaminophen
   NSAIDS
   ±Adjuvants
2. Moderate pain (4–6/10 on self-assessment scale)
   Weak opioids (e.g., codeine, hydrocodone)
   ±Adjuvants
3. Severe pain (>6 on self-assessment scale)
   Strong opioids (e.g., morphine, hydromorphone, oxycodone)
   ±Adjuvants
   Adjuvant drugs include:
   Steroids, anticonvulsants, antidepressants

---

3. With the coming of a variety of sustained-release (SR) oral medications and the newer transmucosal medications, the physician has a variety of choices for optimum pain relief that are appropriate for this group of patients.

C. The usual hospice program is funded as a capitated model.
1. The hospice receives a per diem fee.
2. Therefore the most effective and least costly approaches are encouraged. With the coming of a variety of SR oral medications and the newer transmucosal medications, the physician has a variety of choices for optimum pain relief that are appropriate for this group of patients.

D. Remember to make certain that the pain treatment plan fits the needs of the patient, even if the plan might be somewhat in conflict with your plan.

III. PAIN THERAPY

Here the pain specialist can offer more than the type of drug but can be instrumental in providing a route of administration that is appropriate for the setting. A complete review of these choices can be found in the review by Anderson and Forman. The list includes the following.

A. Sustained-Release Preparations
1. These have been alluded to previously. However, morphine is now available in a 24-hour SR tablet. This simple change to a route that can be given simply and only once a day should be most helpful to the patient.
2. In addition to simplicity, improved compliance can be expected using these oral SR products.

B. Sublingual/Buccal Administration
1. The delivery of drug across the mucosal membrane is a very simple technique and can be used in patients for whom swallowing has become difficult or impossible.
2. Fentanyl is very lipophilic and is a good choice for this route. In particular, its use in breakthrough pain via the sublingual route may prove to be very beneficial.

C. Rectal Administration
1. This route yields good blood levels of a variety of opioids, particularly morphine.
2. This agent delivered in suppositories that melt at body temperature will deliver a constant dose whose level might need adjusting, depending on absorption for the particular patient.
3. Factors that can alter dosing intervals of which the physician should be aware include the following:
   a. Fluid volume in the rectum
   b. Integrity of mucosa
   c. The presence of feces
4. It appears, at least for morphine, that the oral and rectal route offer similar pain relief.

5. Note that the rectal route is not a manufacturer-recommended route of administration, nor is it an approved method of administration. Thus we must urge cautious observation in any patient receiving opioids via this route.

D. Continuous Subcutaneous Infusion

1. This route of drug administration, first described in England in 1979, utilizes all the benefits of intravenous infusion yet affords a simple, less expensive delivery system.

2. Subcutaneous infusion can be utilized for pain control as well as for other medications when the patient cannot tolerate the oral route or the patient/family wishes not to use the rectal route.

3. In addition to being less expensive it is a route that can be easily utilized by less skilled workers than would be needed to attend to the intravenous administration of drug.

4. Both morphine and hydromorphone are the preferred analgesics here because the problems with meperidine, levorphanol, and methadone remain the same as outlined previously.

5. Hydromorphone because of its potency is the agent of choice when large doses are required to relieve pain.

6. One should use the same conversion from oral to continuous subcutaneous infusion as the conversion to intravenous administration.

7. The utilization of this route can be very helpful in the following conditions that affect the terminally ill person.

   a. Intractable nausea and or emesis

   b. Intestinal obstruction

   c. The patient is too weak to swallow.

8. Any site on the chest, abdomen, arms, or thighs can be prepared for infusion.

   a. Select a site, preparing it in a sterile fashion and utilizing a 25- or 27-gauge butterfly needle for infusion.

   b. The site is then covered with a polyurethane film, which will provide a clear view of the needle and surrounding skin.

   c. The site should be observed daily for signs of infection. It is our experience that a properly prepared site can be employed for upward of a week.

IV. SIDE EFFECTS

A. Constipation

See Table 34-2 for pertinent information.

1. In practice, many of these individuals are inactive, take in small amounts of fluid, and have minimal caloric intake. Thus constipation is a major issue that becomes only more relevant when opioids are utilized.

2. The health care worker must make certain that the patient is defecating at least near their normal interval.

TABLE 34-2. *Treatment of constipation in the palliative care patient*

---

1. Diet
   a. Determine frequency of bowel movements
   b. Determine fluid and fiber intake
   c. Rx:
   Increase fluid intake to 2 liters/day. Avoid "diuretic"-type fluids (e.g., coffee)
   If possible, increase fiber intake
2. Treatment to
   Increase fluid load in large intestine
      Sodium docusate
   Increase transit time in large intestine
      Senna product or combination of senna and sodium docusate
   If bowel movements are infrequent or "hard" when produced:
      Oil enema followed by contact cathartic
   Increase transient time:
      Cisapride or metoclopramide

---

      a. It is recommended that combination stimulant laxatives and stool softeners be employed in a dose that will ensure evacuations at least three or four times per week.

      b. If oral agents are ineffective in this regard, then suppositories or enemas must be available.

   3. Constipation is a very common cause of abdominal pain in the person taking opioids. The patient should not have to be hospitalized, as occasionally occurs, to treat this problem.

  B. Other Problems

  Although the pain specialist might not wish to treat the following symptoms, the hospice care team might be involved. The team can be a valuable resource for the pain specialist, especially when that person is the primary physician.

   1. Analysis of the research using the Memorial Symptom Assessment Scale (MSAS) suggests the average number of symptoms per patient is highly associated with quality of life.

   2. As stated earlier in this chapter, an average of 11 symptoms may be present in the terminally ill person. The most common of these in addition to pain are as follows.

     a. Weakness

     c. Fatigue

     d. Anorexia/cachexia/early satiety

     e. Nausea/emesis (Table 34-3)

     f. Insomnia

     g. Cognitive disturbances

     h. Dyspnea

TABLE 34-3. *Treatment of nausea and vomiting in the palliative care patient*

Caused by the initiation of opioids
Haloperidol
Chlorpromazine
Caused by slowed gastric emptying
Metoclopramide
Cisapride
Ondansetron
Caused by "squashed stomach syndrome"
Dexamethasone
Caused by increased intracranial pressure
Haloperidol
Dexamethasone

      i. Xerostomia

      j. Depression/Anxiety

        All these problems are beyond the scope of this chapter and the reader is referred to the bibliography for more information.

  3. Again we remind the reader that the care of people at this stage of life is complex and requires the combined approach of an interdisciplinary team.

RECOMMENDED READING

Anderson RP, Forman WB. Alternate routes of opioid administration in palliative care: Pharmacologic and clinical concerns. *J Pharm Care Pain Symptom Control* 1998;6:5–23.

Doyle D, Hanks GWC, MacDonald N, eds. *Oxford Textbook of Palliative Medicine.* Oxford: Oxford University Press; 1997.

Field MJ, Cassel CK, eds. *Approaching Death: Improving Care at the End of Life.* Washington, DC: National Academy Press; 1997.

Hospice Nurses Association. *Standards of Hospice Nursing Practice and Professional Performance.* Pittsburgh: Hospice Nurses Association; 1995.

Jacox AK, Carr DB, Payne R, et al. *Management of Cancer Pain Reference Guide for Clinicians.* Clinical Practice Guideline No. 9. Rockville, MD: Agency for Health Care Policy and Research; 1994.

Kemp, C. *Terminal Illness: A Guide to Nursing Care.* Philadelphia: JB Lippincott; 1995.

McGuire D, Yarbro CH, Ferrell BR. *Cancer Pain Management,* 2nd ed. Boston: Jones and Bartlett; 1995.

Sheehan DC, Forman WB, eds. *Hospice and Palliative Care: Concepts and Practice.* Sudbury: Jones and Bartlett; 1996.

Waller A, Caroline N. *Handbook of Palliative Care in Cancer.* Boston: Butterworth-Heinemann; 1996.

World Health Organization. Cancer pain relief and palliative care. Report of a WHO Expert Committee. Who Technical Report Series 804, WHO, Geneva, 1990.

The Pain Clinic Manual, Second Edition,
edited by Stephen E. Abram and J. David Haddox.
Lippincott Williams & Wilkins,
Philadelphia, © 2000

35

Radiation Therapy for Cancer Pain

Nora A. Janjan

N. A. Janjan: Department of Radiation Oncology, The University of Texas
M. D. Anderson Cancer Center, Houston, Texas 77030.

I. GENERAL CONSIDERATIONS
  A. Palliative Care in Radiation Oncology
    1. Palliation of symptomatic metastases is a major part of radiation oncology practice.
    2. Radiation therapy is one of the most effective means in relieving cancer pain because it controls the etiology of the pain.
  B. Terminology
    1. Current terminology for delivered radiation is the Gray (Gy) or centigray (cGy). This terminology replaced the familiar term *rad*. The Gy and rad are related as follows: 1 cGy = 1 rad and 1 Gy = 100 cGy = 100 rad.
  C. Dosage
    1. The variables in a course of radiation include (a) the dose per fraction and (b) number of fractions. The dose per fraction is the most important factor in radiation therapy because it affects both the side effects during and after radiation.
    2. Normal tissue tolerance limits the dose of radiation that can be administered. Because of normal tissue tolerance, the total radiation dose that can be administered decreases as the dose per fraction increases. Calculations can be performed that equate different radiation schedules. For example, a radiation course that treats the spinal cord to its tolerated dose can be administered as (a) 40 Gy in 20 fractions or (b) 30 Gy in 10 fractions or (c) 20 Gy in 5 fractions.
    3. Acute Radiation Side Effects
      a. Acute radiation side effects involve rapidly proliferating cells like the mucous membranes of the mouth, the esophagus and bowel, the bladder, and the skin.
      b. Characterized by an inflammatory reaction, acute radiation effects can be minimized by selecting specific techniques for treatment.

       c. Side effects that do occur, such as diarrhea, urinary frequency, and pain, can be controlled with medical management.

       d. Typically, acute radiation side effects are temporary; they occur after the first or second week of radiation and resolve within 2 weeks of completing radiation.

       e. Acute radiation side effects do not predict for late radiation side effects.

    4. Late radiation side effects

       a. Late radiation side effects involve tissues that proliferate slowly or not at all, such as muscle and connective and neural tissues.

       b. Fibrosis and necrosis are characteristics of the dose-limiting late radiation side effects that define normal tissue tolerance.

       c. Careful planning is required to avoid overlap of the radiation fields because a given area can only receive treatment once. This is especially true for dose-limiting normal structures such as the spinal cord that often require palliative radiation.

       d. Late radiation effects occur months to years after the radiation is administered.

II. TYPES OF RADIATION

    A. External Beam Radiation Oncology

      1. All external beam radiation is delivered by either a linear accelerator or, less commonly, a Cobalt unit.

      2. Photon radiation is used to treat tumors that are located several centimeters from the skin surface.

      3. Electron beam radiation is used for superficial tumors that are located usually within 5 cm of the skin surface. The penetration of electron beam radiation is limited to within a few centimeters of the skin surface.

       a. To estimate the depth of penetration of an electron beam the following calculation is often made:

         (1) Eighty percent of the radiation dose is deposited when the electron beam energy is divided by 3.

         (2) Ninety-five percent of the radiation dose is deposited when the electron beam energy is divided by 2.

         (3) For example, if a 9-MeV electron beam is used, 80% of the radiation dose is deposited within 3 cm of the skin surface and 95% of the radiation dose is deposited within 4.5 cm of the skin surface. A structure located 7 cm below the skin surface, such as the lung, heart, and spinal cord, would receive no radiation at all.

    B. Brachytherapy (Implanted Radioactive Sources)

      1. Radioactive implants can be permanent or temporary. The radiation exposure to other parts of the body, hospital personnel, and public is generally very low because of the inverse square law. The inverse square law relates the radiation exposure as the inverse of the square

of the distance from the radiation source: radiation exposure = $1/D^2$, where D = distance. Therefore the radiation emitted from an implant is well localized. For this reason, implants are used to

  a. Deliver extra radiation to sites at high risk for tumor recurrence.
  b. Serve as the only treatment for cancers in an attempt to minimize radiation to other tissues.
  c. Treat a cancer that recurs in a previously irradiated area.
     Another advantage of implants is the abbreviated treatment time, which can range from minutes to days. The tumor must be anatomically or surgically accessible so that the radioactive sources can be placed in and/or around the tumor bed.

2. Permanent implants. The length of time that the patient remains radioactive depends on the radioactive properties of the radioactive source (usually in the form of radioactive seeds) that is placed in the patient's tumor. The radioactive properties include the radiation strength of each seed, the number of seeds placed, and the half-life (time required for half of the radiation dose to decay) of the radiation source. Common examples include implants for prostate cancer.

3. Temporary implants place radiation sources for a specific amount of time to treat a tumor or a surgical bed. Radioactive sources can be placed inside tubes, needles, or catheters. Temporary implants are commonly used to treat soft-tissue sarcomas and gynecologic, lung, and esophageal cancers.

III. CLINICAL APPLICATION
  A. Radiation Schedules
    1. External beam radiation can be delivered as a single large dose (fraction) or several fractions over many weeks. The choice of radiation schedule is dependent on the patient's condition and the area to be treated.
       a. The radiation schedule most frequently used for palliative radiation administers 300 cGy per fraction for 10 fractions (total radiation dose of 3000 cGy). Palliative radiation schedules are designed to
          (1) Shrink the tumor and relieve symptoms quickly.
          (2) Abbreviate the time required for treatment among patients with a limited life span.
          (3) Reduce acute radiation effects, especially over critical structures like the spinal cord and esophagus.
       b. A single large fraction, given as 800 cGy to 1000 cGy, is often used to stop bleeding from cervical cancer or to treat bone metastases.
       c. In contrast, multiple fractions are used for curative treatment. In curative treatment, usually 25 to 35 treatments are administered 5 days per week over 5 to 7 weeks that give 180 cGy to 200 cGy per fraction to treat only microscopic residual disease. Total radiation doses for curative radiation range from 4500 cGy to more than 7000

cGy. Radiation doses in excess of 10,000 cGy are to required to sterilize tumors larger than 1 cm. Total doses in this range result in unacceptable normal tissue effects like fibrosis and necrosis.

    d. The goal of palliative radiation, therefore, is to temporarily shrink the tumor to relieve symptoms for the remainder of the patient's life.

B. Rationale

    1. The focus of palliative radiation is to treat a localized area of tumor involvement causing symptoms or to prevent morbidity with further disease progression, like pathologic fracture, spinal cord compression, or bronchial obstruction. Overall rates of response are 70%.

    2. A multidisciplinary approach that coordinates radiation therapy, systemic therapy, and a surgical intervention may be required. In all cases, prompt medical management of symptoms is needed. Because time is often required to achieve relief of symptoms due to tumor regression, continued medical management of symptoms is generally needed during and after completing radiation and other anticancer therapies. For example, the maximum benefit from radiation to bone metastases is noted 12 weeks after completing radiation; this time corresponds to the time required for recalcification of bone after tumor cell kill.

C. Palliation of Advanced Primary and Metastatic Sites

    1. Bone

        a. The most frequent symptomatic site. Any bone, including the base of skull, can be involved. Base of skull involvement can compromise neural foramina and result in cranial nerve deficits. Nerves are most commonly injured by cancer because they are compressed from metastatic involvement of adjacent bony structures.

        b. Vertebral metastases characteristically can present with a 1- to 2-week history of progressive back pain, and result in epidural tumor extension and spinal cord compression. Spinal cord compression represents a medical emergency that requires prompt initiation of steroids and radiation. Because of exit dose through normal tissues that are in proximity to the vertebral column, such as the stomach and esophagus, 30 Gy in 10 fractions or even more protracted courses of palliative radiation are often prescribed.

        c. Systemic radionuclides or hemibody radiation are effective in treating multifocal bone metastases. Because the activity of systemic radionuclides is confined to bone, their use is contraindicated in the treatment of spinal cord compression.

    2. Lung cancer

        a. Symptoms palliated by lung cancer include hemoptysis, superior vena cava obstruction (resulting from metastatic involvement of mediastinal lymph nodes), pain due to nerve and bone infiltration by a Pancoast tumor, and obstructive pneumonitis.

    b. Typically, 20 Gy in five fractions to 35 Gy in 14 fractions are pre-
scribed. The radiation schedule selected is based on the patient's
clinical condition and concern about adjacent structures like the
spinal cord and esophagus.

3. Pelvic tumors

    a. Control of massive vaginal bleeding from cervical cancer can be
rapidly achieved with 500 cGy fractions over three treatments or a
single 1000-cGy fraction. A superficial x-ray is delivered directly
over the cervix with a cone placed in the vagina. The higher dose
per treatment is possible because the less penetrating x-rays do not
reach the bowel or other pelvic structures.

    b. Other symptoms caused by pelvic tumors include pain, bowel and
ureteric obstruction, and lower extremity edema. These symptoms
can be relieved by shrinking the tumor and by reducing the pressure
on adjacent structures.

4. Central nervous system

    a. Brain metastases can result in nausea and vomiting, and severe
headache due to increased intracranial pressure. Metastases can be
limited to the brain parenchyma but can also involve the skull and
leptomeninges. Because of normal tissue tolerance of the central
nervous system, most radiation schedules include 2 to 3 weeks of
radiation.

    b. Leptomeningeal metastases are rarely treated with craniospinal irra-
diation because of the difficulty in daily treatment set-up, the necessary prolonged course of radiation, and toxicities of treatment.
However, if localized symptoms and nodularity that is documented
on an MRI are present, localized radiation can be given to treat a specific region of the leptomeninges with an understanding of the limited impact on the overall metastatic involvement.

IV. RESULTS

  A. In general, radiation therapy regimens for palliative treatment reduce the
overall time required for therapy to account for the patient's prognosis,
achieve prompt relief of symptoms, and minimize the delay of initiating
chemotherapy or performing a necessary surgical intervention.

    1. Orthopedic or neurosurgical consultation is required if significant bone
destruction is observed and surgical stabilization is considered necessary to avoid pathologic fracture. Pain that persists after radiation can
often be caused by bony instability rather than tumor.

      a. Bony instability can result from compression fractures especially
in the vertebrae and femur. Pathological or compression fractures
are common in the femur if more than 50% of the cortex was
involved by tumor or the metastasis was more than 1.5 cm in size
prior to radiation.

  b. With radiation-induced tumor kill, the bone becomes like an eggshell until recalcification is accomplished.
  c. In the spine, compression fractures can result in severe pain and retropulsion of bony elements that can cause spinal cord compression requiring prompt surgical intervention.
B. Palliation of symptoms can occur quickly in rapidly proliferating or highly radiosensitive tumors such as lymphoma. Other less responsive tumors may require several weeks following completion of radiation to observe an objective response to pain.

V. SUMMARY

Radiation therapy is a highly effective means of eliminating the symptoms of cancer through localized treatment of the disease. The approach to treatment is dependent on patient factors; however, technical advances allow numerous treatment options. The goal of palliative radiation is to minimize treatment-related morbidity while achieving symptom relief. The control of cancer pain has been and will continue to be an important aspect of radiation therapy training and practice.

RECOMMENDED READING

Brady l, Perez CA, eds. *Principles and Practice of Radiation Oncology,* 3rd ed. New York: JB Lippincott; 1997.

Janjan NA. Radiation for bone metastases—conventional techniques and the role of systemic radiopharmaceuticals. *Cancer* 1997;80:1628–1645.

Janjan NA, Weissman DE. Primary cancer treatment: Antineoplastic treatment in pain management. In: Levy MH, Portenoy RK, Weissman DE, Berger A, eds. *Principles and Practice of Supportive Oncology.* New York: Lippincott-Raven; 1998:45–61.

Perrin R, Janjan NA, Langford L. Spinal axis metastases. In: Levin V, ed. *Cancer in the Nervous System.* New York: JB Lippincott; 1996:259–280.

The Pain Clinic Manual, Second Edition,
edited by Stephen E. Abram and J. David Haddox.
Lippincott Williams & Wilkins,
Philadelphia, © 2000

36

Neurolytic Blocks and Other Neuroablative Procedures for Cancer Pain

Pushpa Nambi Joseph and Oscar A. deLeon-Casasola

P. N. Joseph: Department of Anesthesiology,
Kansas University Medical Center, Kansas City, Kansas 66160;
O. A. deLeon-Casasola: Department of Anesthesiology,
Roswell Park Cancer Institute, Buffalo, New York 14263.

I. GENERAL PRINCIPLES
   A. Multidisciplinary approach is essential.
   B. Should be considered an adjunct to other therapies.
   C. Opioid and other adjuvant therapies should be used in conjunction.
   D. Informed consent is mandatory.
   E. Neurolytic blockade can be used to treat somatic (peripheral and intraspinal neurolysis) and visceral pain (sympathetic axis neurolysis).
   F. Prior local anesthetic blockade is desirable to predict prognosis but is not mandatory, because of economic issues.
   G. Cancer pain may have visceral, somatic, and neuropathic components.
      1. Visceral pain is due to activation of nociceptors and produces pain that is poorly localized and is often referred to cutaneous sites. Example is pain due to pancreatic cancer.
      2. Somatic pain is due to activation of nociceptors and is well localized, constant, aching, or gnawing in character. Pain associated with bony metastasis is an example.
      3. Neuropathic pain is mediated by nonnociceptor mechanisms and is constant, dull, squeezing, aching pain with paroxysms of burning, shock-like components; it includes metastatic brachial and lumbar sacral plexopathies. New hypothesis on neuropathic pain involved a nociceptor mechanism (nervi nervorum injury).
II. PHARMACOLOGY OF NEUROLYTIC AGENTS
   Ethyl alcohol and phenol have remained the agents of choice.
   A. Phenol
      1. Various concentrations prepared with saline, water, glycerin, and radiologic dyes are used by mixing phenol with these solvents.

    2. Relatively insoluble in water; supersaturated solutions of 10% phenol are still clinically effective. Phenol in glycerin is hyperbaric.

    3. Biphasic action with an initial local anesthetic effect and a subsequent neurolysis with a possible mechanism of action of phenol through effects on cellular calcium homeostasis.

        a. Its effect is concentration dependent, <5% cause protein coagulation, >5% cause protein denaturation.

        b. Acute complications include neurologic deficits, direct neurotoxic effects, convulsions, CNS depression, and cardiovascular collapse.

        c. It is the agent of choice for peripheral nerve neurolytic blocks.

B. Ethyl Alcohol

    1. It is commercially available in 1-ml ampules and is usually used undiluted.

    2. Alcohol is hypobaric with respect to CSF at a concentration of 35% to 50%, which is frequently used.

    3. It is an irritant to tissue and injection is usually associated with discomfort, which may be reduced with simultaneous injection of local anesthetic.

    4. It is usually readily soluble in body fluids. Thus it needs a larger volume to be effective.

    5. The neurolytic action of alcohol is by dehydration, with the extraction of cholesterol, phospholipids, and cerebrosides and the precipitation of mucoproteins; produces nonselective destruction of nervous tissue.

    6. The use of this agent for peripheral nerve blocks is discouraged as the blocks are painful.

C. Glycerol

    1. Mild agent

    2. Glycerol more specifically affects the damaged myelinated axons implicated in the pathogenesis of trigeminal neuralgia.

    3. It produces perineural damage, myelin disintegration, and Wallerian degeneration.

III. PERIPHERAL NEUROLYTIC BLOCKS

A. Stellate Ganglion Block

    1. In cancer pain following radical neck dissection and postherpetic trigeminal neuralgia

    2. Traditionally, the puncture site is one finger-width lateral and inferior to the cricoid cartilage between the trachea and the carotid sheath. However, CT-guided blockade of the first thoracic ganglion is a better technique.

    3. Needle placement is confirmed using fluoroscopy and a solution of 2.5 ml of 6% phenol, 1 ml of 80 mg methyl prednisolone, and 1.5 ml of 0.5% bupivacaine is injected to provide a final concentration of 3% phenol.

     4. Complications include vascular damage, cerebral infarction, prolonged hoarseness, permanent Horner's syndrome, upper-extremity dysfunction, necrosis, and sloughing of superficial tissues and pneumothorax.

B. Maxillary Nerve Block

     1. Intraoral or extraoral technique can be used.

     2. The entire second division of the trigeminal nerve can be blocked using an intraoral or extraoral approach.

     3. The intraoral technique is less traumatic, has fewer risks, and is less painful to the patient but requires visibility and access to the oral cavity.

     4. For the intraoral approach, the opposite forefinger is placed on the buccal surface of the maxillary molar teeth, moved posteriorly until the bulbous portion is in contact with the posterior surface of the zygomatic process, and a 4-cm, 25-gauge needle is inserted inward, upward, and backward behind the maxillary tuberosity to a depth of 4 cm, taking care to avoid the pterygoid venous plexus.

     5. The entry point of the extraoral approach is at the level of the external auditory meatus, after having identified the coronoid notch of the mandible. An 8-cm, 22-gauge needle is inserted and advanced 1.5 to 2 inches perpendicular to the base of the skull until it strikes the lateral surface of the lateral pterygoid plate; then it is advanced anteriorly until it enters the pterygopalatine fossa no more than 1 cm (Fig. 36-1).

     6. About 2 ml of 2% to 3% phenol should be injected after careful aspiration in the intraoral. Five to 10 ml of phenol will produce profound anesthesia of the midfacial region with the extraoral approach.

C. Infraorbital Nerve Block

     1. Can be done intraorally or extraorally.

     2. Anesthesia of the lower eyelid, lateral nose, and upper lip will be produced by this block.

     3. A volume of 2 ml is sufficient.

     4. Caution is required to prevent injury to the nerve or the accompanying artery.

D. Mandibular Nerve Block

     1. Two intraoral approaches are possible—the closed-mouth and the open-mouth method.

     2. About 2 ml of 2% to 3% phenol may be used.

     3. An extraoral approach is also possible that is similar to the technique for a maxillary nerve block (see Fig. 36-1).

     4. The mandibular division neurolysis by any of these techniques will affect the lower lip and chin as well as the temporomandibular joint, the tongue, and the mandible, gingiva, and teeth.

E. Superficial Cervical Plexus Block

     1. The cervical plexus is formed from C-2, C-3, and C-4 roots.

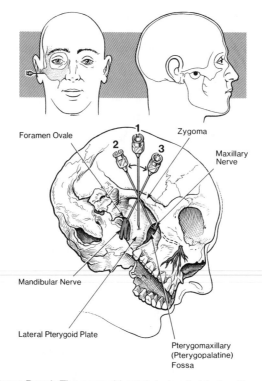

FIG. 36-1. Upper Panel: The coronoid notch is located below the midpoint of the zygoma. A finger is placed at this point and the patient is asked to open his mouth. The condyle of the mandible should be palpable immediately, deep to the fingertip, as the mouth opens. The fingertip should then sink into the coronoid notch as the mouth is closed. Lower Panel: The maxillary and mandibular nerves are approached by way of the coronoid notch below the midpoint of zygoma. **1:** The needle passes through the infratemporal fossa to reach the lateral pterygoid plate. Initial direction of the needle should be medial and slightly anterior. **2:** The needle is then walked anteriorly until it passes into the pterygomaxillary (pterygopalatine) fossa, where the maxillary nerve is blocked. **3:** The needle is then walked from position 1 posteriorly until it passes just posterior to the lateral pterygoid plate to block the mandibular nerve as it emerges from the foramen ovale. The needle point is kept at the same depth as the lateral pterygoid plate to prevent accidental introduction of the needle into the posterior pharynx. (Reprinted with permission from Cousins MJ, Bridenbaugh PO, eds. *Neural Blockade in Clinical Anesthesia and Management of Pain,* 3rd ed. Philadelphia: Lippincott-Raven Publishers; 1997.)

2. The superficial branches pierce the deep cervical fascia just posterior to the sternocleidomastoid muscle.
3. The patient is asked to turn the head away from the side to be blocked.
4. A 22- to 25-gauge needle is inserted subcutaneously just posterior to the sternocleidomastoid and midway between its origin from the clavicle and its insertion on the mastoid.

     5. Five to 10 ml of 2% to 3% phenol is infiltrated subcutaneously after aspiration (Fig. 36-2).

F. Greater Occipital Nerve Blocks

     1. The nerve is best blocked as it crosses the superior nuchal line.

     2. A short 25-gauge needle is inserted near the occipital artery.

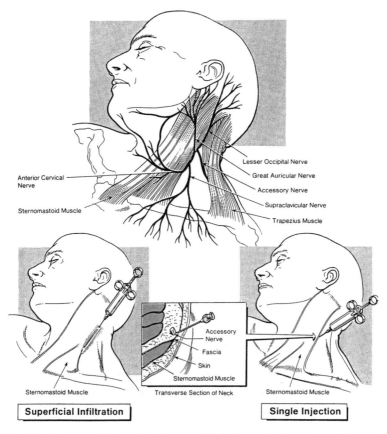

FIG. 36-2. The superficial cervical plexus, which is blocked in the posterior triangle of the neck as it emerges adjacent to the midpoint of the posterior border of the sternomastoid muscle. *Superficial infiltration* is extended along the middle third of the posterior border of the sternomastoid muscle. Note the close relationship of the accessory nerve as it emerges from the posterior border of the sternomastoid muscle at the junction of its middle and upper third (i.e., just above the emerging superficial cervical plexus). *Single injection technique for accessory nerve block.* Note that the accessory nerve lies deep to the deep fascia of the neck and that this needs to be pierced as shown in the "single injection," which is sometimes used as an adjunct to produce muscle paralysis of the trapezius muscle in shoulder operations. Successful block of the superficial cervical plexus results in analgesia corresponding to the C-2, C-3, and C-4 dermatomes shown in Appendix B. (Reprinted with permission from Cousins MJ, Bridenbaugh PO, eds. *Neural Blockade in Clinical Anesthesia and Management of Pain*, 3rd ed. Philadelphia: Lippincott-Raven Publishers; 1997.)

3. Five milliliters of 2% to 3% phenol is infiltrated slowly to produce anesthesia from the occiput to the vertex (Fig. 36-3).

G. Interpleural Block

1. Can be used to treat visceral pain arising anywhere from the head and upper extremity to the abdomen.

2. Especially effective when traditional sympathetic axis blocks are not effective because of tumor involvement or when the anatomy is distorted.

3. The site of somatic nerve block is thought to be the intercostal nerves and sympathetic block by interrupting the sympathetic chain and splanchnic nerves.

4. Technique

a. Position patient with affected site up.

b. Anesthesiologist stands to face the patient's back.

c. The head may be placed up or down 20° to facilitate the spread of phenol by gravity.

d. Skin wheal is raised superiorly to the eighth rib in the seventh intercostal space, 10 cm lateral to midline.

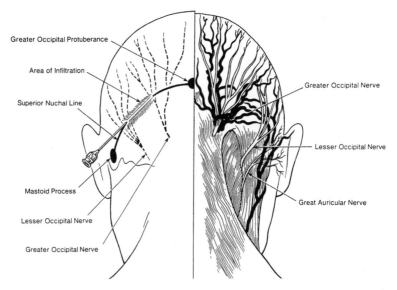

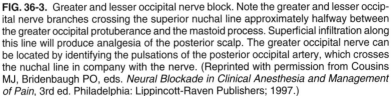

FIG. 36-3. Greater and lesser occipital nerve block. Note the greater and lesser occipital nerve branches crossing the superior nuchal line approximately halfway between the greater occipital protuberance and the mastoid process. Superficial infiltration along this line will produce analgesia of the posterior scalp. The greater occipital nerve can be located by identifying the pulsations of the posterior occipital artery, which crosses the nuchal line in company with the nerve. (Reprinted with permission from Cousins MJ, Bridenbaugh PO, eds. *Neural Blockade in Clinical Anesthesia and Management of Pain*, 3rd ed. Philadelphia: Lippincott-Raven Publishers; 1997.)

     e. Continuous or single-injection technique using epidural needle or short, beveled needle may be done.

     f. Insert syringe filled with 2 ml of saline superiorly to the eighth rib using passive loss of resistance.

     g. Injection will be easy when the needle is in the pleural space.

     h. Thread catheter or give contrast for fluoroscopy and then inject phenol after careful aspiration.

     i. Injection of contrast can determine the volume of anesthetic needed.

5. Contraindications

     a. Relative

          (1) Pleuritis

          (2) Pleural adhesions and fluid

          (3) Bullous emphysema

          (4) Hemothorax

          (5) Pulmonary fibrosis

          (6) Ventilated patients with PEEP

          (7) Recent pulmonary infections

     b. Absolute

          (1) Allergies to local anesthetics

          (2) Extensive infection around insertion site

          (3) Serious bleeding diathesis

6. Complications

     a. Pneumothorax

     b. Systemic local anesthetic toxicity

     c. Pleural effusions and catheter-related problems

H. Celiac Plexus Block (CPB)

1. May be performed in cases of upper abdominal and referred back pain secondary to malignancies involving structures derived from the foregut.

2. The most common indication is pancreatic cancer.

3. Neurolysis of the celiac plexus is effective in treating the visceral component of cancer pain because it contains visceral afferent and efferent fibers and parasympathetic nerve fibers from the upper abdominal viscera.

4. Splanchnic nerve block, retrocrural or "classic" CPB, and anterocrural or "true" CPB method are the most commonly performed techniques.

5. Technique

     a. Anterocrural block

          (1) Patient is placed prone with a pillow under the abdomen to flatten the lumbar lordosis.

          (2) An isosceles triangle is formed by the lower border of the twelfth rib, 7.5 cm from the midline, to the T-12–L-1 vertebral interspace.

      (3) Numbers 20 or 22 Chiba needles are introduced bilaterally to encounter the lower third of the L-1vertebral body and then withdrawn and redirected anteriorly an additional 1.5 to 2 cm.

      (4) After careful aspiration and confirmation of placement of the needle through either fluoroscopy or CT scan, the neurolytic agent is injected, in divided doses of 15 to 20 ml per side (Figs. 36-4 and 36-5). On the right side, a transaortic approach may be used if there is no evidence of peripheral vascular disease.

  b. Retrocrural CPB

      (1) Steps are similar to the anterocrural approach.

      (2) The needles are directed anteriorly to encounter the T-12 vertebral body.

      (3) They are then withdrawn and directed anteromedially an additional 1.5 to 2 cm.

      (4) After careful aspiration and confirmation of placement, the neurolytic agent is injected.

  c. True CPB by anterior approaches

      (1) Can be administered by a surgeon during an operative procedure.

      (2) Ultrasound or computed tomography allow the needle tips to be positioned in the anterocrural location.

      (3) Skinny needles can be passed through the anterior abdominal wall, stomach, intestines, and pancreas.

6. Complications and adverse effects. These are related to the approach utilized:

  a. Anterocrural: If the aorta is pierced (Iscia's technique), aortic dissection or "trash foot" may occur. Diarrhea also appears more frequent with this method also.

  b. Retrocrural: orthostatic hypotension and paraplegia are more frequent with this block. The paraplegia may be related to spasm of the lumbar segmental arteries. Phenol or ethanol toxicity may also occur more frequently with this block due to the volume injected.

  c. Pneumothorax, back pain, and hematuria may occur with any of these approaches.

I. Superior Hypogastric Block

  1. For pelvic visceral pain associated with cancer, the superior hypogastric plexus that contains pelvic afferent and efferent fibers can be blocked.

  2. Patient is placed prone with a pillow under the abdomen to flatten the lumbar lordosis.

  3. The L-4 to L-5 interspace is identified.

  4. Two Chiba needles are introduced 5 to 7 cm laterally and directed anteromedial to the L-5 vertebral body. Eight milliliters of 10% phenol is injected after placement of the needles in the region of

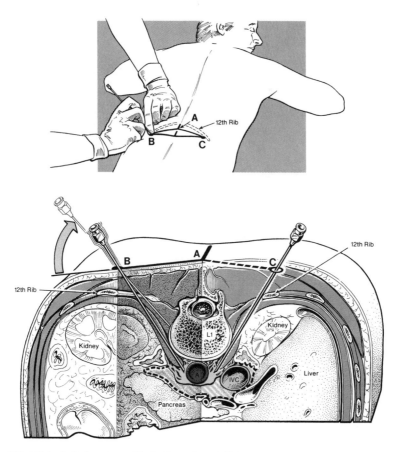

FIG. 36-4. A: Celiac plexus block. Upper Panel: Skin markings, position of patient, and initial insertion of needle. *Note:* Triangle formed by skin marks on lower border of twelfth ribs (**B** and **C**) in line with inferior border of L-1spinous process and joined to inferior border of T12 (**A**). Lower Panel: Needle insertion and deep anatomy. Skin markings and triangle (**A–C**) are still shown. Needle initially is directed in the plane of the line *BA* or *CA*, and at 45° to the horizontal axis of the body, to contact the lateral aspect of the L-1 vertebral body. It passes inferior to the twelfth rib and medial to the kidney. The angle of insertion to the *horizontal axis* of the body is then increased until the needle slips past the lateral aspect of the vertebral body, still in the line *BA* or *CA*, to reach the anterolateral aspect. On the left side, the aortic pulsations will be detected at the needle hub before puncturing the artery. Spread of a test dose of contrast medium (in the approximate area within the *dashed line*) is a valuable guide to correct needle placement prior to diagnostic or therapeutic celiac block. (Reprinted with permission from Cousins MJ, Bridenbaugh PO, eds. *Neural Blockade in Clinical Anesthesia and Management of Pain,* 3rd ed. Philadelphia: Lippincott-Raven Publishers; 1997.)

the hypogastric plexus is confirmed by fluoroscopy and contrast (Figs. 36-6 to 36-9).

J. Ganglion Impar Block

1. May be done through the anococcygeal membrane or through the sacrococcygeal ligament.

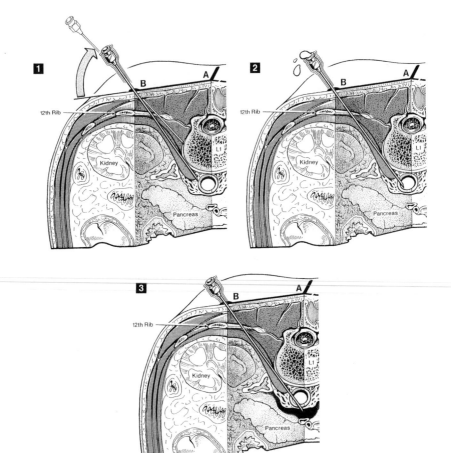

FIG. 36-5. Transaortic coeliac plexus block (see text). (Reprinted with permission from Cousins MJ, Bridenbaugh PO, eds. *Neural Blockade in Clinical Anesthesia and Management of Pain,* 3rd ed. Philadelphia: Lippincott-Raven Publishers; 1997.)

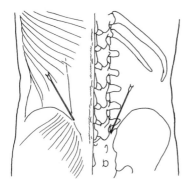

FIG. 36-6. Posterior view illustrating approximate placement of skin wheals, needle trajectory, and relationships among needle path, iliac crests, and fifth lumbar transverse process. (Reprinted with permission from Patt RB, ed. *Cancer Pain.* Philadelphia: JB Lippincott; 1993.)

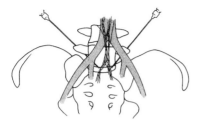

FIG. 36-7. Anterior view of pelvis illustrating location of hypogastric plexus and correct bilateral needle placement. (Reprinted with permission from Patt RB, ed. *Cancer Pain.* Philadelphia: JB Lippincott; 1993.)

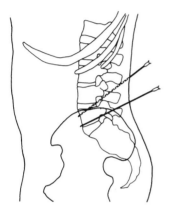

FIG. 36-8. Lateral schematic view of bilateral hypogastric plexus block with paravertebral needles positioned with their tips just anterior to the sacral promontory. (Reprinted with permission from Patt RB, ed. *Cancer Pain.* Philadelphia: JB Lippincott; 1993.)

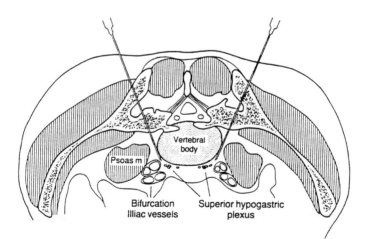

FIG. 36-9. Cross-sectional schematic view illustrating bilateral hypogastric plexus block and needles' relationship to fifth lumbar vertebra, psoas muscle, and iliac vessels. (Reprinted with permission from Patt RB, ed. *Cancer Pain.* Philadelphia: JB Lippincott; 1993.)

    2. Neurolytic agent is deposited in the region of the sacrococcygeal ganglion.

    3. Indications are primarily cancer-related perineal pain (Fig. 36-10).

K. Subarachnoid and Epidural Neurolysis

    1. Effective, inexpensive, quick, with a low incidence of severe morbidity

    2. Use of phenol or ethanol

    3. Indications

        a. Intractable cancer-related pain with failure of antitumor therapy

        b. Failure of more conservative therapies

        c. Limited life expectancy (less than a year)

        d. Somatic pain

        e. Localized pain

        f. Pain responding to local anesthetic blockade

    4. Contraindications

        a. Patient intolerance of positioning

        b. Patient refusal

        c. Pain not responding to local anesthetic blockade

        d. Deafferentation pain

        e. Diffuse pain that is poorly localized

        f. Coagulopathy

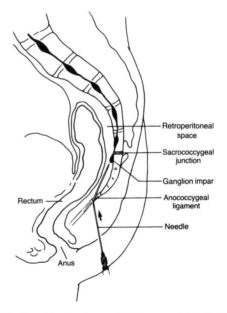

FIG. 36-10. Lateral schematic view demonstrating correct needle placement for blockade of ganglion impar, and anatomic relations. (Reprinted with permission from Patt RB, ed. *Cancer Pain.* Philadelphia: JB Lippincott; 1993.)

5. The nerve roots that innervate the painful area must be identified from dermatomal diagrams.
6. Technique
   a. Similar to standard spinal or epidural techniques
   b. Use of sedation and contrast with fluoroscopy
   c. Phenol or ethanol
   d. The patient is positioned in the normal lateral decubitus with the painful side down.
   e. The spinal needle is directed into the appropriate interspace with the bevel downward.
   f. Care should be taken to avoid injury to the spinal cord.
7. Epidural versus spinal neurolysis
   a. Risk of postdural puncture headache is less.
   b. A broader area can be treated with less incidence of severe complications.
   c. Incremental injections through indwelling catheters can provide a more controlled neurolysis.
   d. Complications of both include the following:
      (1) Inadequate relief of pain
      (2) Temporary or permanent deficits
      (3) Bladder or bowel dysfunction
      (4) Postdural puncture headache
      (5) Pain at the insertion site
      (6) Infection
      (7) Meningitis and neuritis
      (8) Potential anterior and posterior spinal artery thrombosis

IV. NEUROSURGICAL INTERVENTIONS
   A. Pitfalls of Analgesic Neurosurgery
      1. Inadequate or temporary pain relief
      2. Development of neuritis and central dysesthetic pain
      3. Incidental damage to nontargeted structures resulting in neurologic deficit
      4. Likelihood of specific dysfunction and the consequences to the patient must be balanced against the degree of potential benefit.
      5. Multidisciplinary approach is required.
      6. Patient selection and patient expectations are important.
   B. Indications
      1. Intractable cancer-related pain
      2. Failure of antitumor therapy
      3. Failure of more conservative therapies
      4. Longer life expectancy
      5. Pain responding to local anesthetic blockade

C. Current Techniques
1. Peripheral neurectomy—usually avoided due to potential for neuroma formation, incomplete pain relief, motor deficit, and deafferentation pain
2. Sympathectomy. Pain in the lower extremities may be treated successfully.
3. Dorsal rhizotomy
    a. It involves laminectomy and surgical resection of the posterior spinal nerves.
    b. It has a limited role.
    c. Tumor extension beyond the area of denervation limits pain relief.
    d. Possible increase in deficit and disability
    e. High incidence of severe deafferentation pain
    f. More selective rhizotomies also possible
4. Cordotomy
    a. May be accomplished by percutaneously inserted catheters for delivering electric current or thermocoagulation.
    b. Open cordotomy involves cervical or thoracic laminectomy and near complete section of the anterolateral quadrant.
    c. Rarely used because it may cause unintentional destruction of neighboring structures and ataxia, respiratory difficulty, motor paresis, impaired bladder function, and ipsilateral analgesia.
    d. Accurate prognostic neural blockade is impossible.
    e. Percutaneous cervical cordotomy is less risky if the patient's medical condition is poor. Some uncontrolled reports have described good results.
5. Commissural myelotomy
    a. Midline section of the spinal cord intended to interrupt afferent spinothalamic pain fibers
    b. Stereotactic procedure less risky
    c. Useful for pelvic pain
    d. Cingulotomy, which is a stereotactic lesion placed in the cingula
    e. Associated with high psychologic morbidity
6. Pituitary ablation
    a. For intractable bilateral pain secondary to widespread bony metastases when the life expectancy is moderate.
    b. Interference with the endogenous opiate system plays a role in pain relief.
    c. Bone metastases due to prostate or breast cancer respond most favorably.
7. Stimulation techniques
    a. Less destructive
    b. Accomplished with minimal anesthesia and surgical stress

     c. Patient and physician controlled

     d. Dorsal column stimulation useful if the pain is primarily neuropathic

     e. Deep-brain stimulation

     f. Periaqueductal gray matter stimulation

       (1) Associated with the release of endorphins into the third ventricle

       (2) Activates a descending pain inhibitory system originating in the central brain stem and terminating in the substantia gelatinosa

       (3) Analgesia is reversed by naloxone.

       (4) Tolerance can occur with chronic stimulation.

       (5) Analgesia is widespread and bilateral.

       (6) Attractive for pain that crosses the midline and involving the head, neck, or upper extremities.

     g. Thalamic stimulation

       (1) Endorphins are not released.

       (2) Pain relief is strictly contralateral.

       (3) Not reversed with naloxone

8. Techniques specific for malignancy of head and neck

     a. Cervical spine surgery

     b. Trigeminal neurolysis

     c. Cranial nerve rhizotomy or rhizolysis

     d. Medullary tractotomy

     e. Microvascular decompression

PART VI

Techniques

The Pain Clinic Manual, Second Edition,
edited by Stephen E. Abram and J. David Haddox.
Lippincott Williams & Wilkins,
Philadelphia, © 2000

37

Epidural Steroid Injections

Stephen E. Abram

*S. E. Abram: Department of Anesthesiology and Critical Care Medicine,
University of New Mexico, Health Sciences Center—School of Medicine,
Albuquerque, New Mexico 87131.*

Epidural steroid injections are effective for patients with lumbar and cervical radiculopathy. Although the risk of serious complications is low, there is some risk of epidural bleeding, which is higher in patients with intrinsic or drug-associated coagulopathy. Epidural abscess is somewhat more likely among diabetic patients. There may be some risk of aseptic meningitis or arachnoiditis with intrathecal administration of steroids, so it is probably safer to postpone the procedure in the event of an accidental dural puncture. Diabetics are likely to exhibit increased blood sugars and higher insulin needs for at least a few days after injection of deposteroids, and some patients will exhibit cushingoid side effects or adrenal suppression in the postinjection period.

I. PATIENT SELECTION
  A. Inclusion Criteria
    The following criteria are associated with fairly good treatment outcomes. This treatment is not contraindicated for patients who do not meet these criteria, but treatment success is likely to be lower for such patients.
    1. Unilateral radicular pain
      a. Evidence of radiculopathy on the basis of physical exam
      b. EMG evidence of radiculopathy
      c. CT or MRI evidence of disc protrusion at a site compatible with symptoms
        (1) There is some controversy about the need for preinjection imaging. Many physicians feel that history and physical exam evidence of radiculopathy is sufficient. Imaging studies will rule out rare but potentially risky problems (e.g., spinal tumor or abscess).
    2. Relatively recent onset (up to 12 months)
    3. No previous spine surgery
    4. Nonsmoker (treatment success for smokers is significantly lower)

B. Exclusion Criteria
   1. Coagulopathy
   2. Infections, either local or systemic
   3. History of untreated tuberculosis
   4. History of steroid-induced psychosis
   5. Serious substance abuse problem
   6. Multiple spine surgeries
   7. Spinal tumor
      a. Although there is a risk of causing intraspinal bleeding after epi-
         dural needle placement in patients with intraspinal tumors, there is
         some anecdotal evidence for symptomatic improvement following
         epidural steroid injections in patients with epidural metastatic dis-
         ease who have radicular pain. The risk/benefit data for such treat-
         ment are unavailable.

II. PROCEDURE
   A. Drug Selection
      1. The preparations commonly used for epidural steroid injections are
         both suspensions of insoluble acetates (Table 37-1).
         a. Methylprednisolone acetate (Depo Medrol, Upjohn, Kalamazoo,
            MI)—usual dose: 80 mg

TABLE 37-1. *Commercial preparations of methylprednisolone*
acetate and triamcinolone diacetate

Depo-Medrol multidose vials (Upjohn, Kalamazoo, MI)			
Methylprednisolone acetate	20 mg	40 mg	80 mg
Polyethylene glycol 3350	29.5 mg	29.1 mg	28.2 mg
Polysorbate 80	1.97 mg	1.94 mg	1.88 mg
Monobasic sodium phosphate	6.9 mg	6.8 mg	6.59 mg
Dibasic sodium phosphate USP	1.44 mg	1.42 mg	1.37 mg
Benzyl alcohol	9.3 mg	9.16 mg	8.88 mg
NaCl to adjust tonicity			
Depo-Medrol single-dose vials (Upjohn, Kalamazoo, MI)			
Methylprednisolone acetate	40 mg	80 mg	
Polyethylene glycol 3350	29 mg	28 mg	
Myristyl-gamma-picolinium chloride	0.195 mg	0.189 mg	
NaCl to adjust tonicity			
Aristocort Intralesional (Fujisawa USA, Deerfield, IL)			
Triamcinolone diacetate	25 mg		
Polyethylene glycol 3350	30 mg		
Polysorbate 80	2 mg		
Benzyl alcohol	9 mg		
NaCl	8.5 mg		

Reprinted with permission from: Abram SE. Epidural steroid injections for the treatment of lumbosacral radiculopathy. *J Back Musculoskel Rehab* 1997;8:135–149.

TABLE 37-2. *Algorithm for treatment of sciatica with epidural steroid injections*

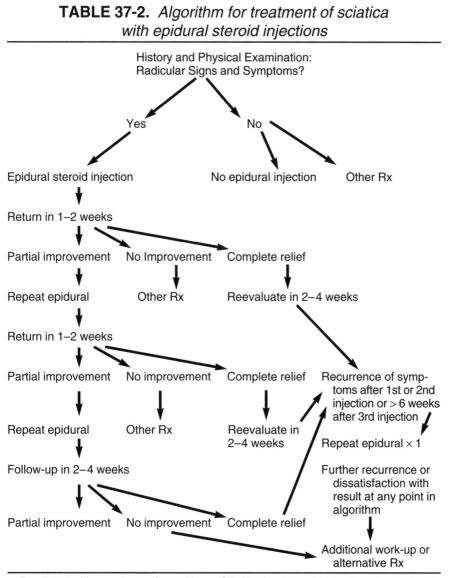

Reprinted with permission from: Abram SE. Epidural steroid injections for the treatment of lumbosacral radiculopathy. *J Back Musculoskel Rehab* 1997;8:135–149.

    b. Triamcinolone diacetate Aristocort Intralesional, (Fujisawa USA, Deerfield, IL)—usual dose: 50 mg

2. Soluble steroid preparations are avoided, as their effects are transient, and they have produced seizures when injected spinally in animals.

3. A short-acting local anesthetic (e.g., 3 to 5 ml, 1% lidocaine) is often added to confirm that the affected nerve root has been contacted by the drug, as evidenced by relief of the pain within 10 to 15 minutes.

B. Site of Injection
   1. Injection should be as close as possible to the site of nerve root irritation (e.g., L-4–5 for L-4 radiculopathy).
   2. Caudal injection (often with 5 to 10 ml added saline) may be effective for S-1 radiculopathy.
   3. For cervical radiculopathy, C-6–7 or C-7–T-1 is usually chosen, as at these sites the procedure is technically easier to perform than at higher levels.

C. Immediate Follow-up
   1. Assess effect of block.
      a. Degree of pain relief
      b. Change in sensation
      c. Presence of motor deficit
   2. Ensure that patient is not driving and has an adult escort.
   3. Inform patient of the possibility of transient exacerbation of pain.
   4. Arrange follow-up visits.
   5. Algorithm for continued treatment (Table 37-2).

RECOMMENDED READING

Abram SE, O'Connor TC. Complications associated with epidural steroid injections. *Regional Anesth* 1996;21:149–162.

Abram SE. Epidural steroid injections for the treatment of lumbosacral radiculopathy. *J Back Musculoskel Rehabil* 1997;8:135–149.

Hopwood MB, Abram SE. Factors associated with failure of epidural steroids. *Reg Anesth* 1993; 18:238–243.

Racz GB, Holubec JT. Lysis of adhesions in the epidural space. In: Racz GB, ed. *Techniques of Neurolysis.* Boston: Kluwer; 1989:133–144.

Rowlingson JC. Epidural steroids. Do they have a place in pain management? *Am Pain Soc J* 1994;3:20–27.

The Pain Clinic Manual, Second Edition,
edited by Stephen E. Abram and J. David Haddox.
Lippincott Williams & Wilkins,
Philadelphia, © 2000

38

Sympathetic Blocks

Stephen E. Abram

*S. E. Abram: Department of Anesthesiology and Critical Care Medicine,
University of New Mexico, Health Sciences Center—School of Medicine,
Albuquerque, New Mexico 87131.*

I. CERVICOTHORACIC SYMPATHETIC BLOCK (STELLATE GANGLION BLOCK)

The two common approaches involve injection of the cervical sympathetic chain at either the C-6 or C-7 levels. With the C-6 approach, there is less likelihood of injecting a nerve root sheath or the vertebral artery, but the needle tip lies closer to the stellate ganglion and, theoretically, there is a greater likelihood of complete sympathetic denervation of the upper limb.

With both approaches the patient is placed supine, head slightly extended, without a pillow. A 10-ml ring control syringe with a 22-gauge 1.5-inch needle is used if the block is done without assistance. Alternatively, the needle can be used with an extension set (immobile needle technique), the injection being done by an assistant.

We generally recommend the use of 1% lidocaine. Longer-acting drugs such as bupivacaine or ropivacaine may be used, but the adverse effects of unintended effects (subarachnoid or epidural spread, recurrent laryngeal block, phrenic block) will be prolonged.

The patient is placed in the sitting or semisitting position after the block to facilitate the caudal spread of the drug.

A. C-6 Paratracheal Approach

Refer to Figs. 38-1 and 38-2.

1. The C-6 anterior tubercle is palpated just lateral to the cricoid cartilage.
2. The carotid artery is retracted laterally using the second and third fingers of the nondominant hand.
3. With the two fingers slightly apart, the tip of the anterior tubercle can usually be felt between the fingertips.
4. The needle is advanced straight downward until the anterior tubercle is contacted.
5. The syringe is aspirated and, if aspiration is negative, 1 ml local anesthetic is injected. If there is little resistance to injection, the remaining

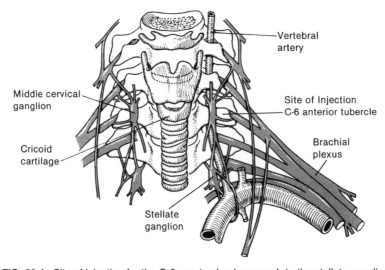

FIG. 38-1. Site of injection for the C-6 paratracheal approach to the stellate ganglion block. Note the relationship of the C-6 anterior tubercle to the cricoid cartilage. The vertebral artery passes anterior to the C-7 transverse process and behind the C-6 anterior tubercle. The lateral portion of the C-7 transverse process lies deep to the prevertebral fascia, adjacent to the C-7 nerve root and the dome of the pleura. (Reprinted with permission from Benumof JL, ed. *Clinical Procedures in Anesthesia and Intensive Care.* Philadelphia: JB Lippincott; 1992.)

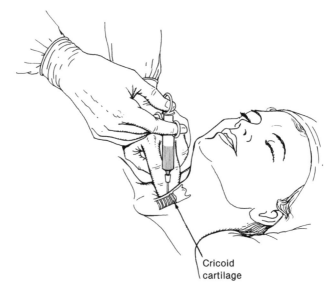

FIG. 38-2. Technique for the C-6 paratracheal approach to stellate ganglion block. The fingertips of the palpating hand straddle the tip of the C-6 anterior tubercle while retracting the carotid sheath laterally. The needle is introduced directly downward onto the tip of the anterior tubercle. (Reprinted with permission from Benumof JL, ed. *Clinical Procedures in Anesthesia and Intensive Care.* Philadelphia: JB Lippincott; 1992.)

10 to 15 ml local anesthetic is injected slowly, with frequent aspiration. If there is some resistance to injection, the needle is withdrawn slightly and aspiration and injection are carried out.

6. Horner's syndrome should become evident within 3 minutes, and the skin temperature on the volar surface of the hand should begin to rise within 5 minutes. Complete sympathetic block to the hand is generally associated with a rise in temperature to 34° to 35°C.

B. C-7 Paratracheal Approach

1. The sternal notch is identified, and a point 3 cm (two finger-breadths) lateral and 3 cm superior to that point is marked.

2. The carotid artery is retracted laterally using the second and third fingers of the nondominant hand.

3. The needle is directed downward and slightly inward until the C-7 transverse process is contacted. Since this transverse process has no anterior tubercle, the needle will be slightly deeper than is optimal, and should be withdrawn about 0.5 cm.

4. The syringe is aspirated and, if aspiration is negative, 1 ml local anesthetic is injected. If there is little resistance to injection, the remaining 10 to 15 ml local anesthetic is injected slowly, with frequent aspiration. If there is some resistance to injection, the needle is withdrawn slightly and aspiration and injection are carried out.

5. Autonomic changes should be the same as those described earlier.

C. Complications

1. Vertebral artery injection
   a. May produce seizures with very small amounts of local anesthetic

2. Subarachnoid block
   a. Caused by injection into a nerve root sleeve

3. Pneumothorax
   a. More common with C-7 approach

4. Phrenic nerve block
   a. Not serious except in patients with respiratory compromise
   b. Produces subjective shortness of breath

5. Recurrent laryngeal nerve block
   a. Produces transient hoarseness
   b. Patients should not eat or drink until symptoms resolve.

II. LUMBAR SYMPATHETIC BLOCK

A. Technique (Figs. 38-3–38-5)

Although this procedure can be done "blind," it is preferable to use a C-arm image intensifier to locate the target site and to confirm needle position. The final needle position should be the anterolateral surface of the L-2 vertebral body, as near the lower border of the vertebral body as possible. The patient is placed in the prone position with a small pillow under the hips and abdomen.

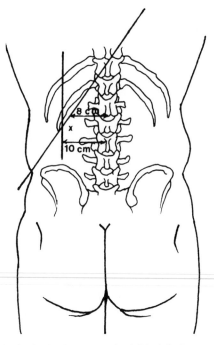

FIG. 38-3. Landmarks for the lumbar sympathetic block (L-2 paravertebral approach).

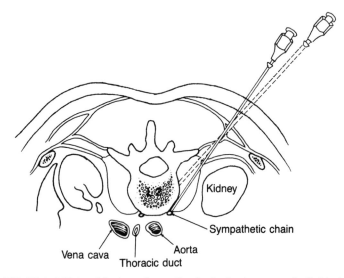

FIG. 38-4. Initial and final needle position for the lumbar sympathetic block.

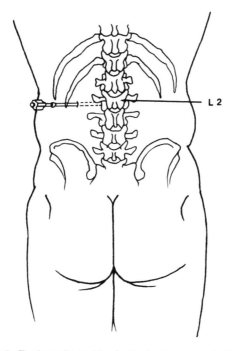

FIG. 38-5. Final needle position for the lumbar sympathetic block.

1. The level of the L-2 vertebral body can be estimated by drawing a vertical line 10 cm from the midline and another line along the lower border of the first rib. Where these lines intersect is generally at the midpoint of the L-2 vertebra.
2. Using the image intensifier, a point is marked 8 cm from the midline, at the level of the lower border of the L-2 body.
3. A skin wheal is raised at this site, and the underlying muscle is infiltrated with 1% lidocaine.
4. A 22-gauge 5-inch (6-inch for heavy patients) needle is advanced through the skin wheal at an angle of about 45°, staying in the coronal plane. The lower portion of the vertebral body is usually contracted at a depth of 3 to 4 inches. Fluoroscopy is used to document the course of the needle. If no contact is made at a depth of 4 to 4.5 inches, the needle is repositioned at a slightly shallower angle.
5. After bony contact is made and fluoroscopy confirms the needle is at the lower one-third of L-2, the needle angle is increased and the needle is redirected until it is tangential to the body and may be advanced anteriorly.
6. Using a lateral view, the needle is advanced until it is even with the anterior border of the body.

7. Following aspiration for blood, 5 ml 1% lidocaine is injected. If there is resistance to injection, the needle is advanced slightly and aspiration is repeated.

8. Skin temperature of the plantar surface of the foot should begin to rise within 3 minutes. Once the temperature has gone up several degrees, a long-acting local anesthetic may be added. Five to 7 ml is generally sufficient. Final skin temperature should be 34° to 35°C.

B. Complications
   1. Intravascular injection
      a. Seizures from local anesthetic toxicity
      b. Possibly significant bleeding in anticoagulated patients
   2. Subarachnoid block
      a. Possible from shallow needle angle with entry into neural foramen
      b. Rare when fluoroscopy is used
   3. Renal or ureteral injury
      a. Small-gauge needle unlikely to cause significant harm

The Pain Clinic Manual, Second Edition,
edited by Stephen E. Abram and J. David Haddox.
Lippincott Williams & Wilkins,
Philadelphia, © 2000

39

Peripheral Nerve Blocks

John W. Luckwitz

J. W. Luckwitz: Mountain West Anesthesia, Salt Lake City, Utah 84117.

Peripheral nerve blocks are used in both the acute pain and chronic pain setting. For instance, intercostal nerve blocks may be used for pain relief following rib fracture or for postherpetic neuralgia. As with all nerve blocks, the key to success involves careful attention to anatomy and meticulous technique.

I. INTERCOSTAL NERVE BLOCK
  A. Anatomy
     See Fig. 39-1.
     1. Intercostal nerves are comprised of primary rami of T-1 through T-11, whereas the subcostal nerve is composed of T-12.
     2. Each intercostal nerve consists of four main branches.
        a. Gray rami communicans
        b. Posterior cutaneous branch (supplies innervation to skin and paravertebral muscles)
        c. Lateral cutaneous division (supplies innervation to skin of much of chest and abdominal wall). This branch arises just anterior to mid-axillary line.
        d. Anterior cutaneous branch
     3. The intercostal nerve lies inferior to the intercostal artery and vein in the costal groove of the rib.
     4. The costal groove is broadest and deepest at the angle of the rib (6–8 cm lateral to the spinous processes).
  B. Indications
     1. Acute herpes zoster of the thoracic region
     2. Differentiating visceral versus abdominal or thoracic wall pain
     3. Pain relief from chest wall trauma, especially rib fracture
     4. Cancer pain
  C. Technique
     See Fig. 39-2.

403

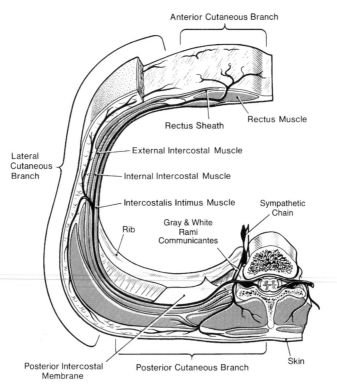

FIG. 39-1. An intercostal nerve and its branches. Approximate area of skin supplied by branches is also shown. There is evidence, however, that local anesthetic injected near the lateral cutaneous branch diffuses posteriorly to reach the posterior cutaneous branch. Note also (**i**) the spinal nerves and dorsal root ganglia in the region of intervertebral foramen, with risk of perineural spread into spinal fluid after intraneural injection in this region; (**ii**) direct injection into an intervertebral foramen may reach spinal fluid by means of a dural cuff; (**iii**) local anesthetic may gain access to epidural space by diffusing into an intervertebral foramen; and (**iv**) close to the midline the intercostal nerve lies directly on the posterior intercostal membrane and pleura. (**v**) Paravertebrally, solution may diffuse to rami communicantes and sympathetic chain. (Reprinted with permission from Cousins MJ, Bridenbaugh PO, eds. *Neural Blockade in Clinical Anesthesia and Management of Pain,* 3rd ed. Philadelphia: Lippincott-Raven Publishers; 1997.)

1. Although intercostal blocks can be performed at several different sites, the most common site is at the angle of the rib.
2. The patient is placed in either a prone or lateral position.
3. Using aseptic technique, a skin wheal is raised at the site of injection.
4. The index finger of the nondominant hand is placed directly over the rib while retracting the overlying skin superiorly.
5. A 22-gauge or 23-gauge, 3- to 4-cm needle is then introduced just off the tip of the palpating index finger to contact the lower margin of the rib.

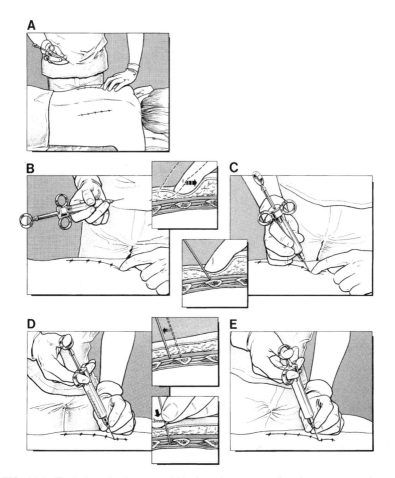

FIG. 39-2. Technique for intercostal block and corresponding deep anatomy (see text). **A:** Skin markings at lateral edge of sacrospinalis muscle (6 to 8 cm from midline). Note the medial curve of the line superiorly to avoid the scapulae. Ribs and interspaces are palpated. The lowest (most inferior) intercostal nerve is blocked first because the lower ribs are easy to palpate. (In **A—E** the diagrams show the second to last intercostal nerves to be blocked in this patient.) **B:** Skin at lower edge of rib retracted superiorly into rib. **C:** Needle inserted onto rib (see also inset). Note finger palpating rib still in place and hand holding syringe firmly braced against back. **D:** The position of the hands now changes. Note left hand now rests on back and holds the needle as it is walked off the inferior edge of the rib and advanced 3 mm. Right hand is free to aspirate and inject. **E:** Injection completed with left hand still firmly against patient's back and controlling the needle. (Reprinted with permission from Cousins MJ, Bridenbaugh PO, eds. *Neural Blockade in Clinical Anesthesia and Management of Pain,* 3rd ed. Philadelphia: Lippincott-Raven Publishers; 1997.)

6. The needle is then walked caudally until the needle just slips under the rib.
7. The needle is then advanced 2 to 3 mm under the rib in a slightly cephalad direction. Care must be taken not to advance the needle more than 3 mm.
8. After negative aspiration, 3 ml of local anesthetic is injected.

D. Complications
1. Pneumothorax
2. Intravascular injection leading to systemic toxicity
3. Subarachnoid block—the dura occasionally extends out a variable distance along the intercostal nerve.

II. LATERAL FEMORAL CUTANEOUS NERVE BLOCK

A. Anatomy
1. Arises from L-2 and L-3 nerve roots at the lateral border of psoas muscle.
2. After coursing along the medial border of the anterior superior iliac spine (ASIS), it pierces the fascia lata 1.5 to 2 cm below the inguinal ligament.
3. Provides sensory innervation to the lateral thigh.
4. No motor innervation

B. Indications
1. Meralgia paresthetica (lateral femoral cutaneous neuropathy)
2. May be caused by obesity or ongoing nerve trauma such as might be caused by wearing a heavy belt low on the hip; or may be idiopathic.

C. Technique
See Fig. 39-3.
1. After placing the patient supine, a skin wheal is raised one finger-breadth (2 to 3 cm) inferior and medial to the anterior superior iliac spine (ASIS).
2. A 22-gauge, 1.5-inch needle is introduced superolaterally through the skin wheal toward the ASIS.
3. A double loss of resistance is felt as the needle passes through the external oblique aponeurosis and the internal oblique muscle.
4. The needle may be passed directly posteriorly through the fascia lata. Drug is deposited both deep and superficial to the fascia.
5. Alternatively, the nerve may be blocked by injecting just medial to the ASIS, again passing through the external and internal oblique.
6. If a paresthesia is elicited, the entire amount of anesthetic is deposited at that site. Otherwise, the drug is injected as the needle is fanned medially and laterally from the initial injection site.
7. A total of 5 to 10 ml of local anesthetic is injected.

D. Complications
1. Because the lateral femoral cutaneous nerve is purely sensory and not located near any major vascular structures, complications are rare.

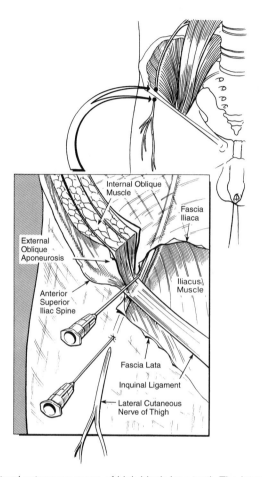

FIG. 39-3. Lateral cutaneous nerve of high block (see text). The lateral cutaneous nerve of the thigh passes inferiorly on iliacus muscle covered by iliacus fascia. Just medial to the anterior superior iliac spine it turns anteriorly to pass just below the inguinal ligament and runs deep to the fascia lata until it emerges subcutaneously. The lateral cutaneous nerve can be blocked (**1**) just medial to the anterior superior iliac spine, when loss of resistance is felt on passing through the external oblique aponeurosis and on emerging through the internal oblique muscle or (**2**) 1 to 2 cm below the anterior superior iliac spine by injecting deep to fascia lata. (Reprinted with permission from Cousins MJ, Bridenbaugh PO, eds. *Neural Blockade in Clinical Anesthesia and Management of Pain,* 3rd ed. Philadelphia: Lippincott-Raven Publishers; 1997.)

2. Rarely, leg weakness may occur as a result of partial femoral nerve blockade.

III. ILIOINGUINAL AND ILIOHYPOGASTRIC NERVE BLOCK
   A. Anatomy
      1. Originates from L-1.

2. Ilioinguinal nerve initially lies between the transversus abdominus and the internal oblique muscle before penetrating the internal oblique muscle medial to the anterior superior iliac spine (ASIS).

3. Iliohypogastric nerve lies slightly superior and superficial to the ilioinguinal nerve.

B. Indications

1. This block may be used intraoperatively or postoperatively following herniorraphy.

2. Ilioinguinal neuralgia may result as a complication of surgical trauma from herniorraphy or from spread of neurolytic agent into psoas muscle during neurolytic celiac plexus blockade.

C. Technique

See Fig. 39-4.

1. Using sterile technique with the patient in the supine neutral position, a 22-gauge, 8-cm, short, beveled needle is inserted 3 cm inferior and medial to the ASIS.

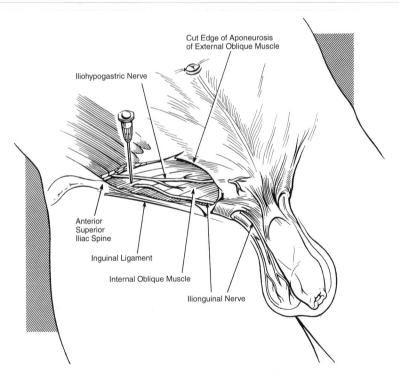

Cut Edge of Aponeurosis of External Oblique Muscle

Iliohypogastric Nerve

Anterior Superior Iliac Spine

Inguinal Ligament

Internal Oblique Muscle

Ilionguinal Nerve

FIG. 39-4. Ilioinguinal and iliohypogastric nerve block (see text). The ilioinguinal nerve emerges through the internal oblique muscle about 1 to 2 cm medial to the anterior superior iliac spine. It lies deep to the external oblique aponeurosis, which can be felt when a short, beveled needle is passed through it. (Reprinted with permission from Cousins MJ, Bridenbaugh PO, eds. *Neural Blockade in Clinical Anesthesia and Management of Pain,* 3rd ed. Philadelphia: Lippincott-Raven Publishers; 1997.)

2. The needle is inserted in a superior and medial direction to contact the inner surface of the ilium.
3. Ten milliliters of local anesthetic is then injected as the needle is withdrawn.
4. A subcutaneous field block may also be added connecting the skin wheal to the umbilicus.

D. Complications

This is a superficial nerve block with no major common complications.

The Pain Clinic Manual, Second Edition,
edited by Stephen E. Abram and J. David Haddox.
Lippincott Williams & Wilkins,
Philadelphia, © 2000

40

Head and Neck Blocks

John W. Luckwitz

J. W. Luckwitz: Mountain West Anesthesia, Salt Lake City, Utah 84117.

Although head and neck blocks are most frequently used for surgical anesthesia, they are also commonly used in the diagnosis and treatment of chronic and cancer pain states. Although technically a head and neck block, stellate ganglion blockade is used in the diagnosis and treatment of upper-extremity pain states and therefore is discussed in Chapter 38.

I. ANATOMY
   A. Cutaneous sensory innervation to face, head, and neck is supplied by the trigeminal nerve and cervical plexus.
      1. Forehead, eyebrows, upper eyelids, and nose are supplied by the ophthalmic division of the trigeminal nerve (V1 or ophthalmic nerve).
      2. Lower eyelid, cheek, and upper lip are supplied by the second division of the trigeminal nerve (V-2 or maxillary nerve).
      3. Lower lip, chin, mandibular, and temporal region are supplied by the third division of the trigeminal nerve (V-3 or mandibular nerve).
   B. Gasserian (trigeminal) ganglion—located in the middle cranial fossa and gives off V-1–3
   C. Cervical plexus consists of the anterior primary rami of C-2–4 that emerge as lesser occipital nerve, great auricular nerve, the anterior cutaneous nerve of the neck, and the supraclavicular nerves.
      1. The skin over the posterior extensor muscles and occiput is supplied by the posterior rami of C-2–4, which comprise the greater occipital nerve.
      2. Pharynx and larynx are supplied by the glossopharyngeal and vagus nerves.
II. INDICATIONS AND TECHNIQUES
   A. Gasserian Ganglion
      See Fig. 40-1.

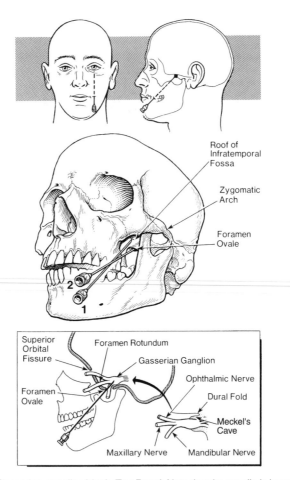

FIG. 40-1. Gasserian ganglion block. Top Panel: Note that the needle is inserted in the cheek about 1 cm posterior to the angle of the mouth as shown and directed toward the pupil in the anterior view and the midpoint of the zygoma in the lateral view. In patients with teeth, needle insertion in the cheek is superficial to the teeth of the upper jaw. In edentulous patients this may lie a variable distance between the angle of the mouth and a line midway between upper lip and nose. A palpating finger in the mouth helps to prevent needle penetration into the mouth. Middle Panel: As the needle is advanced into the infratemporal fossa, it will usually strike the roof of the infratemporal fossa initially (**1**); this is the correct depth to seek the foramen ovale. The needle is then directed slightly posteriorly (**2**) to obtain a mandibular nerve (V-3) paresthesia. Lower Panel: The needle can then be advanced through the foramen ovale into the middle cranial fossa, where it will be adjacent to the gasserian ganglion, as shown. Note the relationships of the dural fold and Meckel's cave, containing cerebrospinal fluid. A needle advanced too far through the foramen ovale can enter the Meckel's cave, and subsequent injections could enter the cranial CSF and produce total spinal anesthesia. (Reprinted with permission from Cousins MJ, Bridenbaugh PO, eds. *Neural Blockade in Clinical Anesthesia and Management of Pain.* Philadelphia: Lippincott-Raven Publishers; 1997.)

1. Technique
    a. An 8- to 10-cm, 22-gauge needle is introduced 2 cm lateral to the angle of the mouth and directed medial and cephalad through the cheek to the midpoint of the zygomatic arch in the lateral plane and the pupil in the frontal plane.
    b. A guiding finger should be placed in the oral cavity to ensure that the needle does not enter the mouth.
    c. The needle is then manipulated until it enters the foramen ovale and is advanced not more than 1 cm until the appropriate paresthesia is obtained.
    d. Fluoroscopic or CT guidance should be utilized to facilitate needle placement.
    e. Very small quantities of local anesthetic (1 ml 1% lidocaine or neurolytic agent) is then injected in 0.25 ml aliquots.
2. Indications
    a. Trigeminal neuralgia
    b. Cancer pain, although this is being replaced by radiofrequency neuroablation
B. Maxillary Nerve
  See Fig. 40-2.
    1. Technique
        a. Patient is placed in supine position with the head rotated to the contralateral side to be blocked.
        b. The mandibular notch is identified by having the patient open and close his mouth.
        c. An 8-cm, 22-gauge needle is passed through the mandibular notch in a slightly cephalad and medial direction until the needle contacts the lateral pterygoid plate at a depth of approximately 5 cm.
        d. The needle is then walked off into the pterygopalatine fossa.
        e. Then 5 ml of local anesthetic is injected in small incremental doses.
    2. Indications
        a. Evaluation of facial neuralgias
    3. Complications
        a. Periorbital hematoma
        b. Temporary blindness from local anesthetic blockade of the optic nerve
        c. Intrathecal injection
C. Mandibular nerve
  See Fig. 40-2.
    1. Technique
        a. Exactly the same approach as that for maxillary nerve (i.e., the needle is introduced through the mandibular notch until the lateral

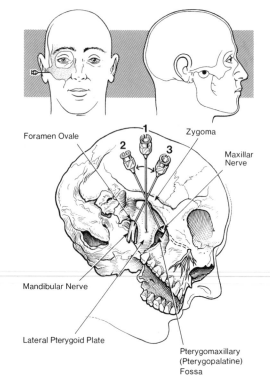

Foramen Ovale

Zygoma

Maxillar Nerve

Mandibular Nerve

Lateral Pterygoid Plate

Pterygomaxillary (Pterygopalatine) Fossa

FIG. 40-2. Upper Panel: The coronoid notch is located below the midpoint of the zygoma. A finger is placed at this point and the patient asked to open his mouth. The condyle of the mandible should be palpable immediately, deep to the fingertip, as the mouth opens. The fingertip should then sink into the coronoid notch as the mouth is closed. Lower Panel: The maxillary and mandibular nerves are approached by way of the coronoid notch below the midpoint of zygoma. **1:** The needle passes through the infratemporal fossa to reach the lateral pterygoid plate. Initial direction of the needle should be medial and slightly anterior. **2:** The needle is then walked anteriorly until it passes into the pterygomaxillary (pterygopalatine) fossa, where the maxillary nerve is blocked. **3:** The needle is then walked from position 1 posteriorly until it passes just posterior to the lateral pterygoid plate to block the mandibular nerve as it emerges from the foramen ovale. The needle point is kept at the same depth as the lateral pterygoid plate to prevent accidental introduction of the needle into the posterior pharynx. (Reprinted with permission from Cousins MJ, Bridenbaugh PO, eds. *Neural Blockade in Clinical Anesthesia and Management of Pain.* Philadelphia: Lippincott-Raven Publishers; 1997.)

pterygoid plate is contacted) except the needle is walked off posteriorly until a V-3 paresthesia is obtained.

   2. Indications

      a. Carcinoma of tongue, lower jaw, or base of mouth

      b. Postherpetic neuralgia

   D. Supraorbital nerve (see Fig. 40-3)

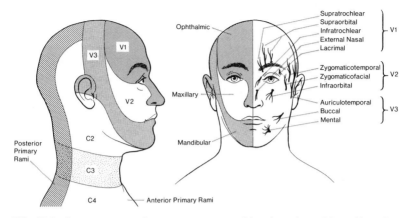

FIG. 40-3. Dermatomes and cutaneous nerves of head, neck, and face. Note that the supraorbital, infraorbital, and mental nerves all lie in the same vertical plane as the pupil, with the eye looking straight forward. The external nasal area is innervated by infratrochlear and external nasal (from anterior ethmoidal n.) branches of V-1 and the infraorbital branch of V-2. The internal nasal cavity is shown in Fig. 40-1. (Reprinted with permission from Cousins MJ, Bridenbaugh PO, eds. *Neural Blockade in Clinical Anesthesia and Management of Pain.* Philadelphia: Lippincott-Raven Publishers; 1997.)

1. Technique
   a. Supraorbital notch is palpated at the junction of the lateral two-thirds and medial one-third of the superior orbital rim, which is located on a vertical line with the pupil when the eye is in a neutral position.
   b. Two to 3 ml of local anesthetic is injected through a skin wheal.
2. Indications
   a. Postoperative neuralgia
   b. Herpes zoster
   c. Cancer
E. Infraorbital Nerve
   See Fig. 40-3.
   1. Technique
      a. A 4-cm, 22- to 25-gauge needle is advanced laterally and cephalad from the junction of the medial one-third and lateral two-thirds of the inferior border of the orbit in the same vertical plane as the pupil and supraorbital notch.
      b. Once a paresthesia is obtained, 2 ml of local anesthetic is injected.
   2. Indications
      a. Evaluation of facial neuralgias
      b. Herpes zoster

F. Mental Nerve

See Fig. 40-3.

1. Technique

a. The mental foramen is palpated over the mandible on a vertical line with the pupil.

b. The needle is angled slightly medially to enter the foramen.

c. Once a paresthesia is obtained, 2 to 3 ml local anesthetic is injected.

2. Indications

a. Evaluation of facial neuralgias

b. Herpes zoster

G. Glossopharyngeal nerve

See Fig. 40-4.

1. Technique

a. A 5-cm, 22-gauge needle is inserted at the midpoint of a line joining the angle of the mandible to the mastoid process and directed medially until the styloid process is contacted.

b. One to 2 ml of 1% lidocaine will produce anesthesia of the glossopharyngeal, vagus, and accessory nerves.

2. Indications

a. Carcinoma of the pharynx or posterior third of the tongue

H. Superficial Cervical Plexus Block

See Fig. 40-5.

1. Technique

a. An 8-cm, 22-gauge needle is inserted subcutaneously immediately posterior and deep to the midpoint of the sternocleidomastoid, and 5 ml of local anesthetic is injected.

b. An additional 5 ml is then fanned superiorly as well as inferiorly.

I. Deep Cervical Plexus Block

See Fig. 40-6.

1. Technique

a. Patient is positioned with neck slightly extended and head turned to contralateral side to be blocked.

b. A line is then drawn between the tip of the mastoid process and Chassaignac's tubercle (transverse process of C-6).

c. A second line is drawn parallel and 1 cm posterior to the first line.

d. 5-cm, 22-gauge needle is then inserted to inject small volumes (1–2 ml) at each level shown in Fig. 40-6.

J. Occipital Block

See Fig. 40-7.

1. The greater occipital nerve is blocked at a point about halfway between the mastoid and the occipital protuberance (inion). A 25-gauge needle is used to infiltrate the subcutaneous tissues at this site. The lesser occipital and great auricular nerves are similarly blocked on this same line but lateral to the greater occipital nerve.

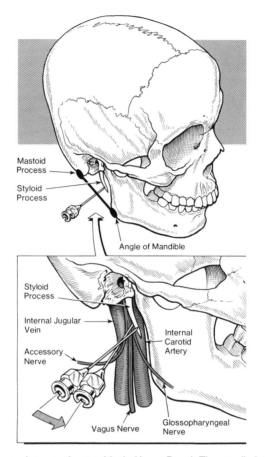

FIG. 40-4. Glossopharyngeal nerve block. Upper Panel: The needle is inserted at a point midway between the mastoid process and the angle of the mandible. Lower Panel: The needle is inserted at a right angle to the skin. At a depth of 2 to 3 cm the styloid process will be contacted (if present). The needle is then walked posteriorly off the styloid process. Local anesthetic deposited at this point will block glossopharyngeal, accessory, and vagus nerves. Note the proximity of the internal carotid artery and the internal jugular vein. (Reprinted with permission from Cousins MJ, Bridenbaugh PO, eds. *Neural Blockade in Clinical Anesthesia and Management of Pain.* Philadelphia: Lippincott-Raven Publishers; 1997.)

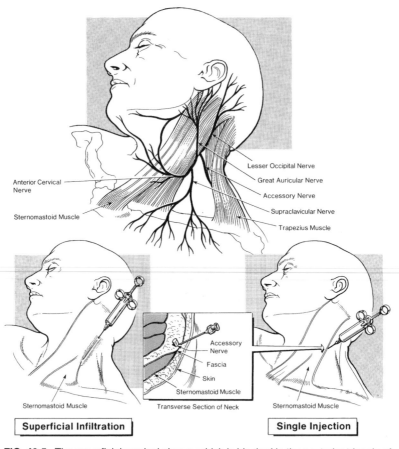

FIG. 40-5. The superficial cervical plexus, which is blocked in the posterior triangle of the neck as it emerges adjacent to the midpoint of the posterior border of the sternomastoid muscle. Superficial infiltration is extended along the middle third of the posterior border of the sternomastoid muscle. Note the close relationship of the accessory nerve as it emerges from the posterior border of the sternomastoid muscle at the junction of its middle and upper third, just above the emerging superficial cervical plexus. Single injection technique for accessory nerve block. Note that the accessory nerve lies deep to the deep fascia of the neck and that this needs to be pierced as shown in the "single injection," which is sometimes used as an adjunct to produce muscle paralysis of the trapezius muscle in shoulder operations. Successful block of the superficial cervical plexus results in analgesia corresponding to the C-2, C-3, and C-4 dermatomes. (Reprinted with permission from Cousins MJ, Bridenbaugh PO, eds. *Neural Blockade in Clinical Anesthesia and Management of Pain.* Philadelphia: Lippincott-Raven Publishers; 1997.)

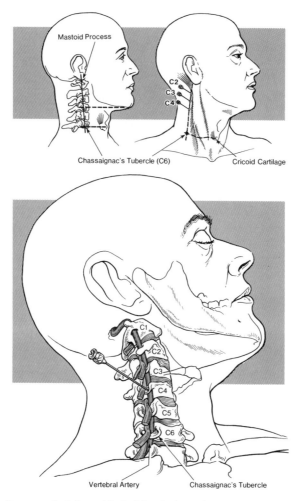

FIG. 40-6. Deep cervical plexus block. A line is drawn from mastoid process to Chassaignac's tubercle (C-6). The latter lies on a line extended laterally from the cricoid cartilage. This line lies over the "gutters" in the superior surface of the transverse processes, upon which the cervical nerve roots pass laterally. The C-4 nerve root is located at the junction of the vertical line and a line horizontally drawn to the lower border of the mandible, with the head in a neutral position. The C-3 and C-2 nerve roots can be located by dividing the distance between the mastoid and horizontal line into thirds (see right upper panel). The C-5 nerve root lies midway between the "C-6 line" and the line above. Individual cervical nerve roots may be blocked by injecting small volumes of local anesthetics, as shown in the upper right. Single injection block of cervical plexus can be obtained by a technique similar to interscalene brachial plexus block, since the cervical nerve roots are contained in a continuous space between scalene muscles. A single needle is inserted on the vertical line at the C-4 level and directed medially and slightly caudad to contact the "gutter" of the transverse process (lower panel). Note that the caudad direction is essential to avoid penetration of an intervertebral foramen, with possible injection into epidural space or dural sleeve (and thus direct entry into CSF). Note also the proximity of the vertebral artery passing through the foramina transversaria of the transverse processes. (Reprinted with permission from Cousins MJ, Bridenbaugh PO, eds. *Neural Blockade in Clinical Anesthesia and Management of Pain.* Philadelphia: Lippincott-Raven Publishers; 1997.)

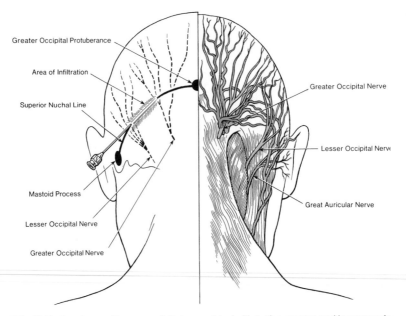

Greater Occipital Protuberance

Area of Infiltration

Superior Nuchal Line

Mastoid Process

Lesser Occipital Nerve

Greater Occipital Nerve

Greater Occipital Nerve

Lesser Occipital Nerve

Great Auricular Nerve

FIG. 40-7. Greater and lesser occipital nerve block. Note the greater and lesser occipital nerve branches crossing the superior nuchal line approximately halfway between the greater occipital protuberance and mastoid process. Superficial infiltration along this line will produce analgesia of the posterior scalp. The greater occipital nerve can be located by identifying the pulsations of the posterior occipital artery, which crosses the nuchal line in company with the nerve. (Reprinted with permission from Cousins MJ, Bridenbaugh PO, eds. *Neural Blockade in Clinical Anesthesia and Management of Pain.* Philadelphia: Lippincott-Raven Publishers; 1997.)

Appendices

The Pain Clinic Manual, Second Edition,
edited by Stephen E. Abram and J. David Haddox.
Lippincott Williams & Wilkins,
Philadelphia, © 2000

Appendix A

Long-Term Epidural Catheter Implantation for Cancer Pain: Patient and Family Reference Material

EPIDURAL HOME CARE SUPPLY LIST

Daily Supplies

12-ml syringes (one per injection time)
Monoject 19- or 20-gauge, 1.5-inch needle with 5-μm filter [Monoject #250] (one per injection)
Duramorph PF

Weekly Supplies

Tegaderm dressing [3M #1626] (two to three per week)
0.22-μm filter [Concord MP-094 or Millex #SLGS0250S] (one per week)

Miscellaneous Supplies

Betadine swabs or swabsticks
Acetone/alcohol swabsticks or alcohol wipes
4″ × 4″ gauze
Porous tape (e.g., Dermacel)

INDIVIDUAL DOSAGE SCHEDULE

For *(patient's name)*

1. Use *only* preservative-free morphine (Duramorph PF), in a strength of _____ mg/ 10 ml. Inject _____ ml every _____ hours.
2. Change dressing every 3 days or more often if required (see "Dressing Change Technique").
3. Change filter once a week (see "Filter Changing Technique").
   Note that some syringes are labeled in milliliters and some are in cubic centimeters. For our purposes, they are the same, so that 10 ml = 10 cc.

NOTE: You are to call us at the pain clinic and/or your physician if any of the following happen:

1. You have an unexplained fever or an extremely sore and tender back.
2. You have inadequate pain relief or the pain returns before the next dose.
3. You require Narcan (naloxone). You should be given Narcan 0.4 mg (one vial) into the thigh or arm muscle if you become *very* drowsy (or unarousable), if you have *severe* nausea and vomiting, or if you have *severe* itching. If you require Narcan you should be taken to an emergency room after receiving it.

INJECTION TECHNIQUE FOR EPIDURAL CATHETER

1. *Wash hands before starting procedure.*
2. Avoid contaminating the filter port, filter cap, needle (including the hub), and tip of the syringe (Fig. A-1). If any of these contact anything that is not sterile (such as the tabletop, fingers, or an area outside of the drug vial), they must be discarded.
3. Assemble the following equipment:
    a. 4″ × 4″ gauze

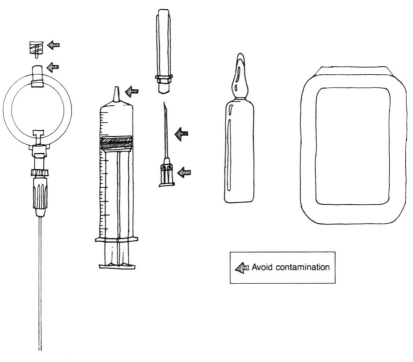

Avoid contamination

FIG. A-1.

   b. The Duramorph vial

   c. One needle

   d. One syringe

4. Take the catheter out of the carrying pouch and place the filter where it can be worked with easily.

5. Open the syringe by twisting the cover and its cap in different directions. Remove the syringe from the cover and lay it down, taking care not to touch the tip.

6. Open the needle by twisting the two parts of its cover in opposite directions. *Do not touch the hub.* Keep a grasp on the needle by holding onto the long part of the cover.

7. Place the tip of the syringe firmly into the hub of the needle: Do not twist (Fig. A-2). Draw 1 ml of air into the syringe through the covered needle to break the plunger seal and then push the air back out.

8. Set the syringe and attached needle down.

9. Using gauze to protect your hands, break the top of the Duramorph vial off by snapping it away from you sharply (Fig. A-3). Beware of glass fragments.

10. Remove the needle cover by pulling it straight off (do not twist) and set the cover down. Carefully insert the needle into the vial and draw up all the Duramorph (Fig. A-4).

11. With the needle pointing up, tap the side of the syringe to get all the air bubbles to the top and then expel the air slowly by gently pushing up on the plunger of the syringe (Fig. A-5). Point the needle at a receptacle (sink, trash can) and watch the top edge of the plunger while pushing gently until the top of the plunger is at the dose indicated on your "Individual Dosage Schedule" (see Fig. A-5).

12. Replace the cover over the needle.

13. With the filter held firmly between the thumb and first two fingers of the left hand, place the needle cover into the left palm and grasp it with the ring and little fingers (Fig. A-6).

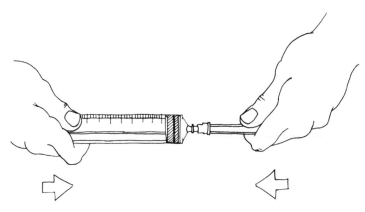

FIG. A-2.

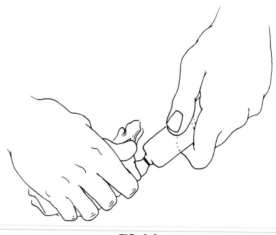

FIG. A-3.

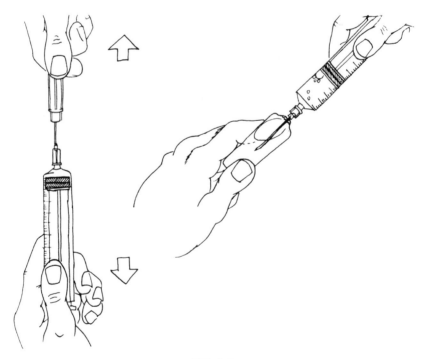

FIG. A-4.

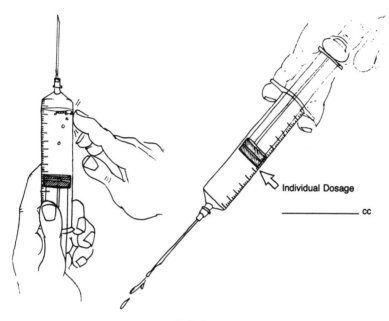

Individual Dosage

_____ cc

FIG. A-5.

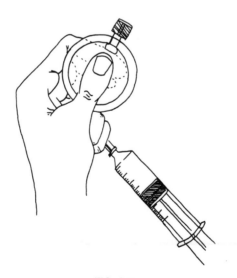

FIG. A-6.

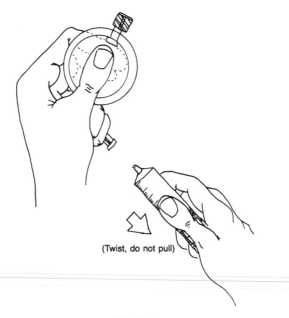

(Twist, do not pull)

FIG. A-7.

14. Twist the syringe out of the needle and place the syringe down on a clean, flat surface, taking care not to contaminate the tip (Fig. A-7).
15. With the right hand, twist the cap off of the filter and place it on the needle hub, giving it a slight twist to secure it (Fig. A-8).
16. Place the tip of the syringe into the filter port snugly without twisting (Fig. A-9).
17. Now hold the syringe in the left hand and pull back on the plunger with the right hand to cause some suction (move the plunger about 1 ml) and hold it there for

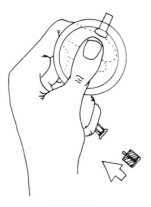

FIG. A-8.

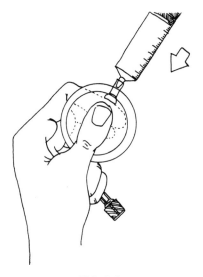

FIG. A-9.

several seconds (Fig. A-10). Watch for blood filling up the catheter or for clear fluid filling up the syringe. A few bubbles are to be expected in the syringe. If either blood or clear fluid appear, recap the filter and call the pain clinic.

18. Push the Dermamorph into the filter by gentle, steady pressure on the plunger (Fig. A-11). If the drug requires excessive pressure to push in or will not go in, call the pain clinic.

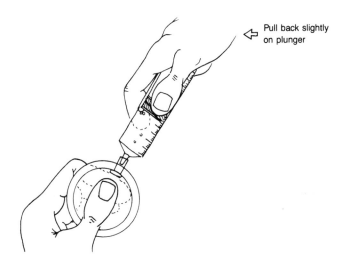

Pull back slightly
on plunger

FIG. A-10.

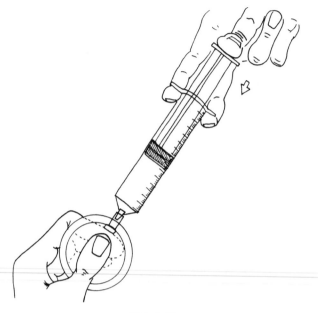

FIG. A-11.

19. When injection is complete, grasp the filter and needle (with the filter cap still attached) in the left hand as before. Remove the syringe and lay it down.
20. Remove the filter cap from the needle hub and place it securely on the filter port, giving it a slight twist.
21. Check to make sure all connections are secure (catheter adapter to catheter, filter to catheter, cap to filter).
22. Discard the needle and all parts of the vial in a container with a lid, such as a plastic milk carton, before placing the container in the garbage.

DRESSING CHANGE TECHNIQUE

1. *Wash hands before starting procedure.*
2. Assemble the following items:
   a. 3 Betadine swabs or swabsticks
   b. 3 Alcohol wipes or acetone/alcohol swabsticks
   c. Gauze
   d. Tegaderm dressing
3. Holding the catheter with one hand, carefully peel the dressing off skin going from front to back. *Be careful not to pull on catheter* (Fig. A-12).
4. Wipe the catheter exit site with a Betadine swab starting at the center of the site and wiping outward in an ever-widening circular spiral motion (Fig. A-13). Do

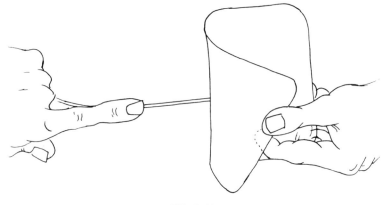

FIG. A-12.

not wipe over the same area twice with the same swab. Repeat with the remaining swabs. Allow the area to dry.
5. Wipe the area in a similar manner with the three acetone/alcohol swabs.
6. Pat the area gently with gauze, touching skin and catheter only with the gauze, not the fingers.
7. Apply the dressing according to the instructions on the package. Remember that the sticky side is also the sterile side, so be careful not to touch it, except at the edges.

FILTER CHANGE TECHNIQUE

1. *Wash hands before starting procedure.*
2. Open a new filter and leave it in the package.
3. Hold the catheter adapter in your left hand, taking care not to pull on the catheter.

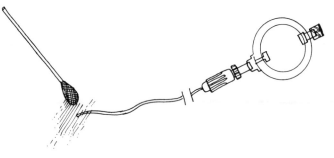

FIG. A-13.

4. Grasp the old filter with your right hand and twist it counterclockwise to disengage the filter from the adapter. Take care not to loosen the adapter from the catheter. Set the old filter down.
5. Pick up the new filter, being careful not to touch the uncapped end.
6. Place the uncapped end into the catheter adapter and twist it clockwise until it is snug.
7. Check to make sure the cap is secure on the filter port.

The Pain Clinic Manual, Second Edition,
edited by Stephen E. Abram and J. David Haddox.
Lippincott Williams & Wilkins,
Philadelphia, © 2000

Appendix B

Dermatome Charts

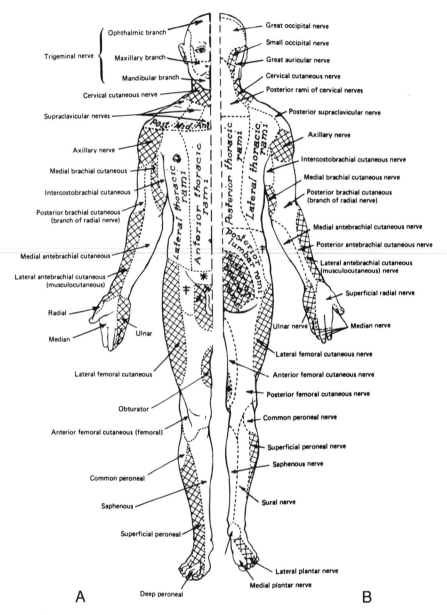

FIG. B-1. Cutaneous innervation. **A:** ventral view; **B:** dorsal view. In ventral view, the nerves represented by symbols are: iliohypogastric (*), ilioinguinal (x), and genitofemoral (‡). (Reprinted with permission from Chusid JG. *Functional Neurology and Correlative Neuroanatomy,* 18th ed. Las Altos: Lange Medical Publishers; 1982: 208–209.)

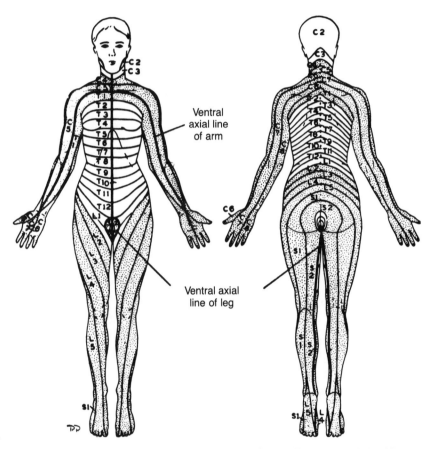

FIG. B-2. Dermatomes according to Keegan and Garrett. These were derived from hypalgesia due to compression of single nerve roots. Compare with Fig. B-3. (Reprinted with permission from Keegan JJ, Garrett FD. Segmental distribution of cutaneous nerves in limbs of man. *Anat Rec* 1948;102:409–437.)

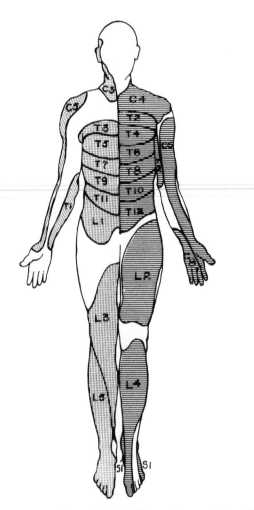

FIG. B-3. Dermatomes according to Foerster. These data were derived by examining remaining sensibility on humans with known nerve lesions. (Reprinted with permission from Foerster O. The dermatomes in man. *Brain* 1933;56:1.)

TABLE B. *Key neurologic landmarks*

Spinal segment	Innervated area	Peripheral innervation
C5	"Shoulder patch"	Axillary nerve
C6	"Six shooter"	Radial nerve (thumb)
		Median nerve (index)
C7	Long finger	Median nerve
C8	Small finger	Ulnar nerve
T1	Medial arm	Medial brachial
		Cutaneous nerve
T2	Sternal notch	Intercostal nerve
T4	Nipples	Intercostal nerve
T6	Xiphoid process	Intercostal nerve
T10	Umbilicus	Intercostal nerve
L1	Inguinal ligament	Ilioinguinal and
		iliohypogastric
		Nerves
L2	Anterolateral thigh	Anterior and lateral femoral
		Cutaneous nerves
L3	Medial knee	Obturator nerve
L4	Anteromedial shin	Saphenous nerve
L5	Dorsum of foot	
	(esp. first web space)	Deep peroneal nerve
S1	Lateral aspect of foot	Sural nerve

The Pain Clinic Manual, Second Edition,
edited by Stephen E. Abram and J. David Haddox.
Lippincott Williams & Wilkins,
Philadelphia, © 2000

Appendix C

Technique for Continuous Opioid Infusion

Continuous infusion of opioid analgesics is a safe and reliable method of achieving continuous pain control for many patients. However, continuous infusions are not always effective, especially for patients with neuropathic or episodic (incident) pain. Indications for continuous infusion include the following:

1. Unacceptability of other routes of administration
2. Concern about poor absorption from alternative sites
3. Opioid toxicity owing to the peak effect of bolus dosing
4. Ease of nursing when frequent repetitive dosing may be impractical
5. Need for rapid titration of opioid effect

The following guidelines should be observed when instituting a continuous infusion:

1. Check with the nursing staff prior to starting an opioid infusion, as most hospitals have established guidelines for such issues as starting doses, frequency of dose adjustments, frequency of blood pressure and respiration checks, and so on.
2. Continuous infusions may be administered intravenously or subcutaneously. Under special conditions and with adequate supervision, infusions may be delivered via catheters into the epidural or intrathecal space. Subcutaneous infusions should be run at <2.0 ml/hr and subcutaneous catheters (use 27-gauge butterfly needles) can usually be left in place for 3 to 7 days before a site change is needed.
3. Short-acting strong opioids, such as morphine or hydromorphone, should be used rather than long-acting opioids. Use a flow-calibrated infusion pump rather than a droprate-calibrated infusion pump.
4. To pick a starting dose, use the equivalency index (see Appendix D) to convert the present 24-hour opioid regimen into the equivalent dose for intravenous infusion of the selected drug. Conversion of the dose given by intravenous/intramuscular bolus to that given by continuous infusion can be done on a milligram-to-milligram basis (e.g., preinfusion regimen of iv morphine 9 mg q 3 hr = 72 mg/24 hr = infusion rate of morphine at 3 mg/hr). If the opioid chosen for infusion is different from the previously given drug, an initial dose reduction of 50% is recommended (e.g., preinfusion regimen of PO hydromorphone 12 mg q 3 hr = 96 mg/24 hr; 96 × 1.33 = 128 mg parenteral morphine; therefore administer morphine as an infusion of 64 mg/24 hr or 2.7 mg/hr).
5. Give a loading dose of a short-acting opioid at the start of the infusion and with each increase in the infusion rate. Administer the loading dose slowly (2 mg/min)

439

and observe vital signs frequently after each bolus dose or increase in the infusion rate. If no loading dose is given when the infusion rate is increased, wait 8 to 12 hours before further rate adjustments to allow for steady-state blood levels. Guidelines for the size of the loading dose are as follows:

Morphine equivalent maintenance dose	Morphine equivalent loading dose
<15 mg/hr	5 to 15 mg
15 to 30 mg/hr	1 hour total of maintenance dose
>30 mg/hr	30 mg

6. Once the infusion is under way, reassess the patient frequently and increase the infusion rate until adequate analgesia is obtained or intolerable side effects develop. One method to ensure proper dose adjustment is to prescribe a prn dose in addition to the infusion. Use the same drug and dose as the loading dose ordered: q 1 to 2 hr prn residual pain. Every 8 to 24 hours add up the additional doses needed and add this to the maintenance infusion rate (e.g., infusion of morphine at 3 mg/hr to 72 mg/24 hr; over 24 hours an additional 60 mg of prn morphine was administered; therefore the calculated 24-hour requirement would increase to 72 + 60 = 132 mg/24 hr = 5.5 mg/hr).

The Pain Clinic Manual, Second Edition,
edited by Stephen E. Abram and J. David Haddox.
Lippincott Williams & Wilkins,
Philadelphia, © 2000

Appendix D

Opioid Conversion Chart

TABLE D. *Pharmacologic equivalence and relevant pharmacokinetic data for opioid agonists*

Drug	Approximate equianalgesic dose		Bio-availability	Relative potency*	Usual starting dose for moderate to severe pain	
	Oral	Parenteral			Oral	Parenteral
Opioid agonists‡						
Morphine§ (MSIR, others)	30 mg q. 3–4 hr. (Around-the-clock) 60 mg. q. 3–4 hr. (single or intermittent dosing)	10 mg q 3–4 hr.	0.3	1.0	30 mg q 3–4 hr.	10 mg
Morphine, Controlled-release§,‖ (MS Contin, Oramorph)	90–120 mg q. 12 hr.	N/A	0.3	1.0	90–120 mg q 12 hr.	N/A
Hydromorphone§ (Dilaudid)	3 mg q. 3–4 hr.	1.5 mg q. 3–4 hr.	0.5	6–7	6 mg q. 3–4 hr.	1.5 mg q. 3–4 hr.
Levorphanol (Levo-Dromoran)	4 mg q 6–8 hr.	2 mg q. 6–8 hr.	0.5	5.0	4 mg q. 6–8 hr.	2 mg q. 6–8 hr.
Meperidine (Demerol)	300 mg q 2–3 hr.	100 mg q. 3 hr.	0.3–0.5§§	0.1	N/R	100 mg q. 3 hr.
Methadone (Dolophine)	12.5–15 q 6–8 hr.	10 mg q. 6–8 hr.	0.7–0.8	1.0	20 mg q. 6–8 hr.	10 mg q. 6–8 hr.
Oxymorphone‖ (Numorphan)	N/A	1 mg q. 3–4 hr.	N/A	10	N/A	1 mg q. 3–4 hr.
Oxycodone (OXYIR, Roxicodone, Percodone)	30 mg q. 3–4 hr.	N/A	0.6–0.7	1.0	10 mg q. 3–4 hr.	N/A

Oxycodone, Controlled-release (OxyContin)	80 mg q. 12 hr. q. 12 hr.	N/A	0.6–0.7	1.0	40–80 mg. q.3–4 hr.	N/A
*Opioid/NSAID combinations***						
Codeine††, ‡/ASA Or APAP (Tylenol #3)	180–200 mg q. 3–4 hr.	130 mg q 3–4 hr.	0.5	0.08	60 mg q. 3–4 hr.	60 mg q. 3–4 hr.
Hydrocodone/APAP‡ (Vicodin, Lorcet, Lortab)	30 mg q. 3–4 hr.	N/A	0.3	1.0	10 mg q. 3–4 hr.	N/A

Modified and adapted from Management of cancer pain: adults clinical practice guideline #9, Agency for Health Care Policy & Research, *J Am Fam Phys* 1997;55:1151–1160

NOTE: Published tables vary according to recommended equianalgesic dosing. Titration to clinical response is therefore necessary for each patient. When changing drugs, it is usually necessary to use a lower than equianalgesic dose and retitrate the response due to incomplete cross-tolerance between different analgesics

* Compared with parenteral morphine.

† Recommended doses do not apply in patients with body weight less than 50 kg.

‡ Recommended doses do not apply in patients with renal or hepatic insufficiency, or other conditions affecting drug metabolism and kinetics.

§ Rectal administration of morphine, hydromorphone, and oxymorphone is an alternative for patients unable to take oral medications. Equianalgesic doses may differ from oral and parenteral doses because of pharmacokinetic differences.

‖ Transdermal fentanyl is an option. Transdermal fentanyl dose is not calculated as equianalgesic to a single morphine dose. See the package insert for dosing calculations. Doses above 25 mcg per hour should not be used in opioid-naïve patients.

** Doses of aspirin or acetaminophen in combinations with NSAID/opioid preparations must also be adjusted to the patient's body weight. Aspirin is contraindicated in children in the presence of fever or other viral disease because of its association with Reye's syndrome.

†† Some clinicians recommend not exceeding 1.5 mg per kg of codeine because of an increased incidence of side effects with higher doses.

‡‡ Total daily dose of acetaminophen should not exceed 4000 mg from all sources, in patients with normal hepatic function.

§§ Oral availability of meperidine is unpredictable, as is absorption after IM administration. Meperidine also has local anesthetic activity and antimuscarinic effects.

The Pain Clinic Manual, Second Edition,
edited by Stephen E. Abram and J. David Haddox.
Lippincott Williams & Wilkins,
Philadelphia, © 2000

Appendix E

Billing Codes

PAIN CLINIC DIAGNOSIS CODES

Back and Neck Pain

724.2 Low Back Pain
724.5 Mechanical Back Pain
724.1 Thoracic Spine Pain
723.1 Neck Pain
724.79 Coccydynia
       Facet Arthropathy
       Sacroiliac Arthropathy
805.8. Vertebral Compression Fx

Postlaminectomy Syndrome

722.81 Cervical
722.82 Thoracic
722.83 Lumbar

Intervertebral Disc Displacement

722.0 Cervical, without Myelopathy
722.11 Thoracic, without Myelopathy
722.10 Lumbar, without Myelopathy
722.71 Cervical, with Myelopathy
722.72 Thoracic, with Myelopathy
722.73 Lumbar, with Myelopathy

Spinal Stenosis

723.0 Cervical
724.01 Thoracic
724.02 Lumbar

Radiculopathy

724.4   Lumbar, Thoracic
723.4   Cervical
724.3   Sciatica, L-5–S-1
353.8   Nerve Root Fibrosis

Neuropathic Pain

356.9   Peripheral Neuropathy
354.8   Mononeuritis Upper Limb
355.8   Mononeuritis Lower Limb
957.9   Peripheral Nerve Trauma, Neuroma
353.0   Brachial Plexopathy
353.1   Lumbosacral Plexopathy
053.9   Acute Herpes Zoster
053.19 Postherpetic Neuralgia
053.12 Postherpetic Trigeminal Neuralgia
350.1   Trigeminal Neuralgia
352.9   Occipital Neuralgia
355.1   Meralgia Paresthetica
250.60 Diabetic Neuropathy (with 357.2)
353.0   Thoracic Outlet Syndrome
355.9   Entrapment Neuropathy

Reflex Sympathetic Dystrophies

337.21 RSD Upper Limb
337.22 RSD Lower Limb
337.20 RSD Unspecified
354.4   Causalgia Upper Limb
355.71 Causalgia Lower Limb
355.9   Other Causalgia

Central Pain Syndromes

349.9   Central Pain
353.6   Phantom Limb Pain

Painful Medical Conditions

577.0   Acute Pancreatitis
577.1   Chronic Pancreatitis
282.60 Sickle Cell Anemia

340   Multiple Sclerosis
729.2 AIDS-Related Pain
729.5 Postphlebitic Pain

Pain, Other Sites

784.0   Headache
307.81 Tension Headache
346.9   Migraine Headache
349.0   Dural Puncture Headache
350.2   Atypical Facial Pain
784.1   Throat Pain
786.50 Musculoskeletal Chest Pain
786.52 Chest Wall Pain
789.0   Abdominal Pain
569.42 Rectal Pain
625.8   Genital Pain, Female
607.89 Genital Pain, Male
625.9   Pelvic Pain
733.90 Bone Pain

Muscle Pain, Spasm

729.1   Myofascial Pain, Fibromyalgia
724.3   Piriformis Syndrome
349.89 Spasticity

Arthritis, Inflammation

715.90 Degenerative Arthritis
714.0   Rheumatoid Arthritis
716.99 Arthritis, Multiple Sites
727.3   Bursitis
720.2   Sacroiliitis
524.60 TMJ Syndrome
733.99 Costal Chondritis

Cancer Pain

174.9   Breast
180.9   Cervix
153.9   Colon
182.0   Endometrial

162.9   Lung
183.9   Ovarian
157.9   Pancreatic
185   Prostate
154.8   Rectal
199.1   Other Cancer

PAIN CLINIC OFFICE VISIT AND PROCEDURE CODES

Outpatient Consultations

99241   Problem focused history/exam, straightforward
99242   Problem focused history/exam, expanded, straightforward
99243   Detailed history/exam, low complexity
99244   Comprehensive history/exam, moderate complexity
99245   Comprehensive history/exam, high complexity

Outpatient-Established

99211   Problem, minimal
99212   Problem-focused history/exam, straightforward
99213   Problem-focused history/exam, expanded, moderate complexity
99214   Detailed history/exam, moderate complexity
99215   Comprehensive history/exam, high complexity

Inpatient Consultation

Initial

99251   Problem-focused history/exam, straightforward
99252   Problem-focused history/exam, expanded, straightforward
99253   Detailed history/exam, low complexity
99254   Comprehensive history/exam, moderate complexity
99255   Comprehensive history/exam, high complexity

Followup

99261   Problem-focused history/exam, straightforward
99262   Problem-focused, expanded, moderate complexity
99263   Detailed history/exam, high complexity

Initial Hospital Care

99221   Detailed/comprehensive history/exam, straightforward/low complexity
99222   Comprehensive history/exam, moderate complexity
99223   Comprehensive history/exam, high complexity

Subsequent Hospital Care

99231   Problem-focused history/exam, straightforward, low complexity
99232   Problem-focused history/exam, expanded, moderate complexity
99233   Detailed history/exam, high complexity

Prolonged Services

99354   Outpatient, face to face (1st hour)
99355   Outpatient, face to face (ea. addt'l. half hour)
99356   Inpatient, face to face (1st hour)
99357   Inpatient, face to face (ea. addt'l. half hour)

Injection Anesthetic

62275   Epidural, cervical or thoracic, single
62278   Epidural, lumbar or caudal, single
62279   Epidural, continuous (any site)
62274   Subarachnoid or subdural, single
62276   Subarachnoid or subdural, differential
62277   Subarachnoid or subdural, continuous

Injection Other Substance

62288   Subarachnoid
62289   Epidural, lumbar/caudal
62298   Epidural, cervical/thoracic
62273   Epidural blood patch

Intravenous Infusion by Physician

36410   IV started by physician
90780   Up to 1   hour
90781   Ea. addt'l. hour, ___hrs. (8 max.)

Destruction by Neurolytic Agent (e.g., chemical, thermal, RF)

62280   Subarachnoid
62282   Epidural, lumbar/caudal
62281   Epidural, cervical/thoracic
64620   Intercostal nerve
64622   Facet joint nerve, single
64623   Facet joint nerve, ea. addt'l. (# sites ___)
64640   Other peripheral nerve
64680   Celiac/hypogastric plexus

Injection, Intralesional, Joint, Muscle

20550 Trigger point (# sites ___)
11900 Injection, intralesional, seven or less
11901 Injection, intralesional, more than seven
20600 Injection, joint, small
20605 Injection, joint, intermediate
20610 Injection, joint, major

Injection, Somatic Nerves

64413 Cervical plexus
64415 Brachial plexus
64402 Facial
64405 Greater occipital
64425 Ilioinguinal, iliohypogastric
64420 Intercostal, single
64421 Intercostal, multiple
64435 Paracervical (uterine)
64440 Paravertebral, single
64441 Paravertebral, multiple
64442 Paravertebral, facet, single
64443 Paravertebral, facet, multiple (addt'l. # ___)
64410 Phrenic
64430 Pudendal
64445 Sciatic
64412 Spinal accessory
64418 Suprascapular
64440 Trigeminal, any branch
64408 Vagus
64450 Other peripheral

Injection, Sympathetic, Visceral Nerves

64530 Celiac, hypogastric plexus
64520 Lumbar, thoracic paravertebral sympathetic
64510 Stellate ganglion
64505 Sphenopalatine ganglion

Implants, Reservoirs and Pumps

62350 Implantation, revision, reposition spinal catheter
62362 Implantation infusion pump
96530 Refill and maintenance

62367   Electronic analysis programmable infusion pump

62368   Electronic analysis programmable infusion pump, with reprogramming

62355   Removal spinal catheter

62365   Removal infusion pump

Implants, Neurostimulators, Spinal

63650   Percutaneous implantation neurostimulator electrodes, epidural

63660   Revision or removal, neurostimulator electrodes

63685   Incision and subcutaneous placement neurostimulator pulse generator or receiver

63688   Revision or removal, implanted spinal neurostimulator pulse generator or receiver

63690   Electronic analysis implanted neurostimulator

63691   Electronic analysis with reprogramming implanted neurostimulator

The Pain Clinic Manual, Second Edition,
edited by Stephen E. Abram and J. David Haddox.
Lippincott Williams & Wilkins,
Philadelphia, © 2000

Appendix F

Patient Pain Questionnaire, Treatment Evaluation Questionnaire, and History and Physical Examination Recording Form

PAIN QUESTIONNAIRE

Date: _____

Name: _____

          Last   First   Middle

1. Sex: [ ] Male   [ ] Female

2. Age: _____ years

3a. When did you first notice the pain for which you are now being treated?

    1 [ ] In the past 2 weeks
    2 [ ] 2 weeks to 3 months ago
    3 [ ] 3 to 6 months ago
    4 [ ] 6 months to 1 year ago
    5 [ ] 1 to 2 years ago
    6 [ ] 2 to 5 years ago
    7 [ ] More than 5 years ago

3b. Have you had this same type of pain before?

    1 [ ] Yes   2 [ ] No

3c. Have you had other painful conditions in the past?

    1 [ ] Yes   2 [ ] No

4. What time of day is your pain the worst?

    1 [ ] Morning, on arising
    2 [ ] Later in the morning
    3 [ ] Afternoon
    4 [ ] Evening
    5 [ ] Bedtime
    6 [ ] Night (during usual sleeping hours)
    7 [ ] Pain is always the same
    8 [ ] Pain varies, but is not worse at any particular time

5. Where is your pain located? Check all areas where you have pain:

    1 [ ] Head   4 [ ] Neck
    2 [ ] Face   5 [ ] Shoulder
    3 [ ] Mouth, throat   6 [ ] Arm

7 [ ] Elbow	15 [ ] Mid back
8 [ ] Hand or wrist	16 [ ] Lower back
9 [ ] Chest	17 [ ] Buttock
10 [ ] Abdomen	18 [ ] Thigh
11 [ ] Multiple joints	19 [ ] Knee
12 [ ] Genitourinary (bowel, bladder, sex organs)	20 [ ] Calf
13 [ ] Groin	21 [ ] Ankle or foot
14 [ ] Upper back	22 [ ] Other

6. What side is your pain mostly on?

1 [ ] Left side   3 [ ] Both sides
2 [ ] Right side   4 [ ] In the middle

7. Would you describe your pain as (check all that apply):

a. Burning [ ]   d. Throbbing [ ]
b. Sharp [ ]   e. Shooting [ ]
c. Aching [ ]   f. Other (describe) [ ] _____

8. Does your pain travel anywhere?

1 [ ] Yes   Where?_____
2 [ ] No

9. Which statement best describes your pain? (Check one)

1 [ ] Always present—Always the same intensity
2 [ ] Always present—Intensity varies
3 [ ] Often present—Have short periods without pain
4 [ ] Often present—Have pain-free periods lasting 1 to 6 hours
5 [ ] Often present—Have pain-free periods lasting over 6 hours
6 [ ] Occasionally present—Have pain once to several times per day, lasting a few minutes to an hour
7 [ ] Occasionally present—Have pain for brief periods, lasting a few seconds to a few minutes
8 [ ] Rarely present—Have pain every few days or weeks

10. On a scale of 0 to 10 (0 being no pain and 10 being the worst pain you can imagine):

What is your usual level of pain? (circle #)   1 2 3 4 5 6 7 8 9 10
What is your highest level of pain? (circle #)   1 2 3 4 5 6 7 8 9 10
What is your lowest level of pain? (circle #)   1 2 3 4 5 6 7 8 9 10

11. Does this pain delay your getting to sleep?

1 [ ] Every night
2 [ ] Almost every night
3 [ ] Some nights
4 [ ] Not at all

12. Does this pain awaken you from sleep?

1 [ ] Every night
2 [ ] Almost every night
3 [ ] Some nights
4 [ ] Not at all

13. Do you usually feel rested after a night's sleep?
    1 [ ] Yes   2 [ ] No
14. Have you had any of the following for relief of your pain? (Check all that apply)
    If used, did it relieve your pain?

1 [ ] Nerve blocks (injections)	1 [ ] Yes	2 [ ] No
2 [ ] TENS (electrical stimulation)	1 [ ] Yes	2 [ ] No
3 [ ] Biofeedback	1 [ ] Yes	2 [ ] No
4 [ ] Acupuncture	1 [ ] Yes	2 [ ] No
5 [ ] Manipulation	1 [ ] Yes	2 [ ] No
6 [ ] Heat therapy	1 [ ] Yes	2 [ ] No
7 [ ] Bedrest	1 [ ] Yes	2 [ ] No
8 [ ] Traction	1 [ ] Yes	2 [ ] No
9 [ ] Massage therapy	1 [ ] Yes	2 [ ] No
10 [ ] Psychotherapy/psychiatric care	1 [ ] Yes	2 [ ] No
11 [ ] Hypnosis	1 [ ] Yes	2 [ ] No
12 [ ] Ultrasound	1 [ ] Yes	2 [ ] No
13 [ ] Exercise	1 [ ] Yes	2 [ ] No
14 [ ] Other_____	1 [ ] Yes	2 [ ] No

15. Have you visited an emergency room for your pain?
    1 [ ] Yes   Approximate # of times: _____
    2 [ ] No
16. Have you been hospitalized for your pain?
    1 [ ] Yes   Approximate # of times: _____
    2 [ ] No
17. Have you had surgery for your pain?
    1 [ ] Yes   Number of operations: _____
    2 [ ] No
18. Do you take medicines for pain relief?

1 [ ] Never (GO TO QUESTION 24)	4 [ ] Yes—One or two times per day
2 [ ] Yes—Less than one time per week	5 [ ] Yes—Three or four times per day
3 [ ] Yes—Several times per week	6 [ ] Yes—Five or more times per day

19. If you take medication for pain, when do you take it?
    1 [ ] When needed for pain   2 [ ] Regularly by the clock
20. Please list all pain medications you are currently taking:

Name of medication	Strength (mg)	Number of times per day
1. _____	_____	_____
2. _____	_____	_____
3. _____	_____	_____
4. _____	_____	_____
5. _____	_____	_____

21. Does your pain medication
    [ ] Relieve all or almost all of your pain?
    [ ] Relieve about 75% of your pain
    [ ] Relieve about 50% of your pain
    [ ] Relieve about 25% of your pain
    [ ] Relieve your pain only slightly
22. For how long do you get relief after taking you pain medication? _____ hours
23. Do you get side effects from your pain medication?
    1 [ ] Yes   2 [ ] No
24. If yes, what are the side effects?
    1 [ ] Nausea   5 [ ] Confusion
    2 [ ] Constipation   6 [ ] Heartburn or abdominal pain
    3 [ ] Drowsiness   7 [ ] Dry mouth
    4 [ ] Dizziness   8 [ ] Other_____
25. Do these side effects limit your use of pain medications?
    1 [ ] Yes   2 [ ] No
26. What is your marital status now?
    1 [ ] Married   4 [ ] Divorced/separated
    2 [ ] Never married   5 [ ] Widowed
    3 [ ] Live with spouse equivalent
27. Who lives with you presently? (check all that apply)
    1 [ ] Live alone   5 [ ] Other relative
    2 [ ] Spouse or   6 [ ] Friend or roommate
        spouse equivalent
    3 [ ] Son or daughter   7 [ ] Other_____
    4 [ ] Parent
28. Is anyone living with you able to help care for you?
    1 [ ] Yes   2 [ ] No
29. Under what circumstances did your pain begin? (Check one box)
    1 [ ] Accident at work
    2 [ ] At work, but not an accident
    3 [ ] Accident at home
    4 [ ] Motor vehicle accident
    5 [ ] Following surgery
    6 [ ] Following illness
    7 [ ] Pain just began, no reason
    8 [ ] Other (describe): _____
30. If you were injured at work, describe how:
    1 [ ] Fall
    2 [ ] Lifting object
    3 [ ] Pushing
    4 [ ] Struck by falling object
    5 [ ] Injury from repetitive activity

6 [ ] Other (describe): _____

_____

7 [ ] Not injured at work

31. What is your current occupation?

1 [ ] Professional specialty (e.g., teacher, nurse)
2 [ ] Executive, administrative or managerial
3 [ ] Technician or related support
4 [ ] Sales-related
5 [ ] Administrative or support occupation, including clerical
6 [ ] Private household service
7 [ ] Protective service occupation (e.g., police, fire)
8 [ ] Service occupation, except protective or household
9 [ ] Farming, forestry or fishing-related
10 [ ] Precision production, craft, or repair-related
11 [ ] Construction-related
12 [ ] Machine operator, assembler, or inspector (e.g., factory-worker)
13 [ ] Transportation or material-moving occupation (bus or truck driver)
14 [ ] Handler, equipment cleaner, helper, or laborer
15 [ ] Military
16 [ ] Student
17 [ ] Homemaker
18 [ ] Vocational rehabilitation or job training
19 [ ] Retired
20 [ ] Disabled
21 [ ] Other _____

Specifically, what do you do at work? _____

32. Are you employed now?

1 [ ] Yes—Full time
2 [ ] Yes—Full time with restrictions
3 [ ] Yes—Full time, but on sick leave right now
4 [ ] Yes—Part time
5 [ ] Yes—Part time with restrictions
6 [ ] Yes—Part time, but on sick leave right now
7 [ ] No—But not because of pain
8 [ ] No—Unable to work or unemployed because of pain

33. Place of employment (if employed): _____

34. Has your job changed because of your painful condition?

1 [ ] Yes   2 [ ] No

35. If your job has changed as a result of your pain, what was your former occupation?

1 [ ] Professional specialty (e.g., teacher, nurse)
2 [ ] Executive, administrative or managerial
3 [ ] Technician or related support

4 [ ] Sales-related
5 [ ] Administrative or support occupation, including clerical
6 [ ] Private household service
7 [ ] Protective service occupation (e.g., police, fire)
8 [ ] Service occupation, except protective or household
9 [ ] Farming, forestry or fishing-related
10 [ ] Precision production, craft, or repair-related
11 [ ] Construction-related
12 [ ] Machine operator, assembler, or inspector (e.g., factory- worker)
13 [ ] Transportation or material-moving occupation (bus or truck driver)
14 [ ] Handler, equipment cleaner, helper, or laborer
15 [ ] Military
16 [ ] Student
17 [ ] Homemaker
18 [ ] Vocational rehabilitation or job training
19 [ ] Retired
20 [ ] Disabled
21 [ ] Other _____

36. Since your pain began, has your income changed?
    1 [ ] No—It has stayed the same
    2 [ ] Yes—It has increased
    3 [ ] Yes—It has decreased slightly
    4 [ ] Yes—It has decreased moderately
    5 [ ] Yes—It has decreased greatly

37. Are you suing because of your pain?
    1 [ ] Yes   2 [ ] No

38. Have you sued because of your pain in the past?
    1 [ ] Yes   2 [ ] No

39. Do you plan to sue because of
your pain in the future?
    1 [ ] Yes   2 [ ] No

40. If are suing or have sued, for what are you suing? Check all that apply:
    1 [ ] Lost wages
    2 [ ] Payment of medical bills
    3 [ ] Payment for pain and suffering
    4 [ ] Other (describe) _____

41. Have you received or are you now receiving any form of financial compensation
for your pain?
    1 [ ] Yes   2 [ ] No
If yes, please indicate the source(s) of payment:
    1 [ ] Worker's compensation
    2 [ ] Government disability
    3 [ ] Insurance or other commercial disability
    4 [ ] Accrued sick leave

5 [ ] Accrued vacation leave

6 [ ] Lump sum disbursement

7 [ ] Other (describe) _____

42. Do you drink alcohol (beer, wine, or liquor)?

    1 [ ] Not at all

    2 [ ] Occasional social drink

    3 [ ] About 1 to 3 drinks per day

    4 [ ] Four or more drinks per day

43. If you drink alcohol, do you drink to relieve your pain?

    1 [ ] Regularly

    2 [ ] Often

    3 [ ] Seldom

    4 [ ] Never

44. Do you smoke tobacco?

    1 [ ] Never smoked

    2 [ ] Formerly smoked

    3 [ ] Smoke less than 1 pack of cigarettes per day

    4 [ ] Smoke 1 to less than 2 packs of cigarettes per day

    5 [ ] Smoke 2 or more packs of cigarettes per day

    6 [ ] Smoke cigars

    7 [ ] Smoke a pipe

If you currently smoke, how many years have you smoked?

Number of years: _____

45. Do you have any of the following medical conditions?

    1 [ ] Heart disease

    2 [ ] High blood pressure

    3 [ ] Diabetes

    4 [ ] Lung disease (asthma, bronchitis)

    5 [ ] Gastrointestinal disease (ulcers, gastritis, colitis)

    6 [ ] Kidney disease

    7 [ ] Liver disease (hepatitis, jaundice, cirrhosis)

    8 [ ] Arthritis

    9 [ ] Neurological disorder (stroke, epilepsy, nerve damage)

    10 [ ] Allergies

    11 [ ] Excessive bleeding or bruising (hemophilia, use of anticoagulants, blood thinners)

    12 [ ] Anemia

46. Are you allergic to any medications?

    1 [ ] Yes   2 [ ] No

If yes, please list _____

47. Please list all nonpain medications you are currently taking:

Name of medication	Strength (mg)	Number per day
1. _____	_____	_____
2. _____	_____	_____
3. _____	_____	_____
4. _____	_____	_____
5. _____	_____	_____

48. Have you ever had treatment from any doctor for anxiety, depression or any other nervous disorder?

    1 [ ] Yes   2 [ ] No

49. Average number of hours you currently spend in a 24-hour day doing the following activities:

    Number of hours:

    a. Sitting _____
    b. Lying down (but not sleeping) _____
    c. Walking _____
    d. Exercising (such as running, swimming, bicycling) _____
    e. Working—not counting employment (such as housework, gardening, washing cars) _____

50. Since your pain began, have you gained weight?

    1 [ ] Yes   2 [ ] No

    If yes, how many pounds? _____

51. Since your pain began, have you lost weight?

    1 [ ] Yes   2 [ ] No

    If yes, how many pounds? _____

52. Please check the aids or devices that you usually use:

    1 [ ] Cane
    2 [ ] Crutches
    3 [ ] Walker
    4 [ ] Wheelchair

53. Please check the number that best corresponds to your ability to do the following things in the past week:

	Degree of Difficulty				
	None	Slight	Moderate	Extreme	Unable to do
a. Dress yourself	1 [ ]	2 [ ]	3 [ ]	4 [ ]	5 [ ]
b. Shampoo your hair	1 [ ]	2 [ ]	3 [ ]	4 [ ]	5 [ ]
c. Stand up from an armless chair	1 [ ]	2 [ ]	3 [ ]	4 [ ]	5 [ ]
d. Get in and out of bed	1 [ ]	2 [ ]	3 [ ]	4 [ ]	5 [ ]
e. Walk outdoors on flat ground	1 [ ]	2 [ ]	3 [ ]	4 [ ]	5 [ ]

f. Climb up 5 steps   1 [ ]   2 [ ]   3 [ ]   4 [ ]   5 [ ]

g. Wash and dry   1 [ ]   2 [ ]   3 [ ]   4 [ ]   5 [ ]
   your entire body:

h. Get on and off   1 [ ]   2 [ ]   3 [ ]   4 [ ]   5 [ ]
   the toilet

i. Bend down and   1 [ ]   2 [ ]   3 [ ]   4 [ ]   5 [ ]
   pick up clothing
   from the floor

j. Open car doors   1 [ ]   2 [ ]   3 [ ]   4 [ ]   5 [ ]

k. Open jars which   1 [ ]   2 [ ]   3 [ ]   4 [ ]   5 [ ]
   before have been
   opened

l. Run errands   1 [ ]   2 [ ]   3 [ ]   4 [ ]   5 [ ]
   and shop

m. Get in and out   1 [ ]   2 [ ]   3 [ ]   4 [ ]   5 [ ]
   of a car

n. Do chores such as   1 [ ]   2 [ ]   3 [ ]   4 [ ]   5 [ ]
   vacuuming or
   gardening

o. Participate in   1 [ ]   2 [ ]   3 [ ]   4 [ ]   5 [ ]
   social activity

p. Participate in   1 [ ]   2 [ ]   3 [ ]   4 [ ]   5 [ ]
   recreational
   activity

NOTE: This section is to be used both as an end-of-treatment evaluation and as a follow-up. When used as an end-of-treatment evaluation, questions 15–18 should be deleted.

TREATMENT EVALUATION QUESTIONNAIRE

Date: _____

Name: _____
       First   Middle   Last

1. Compared to your condition before treatment in the Pain Clinic, has your pain changed?
   1 [ ] Pain has increased
   2 [ ] Pain has stayed the same
   3 [ ] Pain has decreased slightly
   4 [ ] Pain has decreased moderately
   5 [ ] Pain has decreased considerably
   6 [ ] Pain has gone away completely

2. Please evaluate how beneficial your treatment has been at the Pain Clinic by circling the appropriate number below. If you did not have a type of treatment, circle "0" for "Not Appropriate (NA)."

		Made pain worse	Did not help at all	Helped slightly	Helped moder- ately	Helped consid- erably
a.	Injections	0	1	2	3	4	5
b.	Medications	0	1	2	3	4	5
c.	Counseling	0	1	2	3	4	5
d.	Physical therapy	0	1	2	3	4	5
e.	Biofeedback	0	1	2	3	4	5
f.	Relaxation	0	1	2	3	4	5
g.	TENS	0	1	2	3	4	5
h.	Occupational therapy	0	1	2	3	4	5

3. Which statement best describes your pain now? (Check one)

1 [ ] Always present—Always the same intensity
2 [ ] Always present—Intensity varies
3 [ ] Often present—Have short periods without pain
4 [ ] Often present—Have pain-free periods lasting 1 to 6 hours
5 [ ] Often present—Have pain-free periods lasting over 6 hours
6 [ ] Occasionally present—Have pain once to several times per day, lasting a few minutes to an hour
7 [ ] Occasionally present—Have pain for brief periods, lasting a few seconds to a few minutes
8 [ ] Rarely present—Have pain every few days or weeks

4. On a scale of 0 to 10 (0 being no pain and 10 being the worst pain you can imagine):

What is your usual level of pain? (circle #)	1 2 3 4 5 6 7 8 9 10
What is your highest level of pain? (circle #)	1 2 3 4 5 6 7 8 9 10
What is your lowest level of pain? (circle #)	1 2 3 4 5 6 7 8 9 10

5. Does this pain delay your getting to sleep?

1 [ ] Every night
2 [ ] Almost every night
3 [ ] Some nights
4 [ ] Not at all

6. Does this pain awaken you from sleep?

1 [ ] Every night
2 [ ] Almost every night
3 [ ] Some nights
4 [ ] Not at all

7. Does this pain usually awaken you from sleep more than once per night?

1 [ ] Yes
2 [ ] No

8. Most mornings do you feel rested after sleep?

    1 [ ] Yes

    2 [ ] No

9a. Do you take medicines for pain relief?

    1 [ ] Never (GO TO QUESTION 10)

    2 [ ] Yes—Less than one time per week

    3 [ ] Yes—Several times per week

    4 [ ] Yes—One or two times per day

    5 [ ] Yes—Three or four times per day

    6 [ ] Yes—Five or more times per day

9b. If yes, since treatment began, has your need for medication:

    1 [ ] Increased

    2 [ ] Stayed the same

    3 [ ] Decreased slightly

    4 [ ] Decreased moderately

    5 [ ] Decreased greatly

10. If you take medication for pain, when do you take it?

    1 [ ] When needed for pain

    2 [ ] Regularly by the clock

11. Please list all medications you are currently taking:

Name of medication	Strength (mg)	Number per day
1. _____	_____	_____
2. _____	_____	_____
3. _____	_____	_____
4. _____	_____	_____
5. _____	_____	_____

12. Are you employed now?

    1 [ ] Yes—Full time

    2 [ ] Yes—Full time with restrictions

    3 [ ] Yes—Full time, but on sick leave right now

    4 [ ] Yes—Part time

    5 [ ] Yes—Part time with restrictions

    6 [ ] Yes—Part time, but on sick leave right now

    7 [ ] No—But not because of pain (GO TO QUESTION 14)

    8 [ ] No—Unable to work or unemployed because of pain (GO TO Q.14)

13. Since you were last treated for pain in this clinic, how many full days of work have you missed because of pain?

    Number of days: _____

14. Since you were last treated for pain in this clinic, how many times have you arrived late to work or left early from work because of pain?

    Number of times: _____

15. Since you were last treated for pain in this clinic, have you visited the emergency room for pain?

   1 [ ] Yes   Number of times: _____

   2 [ ] No

16. Since you were last treated for pain in this clinic, have you been hospitalized for pain?

   1 [ ] Yes   Number of times: _____

   Total days: _____

   2 [ ] No

17. Since you were last treated for pain in this clinic, have you had any surgical operations for pain?

   1 [ ] Yes

   2 [ ] No

18. Since you were last treated for pain in this clinic, approximately how many physician visits have you had for pain?

   Physician visits: _____

19. Since you were last treated for pain in this clinic, how many visits to health care professionals besides physicians have you had for pain? Include physical and occupational therapists, chiropractors, acupuncturists, nurse practitioners, homeopathic practitioners, etc.

   Other health care professional visits: _____

20. Do you feel the Pain Clinic has helped you with your pain problem?

   1 [ ] Yes, a great deal

   2 [ ] Yes, moderately

   3 [ ] Yes, slightly

   4 [ ] No, not at all

The questions used in this questionnaire were developed by the International Association for the Study of Pain task force on data collection. They are reproduced with permission of the IASP.

HISTORY AND PHYSICAL EXAMINATION RECORDING FORM

History

Chief Complaint:

History of Present Illness:

Description of Present Pain (location, radiation, quality, intensity):

Associated Symptoms (numbness, weakness, autonomic dysfunction, GI or GU dysfunction):

What relieves pain? (activities, rest, position)

When did pain start?

How did pain start? (at work, auto accident, sudden or gradual onset)

How has the pain changed since its onset? (increased, decreased, changed location)

Previous and current medication for pain: (include % relief, duration of effect, adverse effects)

Taking currently:

Not taking currently:

Other interventions (injections, TENS, PT, surgery; include dates, extent, and duration of relief):

Social, vocational history:

Married or single, other person in household:

Daily activity; what activity prevented by pain?

Employment history (current and prior employment, unemployed because of pain? income source):

Level of education:

Use of alcohol, tobacco, street drugs:

Past medical history:

Allergies:

Medications (not already listed, include reason for use; include OTCs)

Other medical problems:

Review of systems:

CNS:

Cardiovascular:

Respiratory:

GI:

GU:

Endocrine:

Family history:

Laboratory Evaluation (give dates, results)

Relevant blood, urine tests:

Neurodiagnostic studies

Imaging studies:

Physical Examination

General appearance:

Gait:

Range of motion:

Tenderness (muscle, bone, tendon, scar):

Provocative test (Tinel's SLR, Spurling's etc.):

Sensory Exam (anesthesia or hypoesthesia, allodynia, or hyperalgesia):

Motor exam (muscle bulk, symmetry, strength, spasm, abnormal movement, reflexes):

Vascular Exam (skin temperature, color, sweating; edema; pulses; venodilation; ulcers, stasis):

Other findings:
    Head and neck
    Chest:
    Abdomen, pelvis:
    Back:
    Extremities:

The Pain Clinic Manual, Second Edition,
edited by Stephen E. Abram and J. David Haddox.
Lippincott Williams & Wilkins,
Philadelphia, © 2000

Appendix G

Pain Glossary[1]

Pain: An unpleasant sensory and emotional experience associated with actual or potential tissue damage, or described in terms of such damage.

Allodynia: Pain arising from stimulus that does not normally provoke pain.

Analgesia: Absence of pain in response to stimulation that would normally be painful.

Anesthesia dolorosa: Pain in an area or region that is anesthetic.

Causalgia: A syndrome of sustained burning pain, allodynia, and hyperpathia after a traumatic nerve lesion, often combined with vasomotor and sudomotor dysfunction and later trophic changes.

Central pain: Pain associated with a lesion of the central nervous system.

Dysesthesia: An unpleasant abnormal sensation, whether spontaneous or evoked.

Hyperanesthesia: Increased sensitivity to stimulation, excluding the special senses.

Hyperalgesia: An increased response to a stimulus that is normally painful.

Hyperpathia: A painful syndrome characterized by increased reaction to a stimulus, especially a repetitive stimulus, as well as an increased threshold.

Hypoesthesia: Decreased sensitivity to stimulation, excluding the special senses.

Hypoalgesia: Diminished pain in response to normally painful stimulus.

Neuralgia: Pain in the distribution of a nerve or nerves.

Neuritis: Inflammation of a nerve or nerves.

Neuropathy: A disturbance of function or pathologic change in a nerve; in one nerve, mononeuropathy; in several nerves, mononeuropathy multiplex; if diffuse and bilateral, polyneuropathy.

Nociceptor: A receptor preferentially sensitive to a noxious stimulus or to a stimulus that would become noxious if prolonged.

Noxious stimulus: A noxious stimulus is one that is damaging to normal tissue.

Pain threshold: The least experience of pain that a patient can recognize.

Pain tolerance level: The greatest level of pain that a patient is prepared to tolerate.

Paraesthesia: An abnormal sensation, whether spontaneous or evoked.

---

[1] Reproduced with permission from Lindblom U, Merskey H, Mumford SM, et al. Pain terms: A current list with definitions and notes on usage. *Pain Suppl* 1986;3:S215–S221.

The implications of some of these definitions may be summarized for convenience as follows:

Allodynia:	Lowered threshold:	Stimulus and response mode differ
Hyperalgesia:	Increased response:	Stimulus and response mode are the same
Hyperpathia:	Raised threshold:	Stimulus and response mode may be the same or different
	Increased response:	
Hypoalgesia:	Raised threshold:	Stimulus and response mode are the same
	Lowered response:	

The above essentials of the definitions do not have to be symmetrical and are not symmetrical at present. Lowered threshold may occur with hyperalgesia but is not required. Also, there is no category for lowered threshold and lowered response if it ever occurs.

Subject Index